Transforming Practice through Clinical Education, Professional Supervision and Mentoring

Editors

Miranda Rose

BAppSc(Speech Pathology) GradDip(Communication Disorders)
GradDip(Health Research Methodology) PhD

Lecturer and Co-ordinator, School of Human Communication Sciences, La Trobe University, Bundoora, Victoria, Australia; Fellow of the Australian Speech Pathology Association

Dawn Best

DipPhysio MEd

Senior Fellow, School of Physiotherapy, University of Melbourne; Consultant in Medical and Health Professional Education, Victoria, Australia

Foreword by

Joy Higgs

PhD MHPEd GradDipPhty BSc

Professor, Faculty of Health Sciences, University of Sydney, Lidcombe, Australia

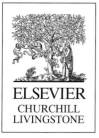

ELSEVIER
CHURCHILL
LIVINGSTONE

EDINBURGH LONDON NEW YORK OXFORD PHILADELPHIA ST LOUIS SYDNEY TORONTO 2005

ELSEVIER
CHURCHILL
LIVINGSTONE

An imprint of Elsevier Limited

First published 2005
Reprinted 2007

ISBN 0 443 07454 2

British Library Cataloguing in Publication Data
A catalogue record for this book is available from the British Library

Library of Congress Cataloguing in Publication Data
A catalogue record for this book is available from the Library of Congress

Notice
Neither the Publisher nor the Editors assumes any responsibility for any loss or injury and/or damage to persons or property arising out of or related to any use of the material contained in this book. It is the responsibility of the treating practitioner, relying on independent expertise and knowledge of the patient, to determine the best treatment and method of application for the patient.

The Publisher

The
publisher's
policy is to use
**paper manufactured
from sustainable forests**

Printed in China

Contents

List of Contributors

Marilyn Baird DCR BA PhD
Associate Professor, Head, Department of Medical Imaging and Radiation Sciences, Monash University, Clayton, Victoria, Australia

Dawn Best DipPhysio MEd
Senior Fellow, School of Physiotherapy, University of Melbourne; Consultant in Medical and Health Professional Education, Victoria, Australia

Louise Brown LACST BAppSc(Sp Path) MEd(Melb)
Senior Lecturer, Human Communication Sciences, La Trobe University, Bundoora, Victoria; Manager of Speech Pathology, Casey Hospital, Victoria, Australia

Megan Davidson PhD BAppSci(Physiotherapy)
Lecturer and Undergraduate Course Co-ordinator, School of Physiotherapy, La Trobe University, Bundoora, Victoria, Australia

Helen Edwards MA PhD
Principal Research Fellow, Academic Development Unit, La Trobe University, Bundoora, Victoria; Consultant, Higher Education, Melbourne, Victoria, Australia

Kerry Ferguson BAppSc(OT) MEd EdD MVAFT
Pro Vice-Chancellor, Equity and Access, La Trobe University, Bundoora, Victoria, Australia

Della Fish MA MEd PhD
Professor of Education (Postgraduate Medicine), King's College, London, UK

Kirstie Galbraith BPharm GradDipHospPharm BCPS
Senior Lecturer, Department of Pharmacy Practice, Monash University, Clayton; Senior Clinical Pharmacist, The Royal Melbourne Hospital, Victoria, Australia

Paul Hagler PhD
Professor and Associate Dean, Graduate Studies and Research, Faculty of Rehabilitation Medicine, University of Alberta, Edmonton, Alberta, Canada

Margaret C. Hodge BP&O(Hons) CPO-AOPA
Lecturer, National Centre for Prosthetics and Orthotics, La Trobe University, Bundoora, Victoria, Australia

Beverly Joffe BA(Speech Pathology and Audiology) MA(Speech Pathology) PhD
Lecturer, School of Human Communication Sciences, La Trobe University, Bundoora, Victoria, Australia

Mary Kennedy-Jones BAppSc(OT) GradDipMgmt St MEd
Doctoral Student, School of Public Health, La Trobe University; Entry-level Curriculum Co-ordinator and Senior Lecturer, School of Occupational Therapy, La Trobe University, Bundoora, Victoria, Australia

Michelle Lincoln PhD
Director of Clinical Education, School of Communication Sciences and Disorders, University of Sydney, Lidcombe, Australia

Jennifer Marriott BPharm PhD GCHE
Senior Lecturer, Department of Pharmacy Practice, Monash University, Clayton, Victoria, Australia

Lindy McAllister BSpThy MA(Sp Path)(Hons) PhD
Associate Professor and Course Co-ordinator Speech and Hearing Science Degree, School of Community Health, Charles Sturt University, Albury, NSW, Australia

Helen McBurney PhD BAppSc(Physio)
GradDipPhysio(Cardiothoracic)
*Associate Professor, School of Physiotherapy,
La Trobe University, Bundoora, Victoria, Australia*

Michael McGartland BSc(Hons) MSc MAPS MACE
*Senior Lecturer, School of Public Health, La Trobe
University, Victoria; Senior Clinical Psychologist,
Primary Mental Health and Early Intervention
Team, The Alfred Hospital, Melbourne, Victoria,
Australia*

Bernie Neville MA PhD
*Associate Professor of Education, La Trobe
University, Bundoora, Victoria, Australia*

Matthew Oates BPod(Hons) MAPodA
*Lecturer, Department of Podiatry, School of Human
Biosciences, La Trobe University, Bundoora, Victoria,
Australia*

Marisue Pickering EdD MEd BA
*Professor, Communication Sciences and Disorders,
Adjunct Professor of Education, University of
Maine, Orono, Maine, USA*

Louisa Remedios BApplSc(Phty) GrandDip(Sports)
Masters by research MAPA
*Lecturer, School of Physiotherapy, University of
Melbourne, Australia*

Maggie Roe-Shaw MPH PostGradDip(Tertiary
Teaching) PostGradDip(HealthPromotion) DipPhty PhD
*Professional Practice Advisor, Ministry of Education,
Wellington, New Zealand*

Miranda Rose BAppSc(Speech Pathology)
GradDip(Communication Disorders) GradDip(Health
Research Methodology) PhD
*Lecturer and Co-ordinator, School of Human
Communication Sciences, La Trobe University,
Bundoora, Victoria, Australia; Fellow of the
Australian Speech Pathology Association*

Magdalen Rozsa BAppSc(Speech Pathology)
*Student Unit Supervisor – Speech Pathology, The
Children's Hospital at Westmead, New South Wales,
Australia*

Susan Ryan PhD MSc BAppSc
*Professor of Occupational Therapy, University
College Cork, Ireland*

Gillian Webb DEd Dip(Physio) GradDip(Exercise for
Rehabilitation) MClinEd
*Deputy Head, School of Physiotherapy, University of
Melbourne, Australia*

Jane Winter BSc GradDip(Nutrition and Dietetics)
MPET(Professional Education and Training)
Consultant Dietitian, Victoria, Australia

Foreword

This book is about professional practice and the important role clinical educators, professional supervisors and mentors play in influencing the quality and evolution of this practice. Because the context is *professional* practice, we expect the quality and transformation of practice to be driven by the insights, responsibilities, learning and innovations of key players, particularly the practitioners themselves. This team of practice transformers includes:

- the students who will become, enthusiastically and with new vision, the next generation of practitioners
- the educators and mentors who shape the learners' paths, while being transformed and tested themselves
- the practitioners, who, although they are 'knee-deep in the "swampy lowlands"' (Schön 1987) of practice, are also actively engaged in transforming that practice and themselves from their own practice wisdom and in the light of workplace and broader environmental drivers
- practice managers, who juggle both environmental constraints and practice imperatives
- and finally, and foremost, the consumers and clients of practice, whose needs and expectations are the principal stimuli for actions that enhance practice.

This book draws on all these voices to focus on the role of clinical education, professional supervision and mentoring in transforming practice. Their messages and issues are explored through the collective wisdom of a range of visionary, experienced authors.

Across the health and social sciences, we have much more in common when it comes to broad principles and strategies of education and practice development than our differences in terminology would imply. Whether you feel more comfortable with the term professional fieldwork than clinical education or educator than supervisor, this book has much to say to you: to enlighten, affirm, challenge and transform.

The four sections in the book provide us with a rich journey of challenges, visions and strategies that assist such transformations: the clinical education process and the role of the clinical educator; teaching and learning; challenges in clinical education; and evaluation and future directions in clinical education and supervision.

Here are some of the key messages that inform the chapters:

- Transforming practice is a dual theme: practitioners are both the source and object of transformation.
- The tasks comprising clinical education, professional supervision and mentoring are complex due to the nature and context of professional practice and the multiple roles that need to be juggled. Part of this challenge is to continue to grow within the roles rather than burn out.
- There are considerable benefits for clients (patients), professionals and health care services in being involved in clinical education, professional supervision and mentoring. Short-term cost savings that limit practitioners' involvement in such activities will inevitably result in long-term limitations to the quality of practice and health care services.

Transformation of practice is both inevitable and desirable. The challenge for education and practice providers is to help make this transformation positive in both the experience of the process and the outcomes for learners and practice participants. This book provides considerable support to meet that goal.

Joy Higgs

REFERENCE

Schön D A 1987 Educating the reflective practitioner. Jossey-Bass, San Francisco

Acknowledgements

This text draws on the collective wisdom of a large group of people and we gratefully acknowledge the privilege of working with and learning from:

- past and present academic staff from Deakin, Monash and La Trobe Universities in Melbourne who presented the Quality Supervision Certificate course, especially those members of the current team who have contributed chapters to this book
- our invited colleagues and overseas authors, who have broadened the perspective of the book and provided insights from North America, the United Kingdom and New Zealand
- participants in the Quality Supervision course and clinical educators, who encouraged and challenged us to reframe our thinking in the light of their experience
- our undergraduate students, who shared with us the demands and joys associated with their developing professional knowledge and expertise.

In addition, we would also like to thank our families who, with great tolerance and unlimited support, assisted us in the development of this book.

Chapter 1

Introduction to clinical education, professional supervision and mentoring

In part one of this chapter the reader is introduced to the terminology and definitions of clinical education, professional supervision and mentoring. In part two, the contexts of these activities are explored from an Australian perspective. In parts three, four, and five, the perspectives of writers from the United Kingdom, the United States of America and Canada are added.

PART 1   Introduction to terminology and definitions

Miranda Rose and Dawn Best

In this text we have purposefully brought together the three partially overlapping but distinct roles of clinical educator, clinical supervisor and mentor, in order to gain a more informed view of the range of activities that are contained within the continuum of supervision practice. It appears to us that at times these three fields, and the research and literature exploring and describing them, have been emerging in parallel rather than in an integrated manner. As a consequence of the somewhat independent nature of the exploration of these three fields, some of the overlap has been ignored. It is our contention that the development of the three fields has perhaps suffered from a lack of cross fertilisation.

In 1996, the academic staff from the Foundation for Quality Supervision, an initiative of the Faculty of Health Sciences at La Trobe University, convened a conference entitled "Expanding Horizons: New directions in clinical supervision, professional supervision and mentoring." It was the intention of the organising committee to bring together a broad range of health- and welfare-related professionals to share knowledge and practice in the fields of clinical education, clinical supervision and mentoring, and in so doing help to foster a better understanding of the similarities and differences across the practices of supervision.

The conference attracted participants from the fields of social work, psychology, physiotherapy, speech pathology, occupational therapy, podiatry, prosthetics and orthotics, nursing, radiography and pharmacy. In delineating the focus for the conference, we were aware that there was ample opportunity for confusion and misunderstanding, particularly with respect to the terminology of supervision and the varied constructs underpinning supervision practice. However, we were motivated to move through any such confusion and work together to find ways to understand and learn from each other. The papers were extremely varied, the participants eager to learn from each other, and the conference was a great success. Quickly though, we came to understand the central importance of clear terminology, and it is with this in mind that we now offer the following section which deals with the challenges of defining the continuum of supervision practice and the recognisable points along the continuum.

When exploring the literature in supervision and clinical education, a plethora of terms to describe the roles are revealed. These include:

- coach
- clinical teacher
- clinical educator
- clinical supervisor
- field supervisor
- preceptor
- mentor
- professional supervisor
- supervisor-mentor
- collaborative peer supervisor.

Each profession appears to favour one or two particular terms and attribute a specific meaning to them. Unfortunately, these varied professional groups do not share a common language so that "clinical supervisor" may mean one thing to psychologists and social workers and something entirely different to physiotherapists and nurses. In pharmacy, the term preceptor is used to denote the same functions ascribed to the clinical educator in speech pathology. Equally, the role confusions and possibilities for role conflict are rife. In some workplaces one experienced employee might be expected to function as line manager, clinical supervisor, mentor and preceptor for a particular newer employee. Thus, such terminological confusions are not "just a question of semantics" but there is also confusion in the actual constructs of practice. Such confusions pose potential limitations on practice and may in some circumstances pose threats to those involved in the various supervisory relationships.

In 2000, Morton-Cooper and Palmer, writing from the field of nursing, provided an extremely helpful framework to assist in the understanding of the various supportive and educational roles of supervision. They suggested that the roles have many of the same inherent qualities but that defining the distinctions between them may help to prevent them being used inappropriately. They suggested that the roles could be distinguished in terms of their relative emphasis on enabling versus ensuring functions. Thus, we offer the following definitions of the roles and then discuss the similarities and differences of each role in terms of the enabling and ensuring dimensions.

CLINICAL EDUCATOR

Clinical education is a term denoting the practice of assisting a student to acquire the required knowledge, skills and attitudes in practice settings (such as health service clinics, field work sites) to meet the standards defined by a university degree structure or professional accrediting/licensing board. In the fields of physiotherapy, speech pathology, occupational therapy, podiatry, prosthetics and orthotics, nursing and radiography, clinical education activity is usually contained within an undergraduate or graduate-entry degree program. It frequently involves students leaving the confines of the university and undertaking practical patient or client activities in a health, welfare or educational setting with the educational support of a qualified practitioner who is employed by the service or agency. McAllister (1997), writing from the perspective of speech pathology, defined a clinical educator as a professional who engages in a:

> Teaching and learning process which is student focused and may be student led, which occurs in the context of client care. It involves the translation of theory into the development of clinical knowledge and practical skills, with the incorporation of the affective domain needed for sensitive and ethical client care. Clinical education occurs in an environment supportive of the development of clinical reasoning, professional socialisation, and life-long learning (p. 3).

The term clinical educator is a relatively new term and is only just gaining widespread acceptance in several allied health professions in Australia. An earlier and commonly used term to denote the role of clinical educator in allied health fields was *clinical supervisor*, and in fact is still the preferred term in the field of physiotherapy. The use of the word supervisor with its origins in the work practices of "overseeing the execution of tasks, superintending" (*The Australian Concise Oxford Dictionary*, 1997, p. 1372), resonated with earlier practices of clinical education which were in fact more didactic and based in an "apprenticeship" model. Therefore, the use of the term supervision had some logic in earlier times, when the more experienced member of the relationship (the supervisor) engaged in telling, modelling and checking behaviours. This contrasts with current concepts of clinical education where facilitative behaviours are highlighted and frequently student-led.

PRECEPTOR

Preceptors, according to Deane & Campbell (1985), "act as agents for their employees, to assist other employees or students in adjusting to their new role" (p. 144). Thus, in precepting, an identified and experienced practitioner provides transitional role support to a newly qualified staff member, within a collegial relationship (Morton-Cooper & Palmer 2000). Specific goals and objectives are usually defined for the relationship, the time course for the relationship is agreed upon, and there may be a formal assessment of the preceptee's acquisition of knowledge and workplace skills. The precepting role differs from the clinical educator role in that both preceptees and preceptors are usually academically qualified or licensed and employed by the same employer, while the clinical educator is a qualified person working with unqualified students. The goals of precepting emphasise adjustment to a particular workplace setting, whereas the goals of clinical education often extend beyond the setting currently at hand and emphasise broad professional functioning.

In the pharmacy profession in Australia, the term preceptor is used to denote both the clinical educator role of a qualified pharmacist facilitating the professional competence of an unqualified student (in undergraduate programmes) as well as the transitional role of the workplace preceptor for graduates of pharmacy degrees who are yet to be licensed. However, in the nursing profession, a distinction is made between clinical educators working with undergraduate preregistration nursing students in health care environments and preceptors who are assigned to individual nurses new to the organisation who need transitional support. To add further fuel to the terminological and role confusion, many allied health professions (for example, speech pathology and physiotherapy) assign what is essentially a precepting role for their more experienced staff to offer support to staff who are new to the organisation but then term the function *mentoring*.

MENTOR

Morton-Cooper & Palmer (2000) define a mentor as "someone who provides an enabling relationship that facilitates another's personal growth and development. The relationship is dynamic, reciprocal and can be emotionally intense. Within such a relationship the mentor assists with career development and guides the mentee through the organisational, social and political networks" (p. 189).

The term mentor is well known and often used colloquially. It originates from Greek classical literature, where in Homer's *Odyssey*, Ulysses (or Odysseus as he is sometimes called) appointed his friend *Mentor,* to care for his home and his son, Telemachus, while Ulysses was away at war. In the story, Mentor became more than a teacher, assuming considerable personal responsibility for Telemachus' development. In the classic mentoring relationship, the mentee seeks a supportive and socially well-networked individual, usually a member of their own profession, who is more experienced than the mentee. Mentors and mentees interact frequently, either in person or in some cases (for example the Speech Pathology Australia Mentor Programme) by telephone, to discuss issues of specific and personal interest to the mentee. Issues of career development and enhancement are central to the mentoring relationship. In classic versions of the relationship, mentors are not part of the mentees' workplace. In more recent and corporate versions, mentors might be on site and even in the same department as the mentee. The role conflicts that can emerge in such "in-house" mentoring relationships are more fully explored in Chapter 19.

CLINICAL SUPERVISOR (PROFESSIONAL SUPERVISOR)

The role of clinical supervisor has been difficult to define, with Butterworth & Faugier (1992) cautioning defining an activity where the field of knowledge is in an early stage of growth. Bond & Holland (1998) commented that there are many definitions of clinical supervision and yet none with widespread acceptance. Various authors have defined clinical supervision as an enabling process that allows the individual being supervised to experience professional and personal growth without penalty (Butterworth & Faugier 1992). Cutcliffe et al (2001) described clinical supervision as:

- supportive
- safe, because of clear, negotiated agreements by all parties with regard to the extent and limits of confidentiality
- brave, because practitioners are encouraged to talk about the realities of their practice
- a chance to talk about difficult areas of work in an environment where the person attempts to understand
- an opportunity to ventilate emotion without comeback
- the opportunity to deal with material and issues that practitioners may have been carrying for many years
- not to be confused with or amalgamated with managerial supervision
- not to be confused with or amalgamated with personal therapy/counselling
- regular
- protected time
- offered equally to all practitioners
- involving a committed relationship (both parties)
- a facilitative relationship
- challenging
- an invitation to be self-monitoring and self-accountable

- at times hard work and at others enjoyable
- involving learning to be reflective and become a reflective practitioner
- an activity that continues throughout one's working life.

Cutcliffe et al also stated that clinical supervision was not to be confused with or amalgamated with managerial supervision or personal therapy/counselling and that it is separate and distinct from preceptorship and mentorship. Cutcliffe et al were keen to distinguish managerial supervision involving controlling standards, and ensuring competency and efficiency, from the more facilitative clinical supervision. In this definition, clinical supervision occurs between a more knowledgeable and experienced practitioner and a less knowledgeable and experienced practitioner and does not involve the assessment and ensuring functions contained in clinical education and managerial or workplace line supervision. However, in the field of nursing, some definitions of clinical supervision have a slightly greater emphasis on consumer protection, for example the definition provided by the UK Department of Health (1993): "A formal process of professional support and learning which enables individual practitioners to develop knowledge and competence, assume responsibility for their own practice and enhance consumer protection and safety of care in complex clinical situations."

Professional supervision is another term used to denote the functions of clinical supervision. In Australia, allied health practitioners might seek the paid services of a *clinical supervisor* outside their organisation, as is the tradition in psychology and social work in this country, to aid them in their ongoing professional growth and enhance their client care. Many allied health practitioners call this role *professional supervision* in order to minimise confusion with the clinical education role, which many still denote as clinical supervision. Thus, in this text we will refer to clinical supervision as professional supervision. The role of professional supervision is dealt with in more detail in Chapter 18.

SIMILARITIES AND DIFFERENCES IN ROLES

As discussed earlier, Morton-Cooper & Palmer (2000) suggested that mentoring, preceptorship and professional supervision could be distinguished according to the relative emphasis each had in the two dimensions of ensuring and enabling functions. They drew on the work of Marchant (1986) who defined ensuring as "making sure the job gets done" and enabling as "assisting practitioners to learn from their experiences and develop practice expertise and personal growth". In order to cover the gamut of supervisory and educative roles addressed in this text, we have adapted Morton Cooper & Palmer's continuum to include the role of clinical educator. An overview of the differences between the four roles is presented in Table 1.1.

Morton-Cooper & Palmer (2000) also provided a much-needed graphic representation of the various complementary but distinct supportive roles that one may encounter across the developmental life span of becoming and being a professional. Their framework is reproduced here (Fig. 1.1) with their kind permission as we believe it adds considerable clarity to the question of defining roles.

Table 1.1 Overview of the differences between mentoring, professional supervision, preceptorship and clinical education (adapted from Morton-Cooper & Palmer 2000)

Mentor	Clinical/professional supervisor	Preceptor	Clinical educator
Intimate, personal enabling relationship	Clinical enabling relationship	Functional enabling relationship	Educative enabling and ensuring relationship
Career socialisation, providing social and political networks	Clinical socialisation, focus on practice	Clinical socialisation in initial post-registration/ transition period	Clinical socialisation in placement period
Unstructured learning support	Semi-structured learning support	Structured learning support	Highly structured learning support
Long-term duration, determined by the needs of those involved	Medium-term duration, determined by clinical partnership and working alliance	Short duration related to clinical allocation, specific period of support	Short duration related to length of clinical placement
Multi-faceted assisting roles but no formal assessment	Clinically and professionally related tasks, and self-assessment	Specific roles with emphasis on role modelling and rehearsal of key skills	Specific education roles, and formal assessment common, gate-keeper assessment role
Chosen by individual	Chosen by individual (or assigned in some "in-house" situations)	Chosen by employee	Chosen by university and clinical site

Figure 1.1 General professional support framework incorporating significant relationships and roles. Reproduced with permission from Morton-Cooper & Palmer (2000).

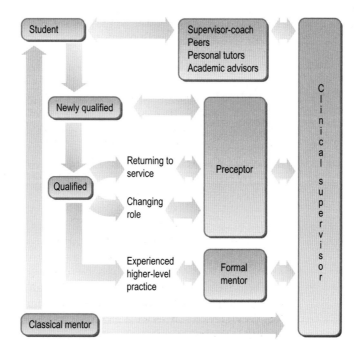

PART 2 Context for clinical education, professional supervision and mentoring

Miranda Rose and Dawn Best

INTRODUCTION

Part one has explored the terminology in use by different professions in order to develop a shared understanding of processes which seek to support the development of professional expertise in health science students and graduates. This section provides the opportunity for a general overview of health care delivery and health science education from writers who represent a variety of health science professions from Australia, Canada, the United Kingdom and the United States of America. Global issues are addressed before an exploration of issues that are specific to particular countries/regions.

Although each profession may seek local solutions for its own individual challenges, it is essential to acknowledge that health care and health science education today are influenced by world issues. Travel, information transmission and technological advances have resulted in the emergence of a changing worldview. Globalisation refers to the increased unification and interconnectedness of the world and its nations (Higgs et al 1999). Neubauer (1998) identified a number of issues which impact on spiralling costs in health and health care within the western world and which impact on third world countries. Physical and national boundaries are no longer barriers to global trade. Multinational companies and world financial trends influence workforce restructuring in both health and education. There is an increasing move towards privatisation with its focus on consumerism.

Higgs & Edwards (1999) identified the following influences on both health and education. Global forces have impacted on:

- the constant need to respond creatively to change
- the exponential growth of information technology on education and health care
- the shift from local to world orientations resulting from globalisation
- increasing demands for accountability and demonstrated outcomes
- decreasing government funding and hence a focus on "user pays" with the need to generate external monies
- the development of managerial structures which are more entrepreneurial and corporate
- increased workload patterns resulting from an increase in client numbers and more diverse populations, as well as the additional responsibility for greater accountability
- a growing emphasis on international and interprofessional links, standards and collaboration
- the emergence of health and education becoming viewed as commodities to be purchased.

It is also important to recognise that, though there are many different models of health, there has been a shift from an illness to a wellness model (Higgs et al 1999). When wellness is also seen as a marketable commodity there are obvious social implications for those who are unable to afford it and a high correlation between low economic status and poor health. The traditional biomedical model, which focuses on diagnosis of client symptoms followed by some management strategy, is no longer able to meet the demands and there is now a shift to incorporate a more holistic approach to health care delivery. The focus has moved from an impairment level to a more functional status. Health promotion activities and patient education to empower people to look after themselves require additional competencies of health care providers. There is a much greater requirement for effective interpersonal skills and team functioning in this approach and hence these have increased importance in health science education programmes today. Although all professions are challenged to address this, different areas of practice and different professions have embraced it to a varying extent (Hunt et al 1999).

Globalisation has resulted in specific changes to health care delivery (Higgs & Edwards 1999, Higgs et al 1999, Higgs & Bithell 2001). There are now:

- growing financial difficulties and workforce shortages within the health sector
- changing patterns of health care delivery with a move from shorter length of stay within acute care facilities to more community- and home-based care
- an expectation that services will be relevant to changing health care needs
- ageing populations
- the impact of technology advances
- a move from the management of acute to chronic conditions
- increased consumer expectations and knowledge.

There is an ongoing challenge to graduate new professionals who have the competencies to meet the future requirements of individual professions, the flexibility to adapt to constantly changing health service delivery models and workplaces, as well as this century's demands for evidence-based and client-centred practice, and with societal demands for greater accountability. There is also the universal recognition that our new graduates will also be prepared to be life-long learners and the future leaders of health service delivery.

Although these global changes have an international impact, each country addresses them in different ways. The following section examines the Australian context.

AUSTRALIA

Health science professional education programmes

Health science programmes in Australia are now located in universities, with the majority offering a bachelor degree. The programmes range from three years in nursing to six years for medicine, with physiotherapy, occupational therapy and speech pathology courses extending over four years. In many programmes there is no allowance for part-time enrolment or minimal tolerance of part-time enrolment only in exceptional circumstances. Until comparatively recently all Australian universities were located within capital cities or large regional cities. However, in the past six years new programmes have begun in the rural sector in response to government initiatives to address workforce deficiencies within rural and remote areas.

The government assists enrolment for Australian residents at university but all students are required to pay course fees under the Higher Education Contribution Scheme (HECS). Payment of the fees may be delayed until the student earns a set taxable income and fees are allocated on predicted income rather than cost of undergraduate education. Some universities have allocated a small number of places to full-fee-paying local students as well as competing for full-fee-paying overseas students. Graduate-entry programmes have been developed for medicine, occupational therapy, physiotherapy, speech pathology and dietetics within the past four years. In most cases these are full-fee-paying programmes, although the cost for courses varies between professions. The complexity of different student enrolments and fee scales has resulted in the development of complicated accounting and administrative processes. This in turn has forced professional courses to comply with set semester dates and credit point values. Administrative processes may conflict with educative trends for more student-centred flexible programmes and are not always sympathetic with clinical education issues.

Higgs & Edwards (1999) summarised the expectations of beginning health science graduates:

- technical and professional competence
- generic skills related to the ability to continue to learn independently and critically self-evaluate
- the ability to interact effectively with people in a variety of contexts – in the last decade Australian university reform has focused on the development of generic graduate attributes as well as discipline-specific knowledge and skills.

Such generic skills relate to:

- a sound understanding of society, including its history and cultural and social issues
- a capacity to consider problems from a range of perspectives, to analyse, to gather evidence, to synthesise and be flexible, creative thinkers
- a capacity for life-long learning
- good oral and written skills (Lowe, as cited in Hunt et al 1999).

This places an additional challenge on curriculum developers, academic teachers and clinical educators, when all are working within tight cost constraints. It also demands ongoing interaction with professional associations who are primarily concerned with meeting demands for technical competence.

The corporatisation of Australian universities has resulted in a competitive environment where there is now open rivalry between universities and programmes for research grants, students, funding and clinical placements. Entire courses, course materials or subjects developed at one university may be sold to another. This marketplace atmosphere may hinder the development of collaborative partnerships with the professions and health care facilities.

There is increasing pressure on universities to ensure that their programmes comply with government regulations and ensure their graduates achieve minimal standards of professional competence. Whether graduation from the programme enables registration to the profession, as in physiotherapy, certification, licensure or credentialing, there is an expectation that some form of internal and/or external accreditation or quality review process is in place. Universities are required to provide details of mission statements, governance, mission, academic programmes, finances, research outcomes, personnel and constituents (Liston 1999). However, Hunt et al (1999) warned that accreditation processes directed at university curricula are set for minimal standards of entry-level graduate competence, so that such scrutiny is only likely to prevent gross incompetence in practice.

Academic teachers

The move to universities from smaller individual private schools and colleges of advanced education has certainly provided considerable benefits for the health science profession. However, the current funding crisis faced by Australian universities raises additional challenges. Academic teaching staff numbers have decreased at a time when student enrolments have increased. There are additional pressures to win grant monies, to research and publish as well as teach. Programmes may have reduced teaching hours but the body of professional knowledge continues to increase. Some universities have accepted full-fee-paying or international students as a way of boosting revenue and these place additional pressures on academic staff. Others have implemented flexible delivery using computer-based programmes. Some programmes have moved from traditional curricula to problem-based learning.

Hidden behind this list of diverse activities is an additional administrative workload related to planning, writing the course and subject documentation to be ratified by the committee structure within the university, staffing implementation and evaluation, and the challenge of maintaining staffing levels commensurate with the responsibility to graduate competent new practitioners. With such an increase in workload, it is not surprising that the supervisory arrangements for students during clinical fieldwork have become a lower priority. Although this text does not set out to explore the complexity of curriculum development and academic teaching, the impact that these issues have on clinical education and supervision must be acknowledged.

Students

The number and diversity of students enrolled in health science education programmes are increasing. Student profiles related to age, gender and cultural background have changed dramatically in the past 10 years. Although school leavers make up the largest group in Australian undergraduate courses, there are increasing numbers of mature-age students. Some of these have prior tertiary experience. In addition, there are an increasing number of graduate-entry masters programmes, which have been specifically designed to attract graduates who already have generic academic skills. Traditional gender balances within the student population have changed so that some courses such as medicine and physiotherapy have achieved a more even gender balance, and others such as occupational therapy, nursing and speech pathology remain female-dominated (Dwyer & Higgs 1999). The impact of Australian immigration policies since 1945 has resulted in a diverse multicultural population amongst local students. In addition, the more recent rise of overseas full-fee-paying students has further increased the number of students who come from different cultural backgrounds. Until recently most students were enrolled in their home state with few travelling interstate.

Students enrolled in health science courses belong predominantly to the middle and upper social strata (Dwyer & Higgs 1999); however, the majority are employed in part-time work. The impact this has on students during their enrolment is considerable and further exacerbated during full-time clinical placements.

Clinical education

Clinical education remains an ongoing issue for professional education. Making the optimal use of the diminished clinical education resource is one of the key issues for professional education today. New universities continue to mount new professional programmes in response to identified future workplace requirements. Masters graduate-entry programmes further increase the numbers of students requiring clinical placements. Students enrolled in northern hemisphere educational programmes e-mail requests to undertake clinical electives within Australian health care facilities.

In most undergraduate programmes the responsibility for arranging the clinical component of the courses rests with the universities. Some have developed in-house clinics, others use simulated patients or simulated clinical activities within on-campus teaching sessions. One of the most critical issues in clinical education is the allocation of clinical hours. There is considerable variation in the number of clinical hours required between health science professions and whether these hours are scheduled before or after graduation from the university. Some courses have up to a third of the course involved in fieldwork. The World Confederation of Occupational Therapy continues to adhere to a minimum of 1000 supervised clinical hours. Meeting this number for the expanded number of programmes and students requires considerable creativity in both the development of clinical student fieldwork places and the supervisory arrangements employed. This has resulted in a move from traditional fieldwork places in acute and rehabilitation facilities to new placements located within the community – these may be within federal, state or local government departments, education systems and public or private companies. Many of these sites may not employ an occupational therapist, so new supervisory arrangements are required (Hummel & Williamson 1999).

Although the majority of health science professional programmes graduate beginning practitioners at the completion of the academic programme, others, such as social work, pharmacy and medicine, defer this requirement until after graduation and the completion of an internship. Table 1.2 provides an illustration of the diversity amongst the professions of members from the teaching team currently involved in the Quality Supervision Certificate course at La Trobe University.

With so much change in both health and education it is interesting to review the goals of clinical education identified by Higgs et al (1991) in an Australian study in the early 1990s. These were:

- understanding of health, illness, holistic health care and the health care system
- understanding of the professional role and personal coping strategies

Table 1.2   Diversity from three local universities and their health professional courses

University	Profession	Award granted	Years of programme	Number of hours in clinical environment	Entry to profession
Deakin	Dietetics	Bachelor of Nutrition and Dietetics	4 years	500 hours	No registration
La Trobe	Occupational therapy	Bachelor of OT; Master of Occupational Therapy Practice – graduate entry	4 years 2 years	1000 hours 1000 hours	Registration required in South Australia, Western Australia, Queensland, Northern Territory
	Physiotherapy	Bachelor of Physiotherapy	4 years	1000 hours	Registration by all state boards
	Podiatry	Bachelor of Podiatry	4 years	1000 hours	Registration by all state boards
	Prosthetics and orthotics	Bachelor of Prosthetics and Orthotics	3.5 years	700 hours	No formal registration
	Speech pathology	Bachelor of Speech Pathology; Master of Speech Pathology – graduate entry	4 years 2 years	750 hours 500 hours*	Registration in Queensland only
Monash	Pharmacy	Bachelor of Pharmacy	4 years	15 weeks in clinical placement in undergraduate course.	Registration required in all states following examination
		Master of Clinical Pharmacy	2 years part-time	Following graduation, 2 × 6-week blocks and 1 year of pre-registration placement	
	Radiography	Bachelor of Radiography and Medical Imaging	4 years	2500 hours	Registration in most states

*Problem-based learning course: significant hours spent in clinical reasoning/preclinical activity in academic subjects.

- awareness of the student's own attitudes, beliefs and responses to health and illness
- understanding of the function of the health care team and the contribution of the professions within the team
- interpersonal skills, including empathy
- specific professional psychomotor and cognitive and affective competencies appropriate to the discipline
- skills in patient or community education
- ability to manage workload and time appropriately

- ability to supervise or liaise with other team members
- ability to process information and record effectively
- ability to self-evaluate his or her own performance
- ongoing commitment to maintaining professional competence
- commitment to professional accountability.

Careful review of the above list will reveal the absence of more recent imperatives for new health professional graduates, such as:

- client-centred care
- evidence-based practice
- outcome measurement
- cultural competence
- economic responsibility
- expertise with information technology (Stephenson et al 2002).

Preparation of clinical educators

It is also increasingly apparent that preparation for the role of clinical educators will result in better outcomes for health care clients as well as learners. Although accreditation for clinicians may be discussed and even documented in position papers in different professions, there is currently no established accreditation process for Australian clinical educators. However, much has changed in the past 10 years. It is now widely accepted that universities have the responsibility to prepare clinicians to support their students' and/or new graduates' learning in the clinical environment. Multiple strategies may be used. These include the distribution of printed text, teleconferencing opportunities, face-to-face workshops and information sessions. Contact hours for preparatory courses range from some that last an hour to accredited certificated and graduate certificate courses. An online programme for Australian Pharmacy Preceptor education has been developed by a national consortium of university pharmacy programmes. In addition, there are now higher degrees specifically for health science educators at universities such as the University of Sydney, University of New South Wales, and Monash University.

The health science professions

Privatisation and restructuring within health care organisations have changed the opportunities for student fieldwork experiences. There has been a move to decentralise services from acute care facilities to community and domiciliary care, with a marked decrease in patient length of stay in the acute sector. Many facilities have also experienced some staffing down-sizing.

There is also an increasing uptake of health insurance and access to private services. Within this consumer focus on health care, there is a greater expectation of clinical expertise (Higgs & Bithell 2001). Private health care placements may be more reluctant to allow students and new graduates the opportunities for practice that are available within the public sector. At a time when there are more students there is also a decrease in placement opportunities.

Professional roles today have broadened to expand to new areas of practice and new roles in response to the demands of society today. Hummel & Williamson (1999) list the diverse practice opportunities of occupational therapy today to:

> include practice with people of all ages with or at risk of developing a variety of physical and psychosocial disabilities through preventative and rehabilitation programs. Consultancies are increasing in number and range from environmental design to art and drama therapy from return to work and employment skills development programs to life style groups for people who are chronically ill (p. 33).

Professional supervision and mentoring

The factors described in the previous section not only relate to the activities of clinical education but many are also relevant to professional supervision and mentoring activities. Indeed, it could be argued that the recent rise in the popularity and adoption of mentoring programmes in allied health and nursing across the globe, and in practitioners seeking professional supervision opportunities for which they are willing to pay personally, is due to the changing contexts of and pressures on their practice. Workplaces concerned about rising employee attrition rates argue strongly for mentoring and supervision programmes. Similarly, the rise in mandatory continuing education for the professions has led to practitioners seeking mentoring and professional supervision at rates higher than ever before. What is of concern, though, is the general lack of preparation practitioners have for their roles of supervisee/mentee or supervisor/mentor. These issues will be more fully explored in Chapters 18 and 19, dealing with the disciplines of professional supervision and mentoring respectively.

CONCLUSION

Although these issues may distract and confuse issues related to clinical education, clinical supervision and mentoring, there is universal acceptance of the importance of a process which supports early and ongoing clinical professional development, even if different professions choose different terminology for the processes and promote a variety of structures to provide the experiences.

REFERENCES

Bond M, Holland S 1998 Skills of clinical supervision for nurses. Open University Press, Buckingham

Butterworth A, Faugier J (eds) 1992 Clinical supervision and mentorship in nursing. Chapman and Hall, London

Cutcliffe J, Butterworth T, Proctor B (eds) 2001 Fundamental themes in clinical supervision. Routledge, London

Deane D, Campbell J 1985 Developing professional effectiveness in nursing. Reston Publications, Virginia

Department of Health 1993 A vision for the future: the nursing, midwifery and health visiting contribution to health care. HMSO, London

Dwyer G, Higgs J 1999 Profiling health science students. In: Higgs J, Edwards H (eds) Educating beginning practitioners. Butterworth-Heinemann, Oxford

Higgs J, Bithell C 2001 Professional expertise. In: Higgs J, Titchen A (eds) Practice knowledge and expertise. Butterworth-Heinemann, Oxford

Higgs J, Edwards H 1999 Educating beginning practitioners in the health professions. In: Higgs J, Edwards H (eds) Educating beginning practitioners. Butterworth-Heinemann, Oxford

Higgs J, Glendinging M, Dunsford E, Panton J 1991 Goals and components of clinical education in the allied health professions. Proceedings of the World Confederation for Physical Therapy 11th International Conference, London

Higgs C, Neubauer D, Higgs J 1999 The changing health care context: globalisation and social ecology. In: Higgs J, Edwards H (eds) Educating beginning practitioners. Butterworth-Heinemann, Oxford

Hummel J, Williamson P 1999 Fieldwork in occupational therapy; close to the edge. Focus on Health Professional Education 1:33–49

Hunt A, Adamson B, Harris L 1999 Community and workplace expectations of health science graduates. In: Higgs J, Edwards H (eds) Educating beginning practitioners. Butterworth-Heinemann, Oxford

Liston C 1999 Curriculum accreditation. In: Higgs J, Edwards H (eds) Educating beginning practitioners. Butterworth-Heinemann, Oxford

Marchant H 1986 Supervision: a training perspective. In: Marten M, Payne M (eds) Enabling and ensuring. Council for Education and Training in Youth and Community Work, London

McAllister L 1997 An adult learning framework for clinical education. In: McAllister L, Lincoln M, McLeod S, Maloney D (eds) Facilitating learning in clinical settings. Stanley Thornes, Cheltenham, p 1–26

Morton-Cooper A, Palmer A 2000 Mentoring, preceptorship and clinical supervision. A guide to professional roles in clinical practice, 2nd edn. Blackwell Science, Oxford

Neubauer D 1998 Some impacts of globalisation on health and health care policy. Occasional paper. Centre for Professional Education Advancement Faculty of Health Science, University of Sydney, Sydney

Stephenson K, Peloquin S, Richmond S et al 2002 Changing educational paradigms to prepare allied health professionals for the 21st century. Education for Health 15:37–49

PART 3   Clinical education, professional supervision and mentoring: a perspective from the UK

Della Fish

INTRODUCTION

I offer the following as my credentials for producing this commentary, because readers are entitled to know the particular viewpoint from which it is written and to be aware of the lenses through which this writer looks.

I am first and foremost an educator, coming from many years' work in teaching and teacher education. My practice is teaching. Originally my practice arena was the classroom. In the last 24 years the clinical setting has gradually become the centre of my work. In the 1980s, I became involved in undergraduate education for a wide range of health care professions in the UK (as advisor in curriculum design to many schools of occupational therapy; as a member of Validation Committees for the College of Occupational Therapists (the occupational therapists' professional body) and as an external examiner for a new joint degree in occupational therapy and physiotherapy). I also carried out some contract research focused on teaching in the clinical setting for the nursing profession (Fish & Purr 1992). Through all this I developed an increasing understanding of the importance of education *in the clinical setting* (which paralleled the importance of classroom teaching practice in teacher education).

Later, as a freelance educational consultant in the 1990s, I ran workshops (on curriculum design and on reflective practice and its assessment) for those who taught in the clinical setting during undergraduate courses in nursing, occupational therapy, physiotherapy, dietetics, radiography, acupuncture and homeopathy. I was also fortunate in being invited to Australia in 2000 by the Foundation for Quality Supervision.

More recently I have moved substantially into postgraduate medical education, and now work directly in the clinical setting observing medical and surgical consultants, as they teach in ward, theatre and clinic, and discussing with them their education and assessment of postgraduate doctors, in an attempt to help them to refine it. I am also joint director of a project investigating the role of theatre teams in providing teaching and assessment for the learning surgeon.

THE TERMINOLOGY

To a large extent, the terminology as defined at the start of this chapter, the lack of cohesion between professions and the global context described are broadly similar between Australia and the UK.

The terms for what were once fieldwork supervisors or student supervisors and are now practice teachers or clinical educators (revealing a change of emphasis) have developed in the UK much as in Australia. (The exception to this is the term preceptor, which is only used by nursing, but in much the way it is defined above.) The increased dimensions of consumer protection (as raised in the definition of clinical supervisor above) have occurred in the UK too in relation to clinical governance.

In fact, by the mid-1990s, each profession had carved its own way through the need to define terms at the start of definitive curriculum documents for courses newly established within universities. And none of them, to my knowledge, consulted other professions about how these might be held in common. Since then little has changed. Professional territory has, until very recently, been more significant than the gains of working across professions. Shared understanding of these terms will be a significant issue in the success of inter-professional team working.

THE CONTEXT

Global forces, by definition, have had an impact in the UK similar to that in Australia. Workload and pressures have increased exponentially in the UK, as in Australia. This is the result of increased numbers of patients/clients and a more diverse population, the demand for international and inter-professional links, the greater use of technology and the requirement for greater accountability. Further, the demand for inter-professional or multidisciplinary team working (which in the UK began quietly in the 1990s) is now in full flood, with an extensive literature of its own developing, including new journals, bringing with it the added pressure for professionals to see themselves as members of a new kind of team. Professionals are under siege (see Fish & Coles 1998).

The prevalence of the demand for competencies, visible outcomes and accountability is ubiquitous. Risk management has become an industry that proliferates protocols in response to the encouragement by the press and lawyers that the public should rush to litigation. Indeed, the insatiable desire in the public for absolute certainty, proof and zero risk, fuelled by the media and the legal profession for their own ends, is rapidly demotivating those left who still cling to the professional ideal of service. And a highly distorted but well publicised version of "evidence-based practice" has given rise to absolutist expectations about treatment. This ignores the original intentions, as stated by those who began it, that medicine (and by association, health care generally) still depends crucially on the judgement of the professional. This (Sackett et al 1997, p. 4):

> requires a bottom-up approach that integrates the best external evidence with individual clinical expertise and patient choice, [and] it cannot result in slavish cook-book approaches to individual patient care. External evidence can inform, but never replace, individual clinical expertise and it is this expertise that decides whether external evidence applies to the individual patient at all, and if so, how it should be integrated into a clinical decision.

UK writers are beginning, however, to be *less* willing to accept the inevitability of much of this, and *more* critical of it; see, for example, Carr & Hartnet (1996) in education and White & Stancombe (2003), in health care. Unease is at last emerging significantly in intellectual quarters about the all-pervasive and all-engulfing nature of competencies (and their twin, "demonstrable outcomes") which emphasise performance to the exclusion of that which drives it. An interest in behaviour is beginning to be recognised as excluding a concern for conduct, and the endless government requirements for more and more paperwork are beginning to be seen as driving out creativity. Further, the deprofessionalising of health care by successive UK governments of both colours together with the media, in the name of accountability, and the (too easily accepted) need to commodify it, and turn professionals into a "workforce" who are no different from all other workers, are beginning to stand accused in the public arena (see O'Neill 2002).

HOW DOES PROFESSIONAL EDUCATION IN THE UK ADDRESS THESE?

The development of health care courses in the UK shows broadly the same response as that in Australia. There is a rapid expansion of undergraduate and postgraduate courses to attend to the education of all kinds of health care professionals. But this expansion has been accompanied by a diminution in the critical edge that used to be developed in universities. Education for all professions has now become university-based. All courses are attending more to government pressures to produce "workers" who are inter-professional (some universities have integrated early parts of health care and medical courses; some new medical schools have set up problem-based learning which takes account of the contributions of other professions). As yet, however, the graduates of both undergraduate and postgraduate courses are being prepared for unquestioning acceptance of the current working context, as described above. This raises grim questions about how and by whom professions will be developed in the future.

Particular trends include postgraduate courses for advanced health care practitioners, and professional doctorates in work-based learning. The National Health Service University is also trying to find its way (as an educational provider for Europe's biggest employer!). And there is an initiative by government (which drives all these things in the background) to "modernise" medical careers. This is making huge changes to postgraduate medical education, and is focusing more on teaching in the clinical setting.

However, universities are in thrall to governments, none of whom can see beyond competencies (in the name of developing technical competence), and so these are still being pushed from the top, as the way to shape courses. Further, market forces together with diminishing resources are forcing corner cutting, particularly in supervisory arrangements, and in the educational support for those teacher-supervisors. Hours in clinical practice are a set requirement, but there is no parallel requirement to provide the resources to support this, and in a number of professions there is a feeling that postgraduates can now cope less well with complex problems than they could in the past.

CONCLUSION

In the light of all this, the significance of clinical education is growing rather than diminishing in the UK, and it will be important for readers to explore the bringing together of the roles described above and expanded on in later chapters.

It should be noted that the ideas and opinions expressed above are entirely my own and do not reflect the views of any institution for which I work.

REFERENCES

Carr W, Hartnet A 1996 Education and the struggle for democracy: the politics of educational ideas. Open University Press, Maidenhead

Fish D, Coles C 1998 Developing professional judgement in health care: learning through the critical appreciation of practice. Butterworth-Heinemann, Oxford

Fish D, Purr B 1992 An evaluation of practice-based learning in continuing professional education in nursing, midwifery and health visiting. English National Board for Nursing, Midwifery and Health Visiting, London

O'Neill O 2002 A question of trust. Cambridge University Press, Cambridge

Sackett D L, Richardson S, Rosenberg W, Haynes R B 1997 Evidence based medicine: how to practise and teach EB. Churchill Livingstone, Edinburgh

White S, Stancombe J 2003 Clinical judgement in the health and welfare professions: extending the evidence base. Open University Press, Maidenhead

PART 4   Clinical education, professional supervision and mentoring: a perspective from the USA

Marisue Pickering

CONTEXT

To begin to understand clinical education, professional supervision, and mentoring in communication sciences and disorders (CSD) in the United

States of America, readers may benefit from having a sense of the field. Perhaps the most significant feature is its size. The American Speech-Language-Hearing Association (ASHA), our national professional organisation, represents over 94,000 certified speech-language pathologists. A number of audiologists and speech, language and hearing scientists are also represented, for a total figure of over 114,000 (ASHA 2004a). The number of accredited university educational programmes is about 250 (ASHA 2004b).

I believe the size of our field makes us parochial in relation to other allied heath fields, a situation I see as different from what is experienced in countries with both fewer professionals and fewer educational programmes (and smaller national populations). Rather than interact with other fields, we are likely to use our time and energy to keep in touch with other CSD university programmes across the country. We are unlikely to pay attention to issues occurring elsewhere, for example, in nursing or physical therapy, which are large themselves. (Physical therapy has over 200 training programmes.) Speech-language pathologists do study, train and work closely with audiologists; historically the two professions have been considered part of CSD and part of ASHA. Audiology, therefore, is the allied health profession about which speech-language pathology programmes would likely know the most.

Another element of our context is that a Master's degree is the expected entry-level degree, the Certificate of Clinical Competence (CCC) the required national credential. (Individual employment institutions may have other standards for specific positions.) To obtain the CCC, individuals must meet several sets of requirements: those of their specific educational institutions, those related to ASHA's accreditation of their educational programmes, and those associated with successfully passing a written national exam and completing a postgraduate clinical fellowship year. Our educational focus occurs within the structure provided by these factors; other professions must work within their own detailed parameters.

CSD in the USA would undoubtedly benefit from interaction with other fields as we consider the issues involved in subsequent chapters. Unfortunately, for the most part, such interaction is not part of our experience. The following comments, therefore, pertain only to CSD.

TERMINOLOGY AND TASKS

The literature related to CSD clinical teaching in the USA goes back at least to 1951 (Moore 1951). Traditionally, university-level clinical teaching has been understood as occurring between individuals termed *supervisee* and *supervisor* (ASHA 1978). Recent CSD literature, however, has introduced the concept of *clinical education* and *clinical educator* (McCrea 2003a, McCrea & Brasseur 2003). Irrespective of terminology, interactions between clinical teachers and students are expected to focus on the development of students' clinical skills.

Students' clinical experiences are supervised by university-based clinical educators or by on-site professionals when students do practica off-campus. Normally students experience a range of service delivery venues, seeing clients who differ in need, age, race, and cultural and linguistic backgrounds.

Supervisors may or may not be specially trained in clinical education; no national professional requirement exists.

Workplace supervision is provided by professionals expected to be appropriately experienced and credentialed; potentially they may be in a field other than CSD. Professional supervision is often understood as separate from clinical teaching (ASHA 1978). Nevertheless, as McCrea & Brasseur (2003) note, supervisory tasks involved in a professional CSD setting can include supervising students placed there for clinical practica as well as speech-language assistants and persons completing their required clinical fellowship year (p. 5). This supervision would be in addition to the primary focus of providing staff evaluations, and monitoring and evaluating services delivered to clients by the professional staff.

Mentoring is not – to my knowledge – officially defined in CSD and is not a significant research focus. Nevertheless, recent texts discussing CSD supervision do include mentoring. McCrea & Brasseur (2003) point to its role in retaining culturally and linguistically minority students in CSD university programmes, and Dowling (2001) mentions its place in supervising people in the workplace. And I have discussed mentoring clinical faculty per se (Pickering 2000).

CURRENT DISCOURSE IN CSD

CSD publications now typically discuss all three types of interactions. The texts noted above are noteworthy in this regard as they both provide a model for the supervisory process as well as tools and strategies applicable across CSD settings (Dowling 2001, McCrea & Brasseur 2003). And, as noted above, mentoring is included. Interestingly, Dowling enlarges the context of her discussion by untypically including a focus on health care professions. Earlier texts in the field, such as mine (Crago & Pickering 1984), tended to limit themselves to supervision as clinical teaching and not venture further. Clearly, the discourse in the field has expanded and become inclusive of other key professional relationships and tasks.

An important contemporary venue for discourse about supervision is ASHA's Special Interest Division 11, Administration and Supervision. Created about 1991, the Division's primary goals are:

- to disseminate state-of-the-art information on leadership skills/styles that are crucial to success of speech-language pathologists and audiologists in the 1990s
- to establish collaboration between university and practice settings
- to develop and promote alternative service delivery models for universities and practice settings
- to establish programme evaluation and quality improvement models across practice settings
- to prepare and establish competencies for supervisors and administrators (ASHA 2004c).

As these goals indicate, the Division's focus goes beyond supervision in the traditional sense. Thus a perusal of a recent issue of the Division's publication,

Perspectives on Administration and Supervision, reveals articles about, for example, telepractices (Elangovan & Givens 2003) and the use of CSD assistants in the workplace (O'Connor 2003). Additionally, since early 2003, the Division has sponsored a "Mentoring Project" whereby members are provided a forum within the publication for sharing knowledge and experience (McCrea 2003b).

Many supervisory issues are under discussion in CSD. Nevertheless, a focus on the development of clinical skills in student clinicians remains a priority. Present-day clinical educators continue to probe issues such as how to help students develop problem-solving skills (McCarthy 2003).

CONCLUSION

At their best, the relationships and tasks of clinical education, professional supervision and mentoring give individuals the sense that someone is watching out for them and helping them. As I have noted elsewhere, we can all benefit from such a sense (Pickering 2000).

REFERENCES

American Speech-Language-Hearing Association 1978 Committee on supervision in speech-language-pathology and audiology. Current status of supervision of speech-language pathology and audiology [special report]. Asha 20:478–486

American Speech-Language-Hearing Association 2004a Welcome to ASHA. Online. Available: http://www.asha.org/default.htm 22 March 2004

American Speech-Language-Hearing Association 2004b ASHA's online guide to graduate programs. Online. Available: http://www.asha.org/gradguide/grad_guide.cfm 22 March 2004

American Speech-Language-Hearing Association 2004c Division 11 administration and supervision. Online. Available: http://www.asha.org/about/membership-certification/divs/div_11.htm 22 March 2004

Crago M, Pickering M 1984 Supervision in human communication disorders. Little, Brown, Boston

Dowling S 2001 Supervision: strategies for successful outcomes and productivity. Allyn and Bacon, Boston

Elangovan S, Givens G 2003 A perspective on telepractices in communication disorders. Perspectives on Administration and Supervision 13(3):5–7

McCarthy M 2003 Promoting problem-solving and self-evaluation in clinical education through a collaborative approach to supervision. Perspectives on Administration and Supervision 13(3):20–26

McCrea E 2003a What's in a name – supervisor or clinical educator? The ASHA Leader 8(22):26

McCrea E 2003b Coordinator's column. Perspectives on Administration and Supervision 13(1):1–2

McCrea E, Brasseur J 2003 The supervisory process in speech-language pathology and audiology. Allyn and Bacon, Boston

Moore P 1951 Supervision of student clinicians. Presentation at the meeting of the American Speech and Hearing Association, Chicago

O'Connor L 2003 The importance of a national credential. Perspectives on Administration and Supervision 13(3):4–5

Pickering M 2000 Mentoring clinical faculty. In: Hargrove P, McGuire R, O'Rourke C, Swisher W (eds) The challenge of change: proceedings of the annual conference of Council of Academic Programs in Communication Sciences and Disorders. Council of Academic Programs in Communication Sciences and Disorders, Minneapolis, p 22–29

PART 5   Clinical education, professional supervision and mentoring: a perspective from Canada

Paul Hagler

INTRODUCTION TO TERMINOLOGY AND DEFINITIONS

The editors' decision to include an introductory section on terminology does more than bring uniformity to this text; it contributes to more meaningful discussions among the professionals and academics who read it. All of us would benefit from more consistent use of terminology in clinical education. In Canada, we face most of the same confusion around commonly used terms, especially when we are talking to members of other professions. It's not that nurses, occupational therapists, dieticians, and pharmacists fail to communicate effectively with one another; it's that communication is more laboured or cumbersome and punctuated by frowns, calls for clarification and occasional misapprehensions that require repair later.

For example, in the process of writing an interdisciplinary, clinical educa-tion, research proposal recently, my co-investigators and I designed an inter-disciplinary survey instrument that needed to be understandable by students and professionals in four disciplines: nursing, occupational therapy, pharmacy and physical therapy. We quickly realised that we refer to some of the same things by different names. A "clinical supervisor" in physical therapy is a "fieldwork supervisor" in occupational therapy and a "preceptor" in nursing. In fact, clinical education placements for nursing students are often referred to as "preceptorships". What you, the reader, may not realise is that Microsoft Word underlines the word "preceptorship" on my computer monitor with a red squiggly line to let me know that it is misspelled. Unfortunately, although this amazing software automatically repairs about 90% of every-thing else I type, it is unable to fix "preceptorship" automatically. Why? Because, not only is "preceptorship" not a word, it's so far from being a real word that the spell-checking feature doesn't even know where to begin.

Why do we do this to ourselves? Make up new words, that is. We certainly don't need them. I don't know about you, but when I open a dictionary, I see more words I don't use than words I do use. So, until I master all the words I don't know – great words like "myrmidon", "esurient" and "pestiferous" – I don't want people making up any more new words and confusing the issue, whatever it may be. The English language provides us with a mind-boggling array of words with which we can communicate the finest nuances of meaning. Do we really need to invent new ones? I have had this conver-sation with some of my linguist friends, and it is at this point that they usually tell me how I fail to appreciate the delightfully dynamic nature of language. If I persist, they begin to scour their own memory banks for various descriptors of me – such as curmudgeon, dilettante or Luddite – frustrated all the while by the realisation that there is a surfeit of even better adjectives, if they could just remember them. But, I digress. It is easy to understand why my co-investigators and I had to define some of the terms introduced above. With ten words for essentially the same activity, the health sciences disciplines need help. Rose and Best are offering us a leg up.

CONTEXT FOR CLINICAL EDUCATION, PROFESSIONAL SUPERVISION AND MENTORING

Historically, the health sciences disciplines were at liberty to be somewhat parochial in their beliefs. That freedom probably caused us to evolve differently in many ways, between disciplines as well as within disciplines, and this included everything from accepted practices to vocabulary. However, as the editors assert earlier in this chapter, world issues influence health care delivery and health sciences educational practices. Instantaneous communication and information exchange have made it not only possible, they have made it imperative, to have a worldview. The health sciences disciplines are now positioned to learn from one another, whether they are on the opposite side of town or on the opposite side of the globe. The editors' observation that there is an increasing move towards privatisation with a focus on consumerism in health care is an example of a change in thinking about what should drive health care services as well as how they should be offered and paid for. This is happening in countries all over the world, including Canada.

PROFESSIONAL EDUCATION IN CANADA

As in Australia, universities in Canada are required to provide mission and vision statements; details of governance, finances and research outcomes; and lists of personnel and constituent groups. Heaven help us if a constituent group disapproves of something we want to do in a post-secondary educational institution. Members of constituent groups are voters, and voters' opinions matter greatly to ministers and deputy ministers. Provincial governments give final approval to implementation of new academic programmes, and in some provinces, they register clinical practitioners and regulate their titles and clinical practices. The warning by Hunt et al (1999) that accreditation of university curricula addresses minimal standards of entry-level graduate competence and, therefore, prevents only gross incompetence in practice, may be true, but that won't last. In Canada, increasing numbers of provinces are accrediting (registering) clinicians, their titles and their scopes of practice. Doing so positions the provincial governance body for each profession (often referred to as a "college") to initiate legal action against individuals who infringe on any of the controlled aspects of their discipline's practice, and one potential catalyst would be incompetence in practice.

In Canada, as in other countries, there has been a corporatisation of universities that has resulted in a competitive environment. Universities compete with one another for students. We compete by offering funding in the form of scholarships, tuition supplements and graduate assistantships. The latter pay students to help professors in their laboratories and classrooms. We even strategically adjust application and admission deadlines to optimise our chances of getting commitments from the best students to attend our graduate programme instead of another one. The central administration offices of Canadian universities generate statistics comparing their own educational programmes with one another in terms of research productivity, grant dollars, number of students, students' grades, average time to degree completion and per capita student success rate with external funding. With a true money-follows-excellence mentality, the programmes with good stats receive more money with which to make themselves even better, and the programmes whose numbers are less impressive end up with even less money, minimising their chances of improvement. This is, one supposes, the "corporate way".

Academic teachers

Unlike Australia, most of Canada's health science professions have been located in major universities for many years, so for some time now, we have faced the same challenges currently confronting our Australian colleagues. The number of academic teaching staff is decreasing as the number of student enrolments is increasing. This phenomenon, discussed in Chapter 3, is reaching near-crisis proportions. There are all the same attendant pressures on academic staff to win grants, publish, teach and do service work in highly competitive environments. Some unfortunate spillover effects can result from entry-level clinical programmes situated in major universities with heavy-duty research expectations. When professors' annual salary increments are tied more to the number of grants and publications they have than to the quality of their teaching and service, it is not difficult to guess where their energies will go. Of course, there are advantages associated with programmes being situated in major universities, such as opportunities to bring the most current research findings directly to the classroom and to involve students in research where it happens as it happens. The important thing is that educators in entry-level programmes do not allow themselves to lose track of why they are there, and that is to prepare the next generation of clinical professionals. This is a noble endeavour that requires a devotion to teaching.

Professional supervision and mentoring

Most professionals tend to agree that they generally lack adequate preparation for their roles as supervisee/mentee and supervisor/mentor. Canadian programmes typically provide limited course content on these topics, and where it exists, it is usually inserted into courses with other, more over-arching objectives. Most Canadian programmes are a long way from being able to offer an entire course in this area, much less make it a programme requirement. As a result, our graduates are ill-equipped to assume any of these important roles with knowledge and confidence. It is arguably appropriate to expect professionals to acquire these skills post-graduation, but with so many pertinent, practice-related continuing education options available, that approach would capture relatively few clinical educators, and it would make it difficult to require such a specialised educational experience. It would be virtually impossible to tie a required credential to it. The American Speech-Language-Hearing Association kicked the idea around for a while and then abandoned it as problematic. So, in my opinion, a certification process for clinical educators is a lofty goal that I predict only the youngest members of the rehabilitation professions will live to see.

CONCLUSION

In summary, I think it is fair to say that, with relatively few exceptions, terminology, educational issues/practices and professional supervision/ mentoring have evolved in remarkably similar ways across disciplines and countries. Perhaps this is partly attributable to globalisation, but to an extent, it may be an inevitable process of evolution. Consider the fact that we are relatively young professions that are in many ways following in the footsteps of professions such as medicine, dentistry and law, all of which have been around much longer and have well-developed governing and credentialing bodies with real clout. More than causing international, interdisciplinary events, globalisation may be serving to keep all of us moving along at about the same pace, which, if you think about it, is a good thing. We can help each other, and no one gets left behind.

REFERENCE

Hunt A, Adamson B, Harris L 1999 Community and workplace expectations of health science graduates. In: Higgs J, Edwards H (eds) Educating beginning practitioners. Butterworth-Heinemann, Oxford

SECTION 1

The clinical education process and the role of the clinical educator

Chapter 2

Models of clinical education

Beverly Joffe

Knowing about models of clinical education has various benefits. Such knowledge empowers clinical educators to enhance the clinical education experience. Informed clinical educators are able to improve overall planning, structuring of sessions, integration and logical progression of the clinical practicum. Advantages to such enhanced, yet streamlined practices (especially in the context of many busy workplace demands) are considerable. Indeed, although not immediately obvious, increased efforts in contemplating clinical education models may well contribute to improved patient care. A carefully considered, seamless clinical education experience could reduce stress for both student and clinical educator, thereby increasing productivity in the clinical setting. Moreover, by facilitating the emergence of competent, fully-fledged practitioners, the informed clinical educator becomes able, in the long term, to contribute indirectly to raising the standard of practice in a particular discipline.

This chapter provides an overview of some models that have application within the field of clinical education for health professional students. Contemplation of some of these models offers insights into why we as clinical educators might favour particular modes of interaction in clinical education contexts. The chapter also suggests why it may be preferable to consider more than one model of clinical education.

WHY LOOK AT DIVERSE MODELS OF CLINICAL EDUCATION?

"Model" as a concept suggests a quality of conduct that is worthy of being copied. Clearly, however, it is unlikely that the notion of one size fits all (or suitability of one model for all individuals and situations) would apply in the clinical education field. Heterogeneity is as probable among clinical educators as it is likely to be across students, and known to be across clients. Diversity might be anticipated with respect to clinical education partners in relation to realities, perceptions, previous experiences and belief systems. Clinical educators (because of their own past learning experiences, or not) may align (consciously or unconsciously), with particular philosophies of education. In a like manner, the students involved in the clinical education situation may be comfortable with distinct learning styles, be at particular learning stages, or exhibit a range of emotions, confidence levels and anxieties.

Similar observations are supported in the literature. For instance, Maloni et al (2003) refer to differences in "prior knowledge, learning styles, cognitive development and culture" (p. 170). It is necessary for clinical educators to be conscious of their clinical education practices and cognisant of associated underlying philosophies. It is also evident that there are implications to tailor clinical education experiences. The extent to which clinical education models take into account, and address such issues, and the manner in which this is done, is worthy of consideration; yet such deliberation is not always made explicit.

There are few empirically tested studies in the health profession literature that provide evidence of what constitutes best practice with respect to models of clinical education. The dearth of rigorous evidence-based research with respect to models of clinical education is unfortunate, especially in light of viewpoints such as those of Nye (2002), who suggests that, if we know what processes contribute to the development of clinical skills, we can attempt to utilise these processes on a more conscious level. The notion of practice outpacing research in the field of clinical education has been broached in the literature. Zungaloo (2003), for instance, refers to "the powerful influence of a strong tradition supported by a very limited database " (p. 166), with respect to clinical education practices for nurses. A perusal of the literature suggests that a similar state of affairs exists across other health profession disciplines. Nonetheless it is instructive for the clinical educator to consider some models of clinical education that are presented in the literature, notwithstanding that the outcomes for all may not necessarily have been empirically tested.

SOME MODELS OF CLINICAL EDUCATION

Goldhammer and his colleagues' (1980) early work in education includes a model that incorporates the main stages of a pre-observation meeting, in which educator and student establish rapport and review plans, as well as discuss and rehearse changes. The next stage involves the educator observing the session, then noting issues for future discussion. A subsequent phase incorporates the educator analysing data collected in relation to the observed session and planning a strategy for feedback. In the following stage the clinical educator provides feedback and recommendations for improvement. This phase may also incorporate elicited self-evaluation from the student. Finally, both educator and student conduct independent analyses and devise plans for modification.

By addressing the need to establish rapport, this model considers affect within educator–student encounters. This education model gives credence to interpersonal and emotional aspects. According to Decleva (1994), integrated and holistic understanding on the part of the student is assisted by the clinical educator's sincerity, warm rapport, a mutually trusting relationship, empathy for the student's point of view and unconditional acceptance. Decleva (1994) posits the potential for the quality of clinical educator–student interactions to change students' attitudes, and also the likelihood of educators' attitudes influencing student attitudes within the learning experience and towards their clients. Pickering (1984) highlights the need for supervisors to go beyond only cognitive responses to items that students raise for discussion.

Goldhammer et al's model does not specifically prescribe students' observation of educators; neither does it explicitly specify substantial, structured reflection tasks. Yet the premise that it is worthwhile providing opportunities for students to observe educators in action is illustrated in the following quotation: "throughout history and still today, the observation of exemplary practice serves an important function in the mastery of skills necessary for competent practice of a profession" (Goldberg 1997, p. 310). The value of providing students with opportunities to observe is also supported by Schön (1987), who considers learning in relation to what can be gained "from a careful examination of artistry, that is, the competence by which practitioners actually handle indeterminate zones of practice" (p. 13). Whereas it is possible to argue that observation of the clinical educator may be outmoded because of paradigms that have moved some way from didactic teaching models, there is undoubtedly some merit in such practices.

A model in speech pathology proposed by Mandy (1989) extends Goldhammer et al's model by adding a reflective component, and being explicit about learning styles as well as clinical education models (Fig. 2.1).

Mandy suggests that within the pre-observation stage, clinical educator and student clinician first discuss the clinical education model, and also the student's prior learning experiences. As an aside, it would seem that such meta-analysis of the clinical education process could be an empowering experience for students and assist them in gaining autonomy in clinical learning. It also makes the expectations of the clinical education interaction and the opportunities for negotiation within the relationship clear for the student.

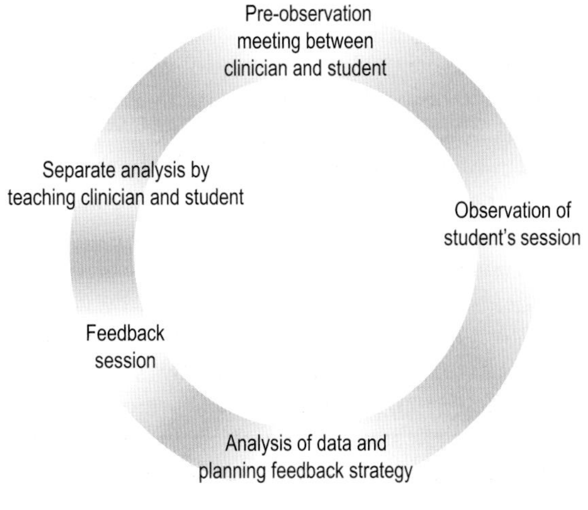

Figure 2.1 Illustration of Mandy's depiction of Goldhammer et al's (1980) supervision cycle. Reproduced with permission from Mandy (1989).

Pre-observation meeting between clinician and student

Separate analysis by teaching clinician and student

Observation of student's session

Feedback session

Analysis of data and planning feedback strategy

Subsequently (within Mandy's model) client management plans are contemplated. Following this discussion, and still within this stage, the clinical educator considers the student learning styles, whilst simultaneously making adaptations to proposed clinical education styles. Hence, there seems to be a dynamic tailored component within this model, albeit a lack of opportunity within this framework for students to observe the skilled practitioner at the outset.

The next stage in Mandy's model, that is, where the clinical educator engages in observation of students in the clinical practicum setting, is similar to that described for the approach of Goldhammer et al. Mandy is of the opinion that data collected by the clinical educator during observation may assist students' recollection and contemplation of the clinic session. According to McCrea & Brasseur (2003), who provide helpful strategies for observation, "data collection on clinician behaviour is so important that supervisors must make a great effort to perfect systems for recording that they can use easily and efficiently" (p. 165).

Mandy (1989) suggests that the analysis and strategy phase (stage 3) include both student and clinical educator independently deciding on a topic for discussion and the manner in which to approach such dialogue. Here again, a process such as this suggests some equality in the clinical educator–student relationship. Additionally, the clinical educator structures the next phase so as to encourage reflection on the part of the student. Stage 4 of Mandy's model encourages student practitioners to recall their experiences, whilst withholding self-judgement. Furthermore, clinical educators are encouraged to listen actively. This is in line with proposals within supervision in education to "listen more, talk less" (Acheson & Gall 1997, p. 161).

Mandy suggests further that clinical educators accept student recollections, and at the same time refrain from judging or negating any of the emotions verbalised by the students. Hence, the emotional variable appears also to be taken into account in this model. The potential of videotaping to enhance self-evaluation is also considered. Stage 5 within the model advocated by Mandy involves further reflection and insights, in order that clinical educator and student both move toward increased awareness of their clinical practices. According to Mandy, in some instances applying the model with a single case for the student may suffice. Mandy suggests further that advanced students may be given the opportunity for more self-evaluation, a view shared by Anderson (1988). The model advocated by Anderson proposes a progression from evaluation-feedback to student self-appraisal (according to students' stage of training and level of competence).

A model proposed by Cox (1993), for medical education, addresses the importance of building in a reflective process and creating opportunities for students to pursue further knowledge from other sources, e.g. texts and peers. This model, presented in Figure 2.2, also highlights the merit of enabling students to learn both away from and with the clinical educator.

Cox's model would presumably allow for demonstration by clinical educators, and hence observation by student clinicians. Yet authors such as Goldberg (1997) put forward a notion that such a process rarely happens within a field such as speech pathology and that, instead, "learning is often by trial and error" (p. 310). Nonetheless, tacit knowledge is eventually likely

Figure 2.2   Diagram of
clinical education model
(modified from Cox 1993).

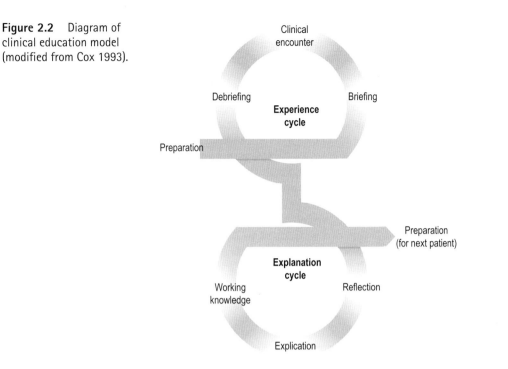

to emerge from experience within clinical encounters, as depicted in Cox's
clinical education model.

McLeod et al (1997) propose five partitions to categorise various models –
descriptive, integration, developmental, interactive and collaborative – which
are summarised as follows. Within the integration models, the authors
include the conceptual model and the integration model. In such models
there are connotations of the responsibility of various educators to ensure
integration across learning contexts within a curriculum, so as to assist the
student progress toward achievement of requisite knowledge, skills and
attitudes (McLeod et al 1997, Pickering et al 1992). The third partition, or developmental models, according to McLeod et al (1997), pertains to progressive
levels of ability and assumptions of meeting associated needs in the clinical
education process. Hence the notion of continuum of clinical education,
according to Anderson (1988), is cited (McLeod et al 1997) and encompasses
"evaluation-feedback, transition, and self clinical education" (p. 33).

Fletcher (1993, p. 6) suggests that models such as those described by
Brady (1985) are pertinent to clinical education. These include: the expos-
ition model, behavioural model, cognitive developmental model, interaction
model and transactional model. Specific strategies to enhance learning are
also described in the literature, for instance the use of field journals together
with the literature to assist integration and application for students in the field
of social work (Dettlaff & Wallace 2002). At a macro level, Burnard (1995)
outlines a model for nursing education that encompasses stages that include:
self-assessment plus input from the syllabus; negotiation of the timetable;
the learning process incorporating theory and skills via various methods
and the use of the experiential learning cycle; and then self-evaluation, peer
evaluation and tutor evaluation (p. 77).

Some authors assign equal weight in responsibility to clinical educator and student for assisting optimal clinical learning environments. Neary (2000), for instance, considers both the quality of the teaching itself and the teacher, as well as "the quality of the students and their willingness and motivation to learn … and also … the construct of active learning time, i.e. how much time is spent on outcome-related activities" (p. 92). Neary also emphasises the need for engagement on the part of the student, and "a stimulating environment for active learning to take place" (p. 94).

Multiple suggestions can be confounding. It is also not enough merely to adopt prescribed practices in an ad hoc manner. What may be more helpful is to consider assumptions that might potentially underlie some models. For instance, Rowland (1993) outlines practices anticipated in didactic versus exploratory models. Hence, within didactic frameworks it is expected that "the role of the tutor is to impart a body of prescribed professional knowledge (or skill) to the learner" (Rowland 1993, p. 18). The alternative model would involve creation of a context for exploration and learning to occur. Rowland outlines yet another model which combines both these approaches. Given unique facets of individuals, such general philosophies and the potential to combine or "mix and match" have much to offer participants in the clinical education process. Best & Rose (1996) highlight the need for clinical educators to be flexible with respect to clinical education style and process.

Lazar (1991) suggests that "the old Chinese proverb that questions whether it is better to give a man a fish for today or teach him the art of fishing to prepare him for a lifetime applies well to the contemporary task of education" (p. 109). So too is such a perspective pertinent to the notion of models of clinical education. The intention of this chapter has been to empower clinical educators with the knowledge that there can be many ways to approach clinical education and that further exploration of models and apparent underlying philosophies, together with analysis, reflection and integration, has the potential to enrich and extend the clinical education process.

REFERENCES

Acheson K A, Gall M D 1997 Techniques in the clinical supervision of teachers, 4th edn. Longman, New York

Anderson J 1988 The clinical educatory process in speech-language pathology and audiology. Little, Brown, Boston

Best D, Rose M 1996 Quality supervision. Theory and practice for clinical supervisors. W B Saunders, London

Brady L 1985 Models and methods of teaching. Prentice Hall, Melbourne

Burnard P 1995 Learning human skills: an experiential and reflective guide for nurses, 3rd edn. Butterworth-Heinemann, Stockholm

Cox K 1993 Planning bedside teaching: 5. Debriefing after clinical interaction. Medical Journal of Australia 158:571–572

Decleva V 1994 An exploration of teachers as role models and the effects of humanistic teaching on students'/patients' relationships: an integrated humanistic Rogerian-personal construct approach. Unpublished Masters dissertation. La Trobe University, Bundoora, Australia

Dettlaff A, Wallace G 2002 Promoting integration of theory and practice in field education: an instructional tool for field educators. The Clinical Supervisor 21(2):145–160

Fletcher D P 1993 The influence of clinical supervisory style on perceptions of the efficacy of clinical education of final year speech pathology students. Unpublished Masters dissertation. La Trobe University, Bundoora, Australia

Goldberg S A 1997 Clinical skills for speech-language pathologists. Singular Publishing Group, San Diego

Goldhammer R, Anderson R, Krajewski R 1980 Clinical education: special methods for the clinical education of teachers. Holt, Rinehart and Winston, New York

Lazar D 1991 Seven ways of teaching: the artistry of teaching with multiple intelligences. Skylight Publishing, Illinois

Maloni J A, Garvin A H, Garvin C F et al 2003 Take time to teach thoughtfully. Nursing Education Perspectives 24(4):170–171

Mandy S 1989 Facilitating student learning in clinical education. Australian Journal of Human Communication Disorders 17:83–93

McCrea E S, Brasseur J A 2003 The supervisory process in speech-language pathology and audiology. Pearson Education, Boston

McLeod S, Romanini J, Cohn E S et al 1997 Models and roles in clinical education. In: McAllister J L, Lincoln M, McLeod S et al (eds) Facilitating learning in clinical settings. Stanley Thornes, London

Neary M 2000 Teaching, assessing and evaluation for clinical competence: a practical guide for practitioners and teachers. Stanley Thornes, Gloucester

Nye C H 2002 Using developmental processes in supervision: a psychodynamic approach. The Clinical Supervisor 21(2):39–53

Pickering M 1984 Interpersonal communication in speech-language pathology supervisory conferences: a qualitative study. Journal of Speech and Hearing Disorders 49:189–195

Pickering M, Rassi J A, Hagler P et al 1992 Integrating classroom, laboratory, and clinical experiences. Asha 34:57–59

Rowland S 1993 The enquiring tutor: exploring the process of professional learning. The Farmer Press, London

Schön D A 1987 The reflective practitioner: how professionals think in action. Temple-Smith, London

Zungaloo E 2003 Challenges in nursing education research: examining clinical learning experiences. Nursing Education Perspectives 24(4):166

Chapter 3

Costs of clinical education

Paul Hagler

INTRODUCTION

Whenever people engage one another in an active, time-intensive, interpersonal endeavour, like the clinical education process, there are inevitable costs associated with getting the job done. These may include physical, temporal, emotional and monetary costs that, in the extreme, can deplete the participating human and organisational systems. However, it may be equally true to say that the same active, time-intensive, interpersonal endeavour, with all its acknowledged cost-related implications, can yield desirable outcomes or benefits that nurture the system and pay off in ways that make it all worthwhile. This is especially true when right-minded people implement the process in constructive ways (see Chapter 21). Therefore, this chapter is about both the costs and benefits of clinical education, for if we focus solely on costs or solely on benefits, the story is only half told.

All education programmes in the allied health disciplines rely on one or more structured practica or preceptorships to train the next generation of clinical professionals, but a commensurate commitment by clinicians and administrators in clinical service facilities to provide these experiences does not always exist. Clinicians and administrators do not necessarily see practicum students as a complementary presence. Several possible explanations exist. One is the assumption that student-provided services are of lower quality than services provided by fully qualified and credentialed professionals. Another is the belief that students provide less service than more experienced professionals, because they are less efficient than professionals. For example, students may take longer to do assessments and interpret the results or spend more time planning interventions. Maybe their clients do not progress as rapidly, resulting in lower discharge rates by students. As a result of their inexperience, students may take longer to write reports and carry out their non-patient care responsibilities. These are possible explanations for clinicians' and administrators' negative attitudes. Some of them may be well founded, but others may not. Therefore, this chapter is also about what we know and what we do not know.

IMPLICATIONS

Why is it so important to understand the issues around the costs of clinical education? The answer is because people make important decisions based on their beliefs about these issues. When the decision-makers are upper-level administrators and unit managers in clinical service facilities and their decision is to reduce the number of students at their institution or to discontinue taking students altogether, there are serious implications. Before listing the potential problems, however, we should examine why decision-makers sometimes want to distance themselves from students in training.

Clinical service facilities have a mandate to provide high-quality patient care and they usually express their mandates in organisational mission statements. When clinicians and administrators involved in service delivery in health care settings perceive students to have a deleterious effect on patient care, it is not surprising to see them pull back from their commitment to participate in the education of the next generation of professionals and, in so doing, use their institutional mission statement as the explanation for doing so. Such decisions have long-term adverse effects on service delivery, on the life cycles of the health sciences professions, and on the efficacy of the current move to foster evidence-based practice by clinicians.

Effects on service delivery

When decision-makers in clinical service facilities decide to reduce or curtail their involvement in clinical education, they may be creating service delivery problems for everyone, even themselves. As Hancock & Hagler (1998) pointed out, the health sciences professions need clinical service facilities to provide practical experiences for students, because educating students in classrooms, even when an on-site clinic is one of the classrooms, will not provide the breadth and depth of education required to produce competent new professionals. There are aspects of education that only occur in health care facilities and not in university classrooms and clinics that are critical in the preparation of new professionals. Clinical settings are a necessary part of the education of the next generation of clinical professionals, as is the enthusiastic participation of administrators and clinicians in those settings. Unfortunately, administrators and clinicians are not always enthusiastic about taking students.

Effects on the life cycle of the health sciences professions

When decision-makers in clinical service facilities decide to reduce or curtail their involvement in clinical education, they adversely affect the life cycle of the health sciences professions whose students they were helping to educate. Hancock & Hagler (1998) went on to say that health care funding cutbacks and restructured service delivery paradigms have not only resulted in heavier workloads for professionals but they also have made it increasingly important for professionals to provide efficient, high-quality patient care. If the situation is problematic in public health care facilities, it may be even worse in privatised health care facilities, where administrators monitor costs even more closely.

Under these conditions, service providers very carefully scrutinise requests from university programmes to accept students, and they do so from a cost/benefit perspective. If they view students as a liability, the number of available practicum assignments and the variety of potential experiences within that facility are likely to decrease. If administrators and clinicians see students as an asset, they will probably offer more placement choices for more students. More opportunities for more students give university-based placement coordinators more placement options that enable them to arrange better matches between students' experiences and certification requirements and ultimately yield better-prepared future professionals. Fewer options will seriously compromise the skills and abilities of new graduates at a time when the profession can ill afford educational compromise.

A compromised educational system can have far-reaching implications and do long-term damage to a profession, especially now. Interdependence exists among the activities of professional education, clinical practice and research in the health sciences. This interdependence is cyclic and, like any chain of events, a weak link can spell disaster.

For example, a shortage of health sciences practitioners results in clinical job vacancies in acute care hospitals, private practices, rehabilitation centres, workers' compensation boards, community facilities, extended care facilities, schools and special schools. Job vacancies mean reductions in clinical services, which make for frustrated patients/clients and family members, over-worked clinical professionals, frazzled administrators and fewer practicum placements. Citizens tell their governments to develop long-term human resources strategies in health care and to increase funding to programmes in post-secondary institutions to educate students who they hope will replenish the ranks of clinical professionals and eventually take practicum students of their own. A few of those clinical professionals will elect to return to school to become the next generation of academics – and they will be the teachers and researchers who inspire another generation of students. This is the life cycle of the health sciences professions. If it is to work, there must be volume turnover and an intact chain of events. Break the chain, and the system breaks down. It may take years to see the full effects, but see them we will.

Clinical professionals are not the only commodity in short supply. Most academics in rehabilitation science are members of their professions first and become academics later, so we can never have enough researchers/academics without first having enough clinical professionals. This situation is a Catch 22, insofar as we can never have enough clinical professionals without first having enough researcher/academics. Universities are currently in dire need of more health sciences researchers to accommodate impending retirements by the last of the professors from the baby-boomer generation. There is an alarming tendency lately for vacant positions in the professoriate to remain open for two years or longer, and some searches last for up to eight years. Many administrators express grave concern about their ability to recruit and retain faculty over the next 5–10 years, when an estimated 25–40% of current faculty members will retire. Throughout North America, universities are facing a steady stream of retiring academics. Given this demographic imperative, it is essential that individuals be educated not only to fill clinical job vacancies but also to replace retiring researchers and to expand the number needed to meet the disciplines' requirements for basic, applied and clinical research to support best practice. First, however, a healthy proportion of future researchers must be educated as clinical professionals.

John Bernthal (2001a), president of the American Speech-Language-Hearing Association, wrote:

> *The number of research doctoral candidates [in speech pathology and audiology] available to assume academic positions has reached a crisis level and, based on all available data, the situation is only going to get worse unless something is done to increase their number.*

To support his assertion, Bernthal (2001b) cited some alarming statistics. For example, during the 1997–1998 academic year, there were 2.3 applicants for each tenure-track, doctoral-level academic position available in the USA. It is generally accepted that candidates apply in several places simultaneously, therefore it is probably safe to assume that the applicant pool was much smaller even than the reported figure implies. He also observed that the majority of external funding is currently obtained by researchers 55 years of age and older, many of whom will be retiring in the next decade. Reid (2002) reported that about one-third of Canada's 34,000 faculty members are over the age of 55 and rapidly nearing retirement and that the growing shortage of academics is compounded by the relatively small percentage of students who go on to complete graduate degrees. These factors have led to a predicted shortfall of 30,000 to 35,000 professors within about 10 years (Giroux 2000). To the extent that these figures are mirrored in other countries, there may even be an imminent global shortage in the professoriate.

Effects on the future of evidence-based practice

When decision-makers in clinical service facilities decide to reduce or curtail their involvement in clinical education, they adversely affect the future of evidence-based practice and ultimately compromise the very thing they are mandated to provide – high-quality clinical services. There exists an increased emphasis on the need for improved evidence to support clinical practice in the health sciences. If practitioners are to engage in up-to-date, efficient, clinical practice, the professions must increase their research capacity. As economic pressures continue to build, health care services must focus more on prevention, early discharge, home care and cost-efficient service delivery.

Health care consumers are actively participating in their own care and that of their family members and are demanding more facts and comparative information about their options for care. Increased survival rates from pre-term birth, serious injuries and illnesses lead to increased rehabilitation needs post-injury/post-illness, and an ageing population will place increased demands on rehabilitation services. In addition, health care professionals themselves are calling for more scientific foundations and holistic approaches for their clinical practices across the life span. Rehabilitation professionals tend to practise in a client-centred model that emphasises natural "fit" in the community, but relatively little research has been done to help guide the integration of these complex factors.

Therefore, it is important to ensure the continuation of a comprehensive, dynamic educational base, one that produces clinical professionals who will be evidence-based practitioners from whose ranks we can attract the next generation of researchers (see Chapter 9). We must appreciate the cyclic, interdependent nature of professional education, clinical practice and research, and we must understand the ways in which they complement one another, if we are to nourish the health sciences professions.

Underlying implications of non-participation by clinical service facilities

The above discussion focused on the over-arching effects of decisions by clinicians and service facility administrators to pull back from student placements. They were: compromised service delivery, broken chains of events in the life cycles of the health care professions and stagnation in the area of evidence-based practice. However, several more subtle consequences are associated with a shortage of clinical placements. As indicated above, one is fewer choices for students. On the surface, this might seem acceptable, because someone else will always take the student. However, on closer inspection, that does not always work. To begin with, there seems to be a chronic shortage of placements. At least university placement coordinators are usually quick to confirm this. However, even when there are enough placements to find something for each student, it still may not be an acceptable situation, especially in the long term.

Placement shortages cause some students to fail to get what they want in terms of clinical experience and may result in disenchantment with their career choice and an eventual decision to leave the field. Similarly, they may not get what they need in terms of experience and will eventually graduate with seriously compromised clinical skills. A third drawback is the lost opportunity for clinical service facilities to get to know prospective new employees in ways that simply cannot be matched even by the most sophisticated interview techniques. The spillover effects of this lost opportunity may be bad hires, disgruntled new employees, higher employee turnover rates, reduced job satisfaction, employee time lost to the search and selection process, reduced quality of care for patients/clients and higher costs for employers.

PRACTICUM STUDENTS MAY BE AN ASSET

On the other hand, some administrators and professionals involved in the delivery of rehabilitation services encourage student practicum placements in their institutions. They value students for a variety of reasons. They see them as potential new employees whose technical and interpersonal skills they could never hope to assess so thoroughly during a typical job interview. From their students' ranks, they can hire with increased confidence, and they enjoy the opportunity actively to pursue the most promising applicants. They are assured of a goodness of fit between the new employees' skills and abilities and their own staff requirements. New employees are more likely to be satisfied with their jobs and remain on staff longer, and if that happens, the institution spends less time in the costly search and selection process. Most important, these administrators believe that well-chosen, contented staff members provide a higher quality of care for patients/clients.

Finally, and perhaps most importantly, these administrators and professionals believe well-supervised students provide their patients/clients with service that is comparable in quality to that provided by fully credentialed professionals. When circumstances are just right, the student's presence frees up some of the supervising professional's time to see other patients. This means the institution can provide more patient care than would have been possible without the student on site. Thus, some employers believe students are good for patients/clients, good for the institution and good for the professions.

How can such disparate views of the value of students prevail? Only one of these perceptions may be accurate or, depending upon the circumstances surrounding the practicum experience, certain aspects of both views may prove to be true. Research has improved our understanding of how students affect productivity, and a few well-designed research projects have begun to explain some of the specifics of how students affect service delivery, but more research is needed.

What we know

Research regarding the impact of practicum students on service delivery in the health sciences can be divided into two categories: cost–benefit research and productivity research. The cost–benefit literature fails to provide conclusive evidence to indicate that students are either an asset or a liability during clinical education. One study (Hammersberg 1982) found that students were a financial liability but other research found students were a financial benefit (Pobojewski 1978, Porter & Kincaid 1977). Historically, cost–benefit studies have taken a too simplistic approach to the process of determining the effects in monetary terms of practicum students in clinical service facilities. Although current approaches to cost–benefit analysis are sophisticated by comparison, none of them have yet been applied to practicum students in the rehabilitation professions. However, even the most well-done cost–benefit analyses are not able to translate important variables such as employee and patient/client satisfaction into dollars. Rather than approaching the issues around the effects of practicum students from a monetary perspective, some investigators have tried to provide information on how students affect the amount of patient care (productivity). Historically, this has been a meaningful variable for administrators of clinical service facilities.

Productivity cost–benefit research explores the service delivery outcomes associated with hosting students for their clinical placements. This approach asks how students affect patient care. It has the advantages of obviating the conversion of everything to dollars, and it maintains the focus on the mandate of most service-oriented institutions, which is to provide patient care. It also has relevance to frontline health care providers, patients or clients, and their families, and the outcomes are relatively easy to measure. Sometimes the outcome variables even pre-exist in institutional databases, making active data collection unnecessary. However, there are some disadvantages. The bean counters who sit at the right hand of most health care administrators today are not as interested in patient care as they are in the financial bottom line. Another disadvantage is that a research focus on amount of patient care (usually expressed in terms of patient visits or time charges to various types of patient care) fails to examine other important variables such as consumer satisfaction, quality of care and duration of intervention.

For the most part, early findings of productivity studies suggested that facilities benefited from having students in terms of increased patient visits and increased service delivery (Leiken 1983, Leiken et al 1983, Lopopolo 1984, Cebulski & Sojkowski 1988, Bristow & Hagler 1994, 1997, Ladyshewsky 1995). Although results indicated that students are an asset, there was a need for further research to discover what qualities or mixes of qualities among internship environments, students and clinical educators were needed to enhance productivity. Length of practicum, student experience, clinical educator work and supervision experience were potentially influential variables on the amount of patient care provided in facilities offering speech-language pathology treatment.

Hancock & Hagler (1998) investigated the effects of two of those variables, clinical educator work experience and clinical educator supervision experience, on student productivity, and a few years later the same authors carried out a follow-up data analysis that explored the effects of co-existing student variables (Hancock & Hagler, unpublished). In the original study, they learned that speech-language pathology students maintained the amount of patient care and increased the amount of non-patient care at a rehabilitation hospital. In the subsequent data analysis, they found that students had a positive effect on productivity in the institutions in which they did their clinical placements. The subjects were 11 speech-language pathology clinical educators and their 11 student interns. Data related to patient care and non-patient care activities were obtained from the participants. The results indicated that students were an asset in terms of both patient care and non-patient care.

Supplementary analyses revealed significant relationships between students' clinically related pre-programme experience and the two indices of productivity. A positive relationship existed between the amount of student experience and the amount of patient care the students were able to provide during their placements. They attributed this outcome to the possibility that previous experience may lead to increased confidence, which, in turn, may enable students to perform patient care more independently, that is with less extensive direct supervision. The relationship between previous related experience and amount of patient care suggests that productivity might be increased even more if students had more such experience before entering their programmes and/or acquired related clinical or teaching experience during their programmes prior to their practicum experiences.

What we need to understand better

Much of the previous research fails to examine other important variables such as consumer satisfaction, quality of care, duration of intervention, length of practicum, types of patients/service delivery programmes to which students are assigned, the influences of context-based or problem-based learning, and graduate-level versus undergraduate-level education. It is reasonable to believe that these variables may also influence the costs and benefits of students in practicum.

CONCLUSION

In conclusion, there is mounting evidence to suggest that the costs of educating students in health care settings is more than offset by the advantages that accrue to the host institutions, the amount of care the students provide while on site and the long-term benefits to the professions. As more research is completed, we will come to an improved understanding of the complex relationships that explain why so many clinicians and administrators have such divergent views of the ways in which this process affects their institutions and the care they are mandated to provide for their patients/clients. It is important that investigative work of this type continue, because without it decision-makers will continue to implement policies that have long-term adverse effects on service delivery, on the life cycles of the health sciences professions and on the efficacy of the current move to foster evidence-based practice by clinical professionals.

REFERENCES

Bernthal J E 2001a Discipline and professions face critical shortage of research doctorates. The ASHA Leader May 29

Bernthal J E 2001b Strategies to recruit and retain doctoral-level teacher scholars. The ASHA Leader June 26

Bristow D, Hagler P 1994 Impact of physical therapy students on patient service delivery and professional staff time. Physiotherapy Canada 46:275–280

Bristow D, Hagler P 1997 Comparison of individual physical therapists' productivity to that of combined physical therapist–student pairs. Physiotherapy Canada 49:16–23

Cebulski P, Sojkowski M 1988 Clinical education and staff productivity. Clinical Management in Physical Therapy 8:26–29

Giroux R J 2000 The changing face of academe: the challenge of graduate studies in a university in transition. Speech at the annual conference of the Canadian Association of Graduate Studies in Winnipeg, Manitoba

Hammersberg S 1982 A cost/benefit study of clinical education in selected allied health programs. Journal of Allied Health 1:35–41

Hancock J, Hagler P 1998 A pilot study of the effects of S-LP practicum students on service delivery. Journal of Speech-Language Pathology and Audiology 22(3):141–150

Hancock J, Hagler P unpublished Secondary analysis of data collected in a previous study of the effects of S-LP practicum students on service delivery

Ladyshewsky R 1995 Enhancing service productivity in acute care inpatient settings using a collaborative clinical education model. Physical Therapy 75:503–510

Leiken A 1983 Method to determine the effect of clinical education on production in a health care facility. Physical Therapy 63:56–59

Leiken A, Stern E, Baines R 1983 The effect of clinical education programs on hospital production. Inquiry 20:88–92

Lopopolo R 1984 Financial model to determine the effect of clinical education programs on physical therapy departments. Physical Therapy 64:1396–1402

Pobojewski T 1978 Case study: cost/benefit analysis of clinical education. Journal of Allied Health Summer:192–198

Porter R, Kincaid C 1977 Financial aspects of clinical education to facilities. Physical Therapy 57:905–909

Reid M 2002 Retired university profs find new life at U of C. Edmonton Journal

Chapter 4

Exploring the roles of the clinical educator

CHAPTER CONTENTS

PART 1 Introduction

Dawn Best

One of the aims of this text is to prepare clinical educators for the important task of assisting student learning in their clinical practice. We acknowledge that there may be considerable variation in the individual job descriptions of clinical educators and that different professions and workplaces may have different responsibilities. However, it is useful to spend some time considering the potential roles associated with being a clinical educator. We all bring our own interpretation of the role and this will influence our activities. My energies in my early days of being a clinical educator focused strongly on my perception of the role of protector of patients and to a lesser extent protector of students. Thinking back, this was grounded on the ethical principle of non-maleficence, that is, above all do no harm! However justifiable, it must be acknowledged that this was a very limited view of the role and failed to acknowledge other important aspects that needed to be addressed.

Farmer & Farmer (1989) identified the following five roles for speech pathologists working within the USA:

1. Professional (this involves activities related to membership of professional associations at local, state or national levels)
2. Researcher (this relates to clinical or educational practice)
3. Administrator
4. Clinician
5. Educator.

More recently, McLeod et al (1997) identified that clinical educators undertake the following seven roles:

1. Role model
2. Colleague
3. Teacher
4. Evaluator
5. Administrator manager
6. Counsellor
7. Researcher.

It is interesting that the first two roles of their list make explicit the important influence clinical educators have on students in the professional social-isation process. Sometimes we may forget in the busy activities associated with the other roles that these first two will influence all of the other more task-oriented roles.

The following introductory activity from Best & Rose (1996) can be used as an individual personal exploration or as a group activity. It aims to help you understand the roles of clinical educator and to explore potential role overlaps.

- Think about the type of clinical facility in which you work and list down one side of the page the roles that you have within your own job description.
- Compare the list of roles that you have generated with those suggested by Farmer & Farmer (1989). Perhaps your particular situation demands add-itional roles. Perhaps not all items in their list are applicable to you.
- On the opposite side of the page list the roles you have in your personal life.

It is important to acknowledge these roles as well as those associated with our work.

- Look at this profile of your roles and reflect on your work day. As you reflect on your list, designate the approximate percentage of your total work time allocated to each role:
  - when you do not have students in your facility
  - when students are in your facility.

- What happens to the time allocation when you include student supervision in your responsibilities?
- What strategies do you use to accommodate the role of student supervisor?
- Which aspects of this are you happy with?
- Which aspects would you like to improve?

Our supervision is influenced by personal factors. It is important to recognise that each of these roles has its own pressures, obligations, pleasures and rewards. It is also essential to realise that each interacts with another at either a conscious or unconscious level. For example, stresses at home related to our parenting role may influence our attitude to students at work. Our own experience of teachers will have an impact on our own teaching. Our successes in one part of our life will have a positive influence on our clinical education activity. We must be aware that it is very easy for stresses related to one of our roles to overflow into another area.

> Being a quality clinical educator is about taking a good look at ourselves

- Take the time now to reflect on *all* of the roles for which you currently take responsibility.
- What are the conflicts in the roles you undertake?

Most clinical educators immediately see that their role in providing health care service delivery may be in conflict with their educative role. It is important to acknowledge this fundamental conflict in student education (see Chapter 10).

Some of the literature talks about the triad formed between the student, supervisor/clinical educator and client. This threesome adds a dimension to clinical teaching that is both a strength and a weakness. Its greatest strength is its reality. This is the real world – a real client with a real clinical problem in a real clinical setting. No matter what happens in the interaction it is the real thing. It is a weakness because it is complex. It is frequently difficult to coordinate the timing of the interaction, which is often unpredictable and often impossible to find an appropriate space away from distractions. It is also intensely rewarding but often draining!

Turney et al (1982) suggested that the supervisory or clinical education process may be divided into the following roles:

- manager
- instructor
- counsellor
- observer
- giver of feedback
- evaluator or assessor.

These authors write about teacher education but the roles they identify also apply to health science education. This resource uses the above breakdown of roles to investigate specific skills and strategies for effective supervision. You may like to read through them all or only select those sections that contribute to your specific learning needs.

All clinical education requires components from these six areas. In different health care environments and in different situations throughout the placement, one of the roles may become more important.

Sometimes the relative importance of each role relates to the timing of the clinical education. Most clinical educators would see the manager role take precedence early in the placement and the evaluator role at the end of the unit as assessment papers are filled out. As some clinical educators have discovered, it is impossible to fill in an end-of-unit assessment form without taking the role of the observer seriously throughout the unit. Many clinical educators engaged in a counselling role mid-placement may discover that much time could have been saved and anxiety reduced with a greater emphasis on the manager role early in the placement.

ROLE CONFLICT

Analysis of the separate roles also provides a useful framework to help us become aware of some of the inherent contradictions hidden behind supervision and clinical education. It is impossible to be both counsellor and assessor at the same time. On the other hand it is very difficult to instruct without also giving feedback on the student's attempts to follow that instruction.

Turney et al (1982) depict the relationship between the different roles in teacher education as shown in Figure 4.1. Notice how Turney et al depict the manager role differently to all the other roles by encircling them within the boundaries of management.

■ Which roles articulate with each other?
■ Which roles are isolated?
■ Which roles are given special significance?

Does this model match your clinical education experience in health science education – either as a student or a clinical educator? Take the time to develop a model that better fits your own situation. Share this with a diagrammatic representation or drawing with your colleagues for discussion. Consider using mime, dance or three-dimensional models to illustrate your key points.

Figure 4.1   Role relationships according to Turney et al (1982)

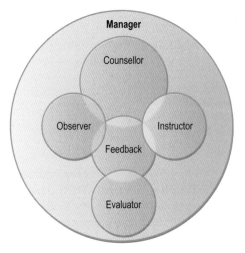

Parts two to five of this chapter look in more detail at each of these roles: manager, instructor, counsellor and assessor.

REFERENCES

Best D, Rose M 1996 Quality supervision. Theory and practice for clinical supervisors. W B Saunders, London

Farmer S, Farmer J 1989 Supervision in communication disorders. Merrill Publishing, Ohio, p 123–125

McLeod S, Romanini J, Cohn E et al 1997 Models and roles in clinical education. In: McAllister L, Lincoln M, Mcleod S et al (eds) Facilitation learning in clinical settings. Stanley Thornes, Cheltenham, p 53–61

Turney C, Cairns L, Eltis G et al 1982 Supervision development programs role handbook. Sydney University Press, Sydney

PART 2 The manager role

Louise Brown and Mary Kennedy-Jones

INTRODUCTION AND AIMS

There are many levels of management that may occur within a clinical education setting. In the Turney et al (1982) model, the manager is seen as the encompassing role for all other roles (Fig. 4.1).

In this part, we identify a broad view of the "manager" role and function within clinical education. Some of this function may reside with the departmental manager or the overall manager of the clinical education process in the organisation. Some may relate specifically to the manager of a particular placement or clinical education experience. In some organisations, the responsibility rests predominantly with one individual; in others there may be multiple layers of responsibility. It may even be intended that the student learn some components of management during the placement (e.g. caseload management, protocol development).

It is intended for readers of this text to identify the actual management roles and responsibilities that are relevant to their particular clinical education situation. You can then see if the reflection questions we have posed help refine the management process during a placement or in anticipation of a future placement.

Some aspects of the format of this chapter may look familiar to all those managers who participate in accreditation processes and quality improvement programmes. This familiarity comes from the process of identifying roles and tasks and ensuring that evidence is available to demonstrate achievement of the roles and tasks. The format we have followed is also consistent with the Kolb (1984) experiential learning process discussed in Chapter 6 that describes phases of abstract conceptualisation, active experimentation, concrete experience and reflection. In this chapter, we identify the underlying theory, assumptions or needs which will ensure a well-managed clinical learning experience (abstract conceptualisation). We then suggest a plan of action which will meet those needs and which is consistent with the theoretical assumptions (active experimentation). Next we provide some examples of the actual evidence that would demonstrate that you have followed through with the plan (concrete experience). Finally, we suggest that you will need to reflect on this evidence and action to see if it has met the requirements you initially identified (reflection).

We are very aware that this chapter only touches on some of the managerial roles and responsibilities that are required for successful clinical education. We hope that the format we have used will help you identify and develop plans for the many issues not specifically covered here. A complementary view of the educator or teacher-manager is covered very effectively and thoroughly elsewhere (Higgs 1992, 1993, McLeod et al 1997) as well as being the focus of other parts in this chapter relating to the roles of clinical supervision.

PREPARATION AND ANTICIPATION

Learning environment

The key assumption here is that optimal student learning will occur in a place that values learning for all (Box 4.1). It is assumed that visionary leaders or managers will ensure staff members are prepared and able to facilitate student learning. They will have a positive attitude to learning for themselves, their colleagues, their students and their clients. It is an empowering and active view of the centrality of learning to effective clinical and workplace practice. Many of these notions are described by Knowles et al (1980, p. 66): "an organisation is not simply an instrumentality for providing organised learning activities for adults; it also provides an environment that either facilitates or inhibits learning". The characteristics of static learning and working environments are compared with those of innovative organisations which facilitate change and learning in Table 4.1.

Box 4.1   How have you planned to achieve a working environment in which learning is a corner stone, as well as being truly valued? What is the evidence that you have done this?

For example:

- When you interview new staff, do you attempt to ascertain if they are life-long learners?
- Do your staff appraisal and development processes ensure that you understand the learning aspirations of staff in your area?
- Do you understand your own learning aspirations?
- Do you have a reasonable budget for professional development?
- Do you have an accessible and well-used professional library?
- Do you have a professional development or in-service plan for the department and the whole agency?
- Do you use processes such as client reviews, critical incident reviews (see later in this chapter) and debriefing to encourage supported learning by all staff members?
- Other evidence:

Table 4.1   Some characteristics of static versus innovative organisations (Knowles et al 1988, p. 11)

Dimensions	Characteristics	
	Static organisations	**Innovative organisations**
Structure	Rigid – much energy given to maintaining permanent departments, committees; reverence for tradition, constitution and by-laws	Flexible – much use of temporary task forces; easy shifting of departmental lines; readiness to change constitution; depart from tradition
	Hierarchical – adherence to chain of command	Multiple linkages based on functional collaboration
	Roles defined narrowly	Roles defined broadly
	Property-bound	Property-mobile
Atmosphere	Task-centred, impersonal	People-centred, caring
	Cold, formal, reserved	Warm, informal, intimate
	Suspicious	Trusting
Management philosophy and attitudes	Function of management is to control personnel through coercive power	Function of management is to release the energy of personnel; power is used supportively
	Cautious – low risk-taking	Experimental – high risk-taking
	Attitude to errors: to be avoided	Attitude to errors: to be learned from
	Emphasis on personnel selection	Emphasis on personnel development
	Self-sufficiency – closed system regarding sharing resources	Interdependency – open system regarding sharing resources
	Emphasis on conserving resources	Emphasis on developing and using resources
	Low tolerance for ambiguity	High tolerance for ambiguity
Decision-making and policy-making	High participation at top, low at bottom	Relevant participation by all those affected
	Clear distinction between policy-making and policy execution	Collaborative policy-making and policy execution
	Decision-making by legal mechanisms	Decision-making by problem-solving
	Decisions treated as final	Decisions treated as hypotheses to be tested
Communication	Flow restricted	Open flow – easy access
	One-way – downward	Multidirectional – up, down and sideways
	Feelings repressed or hidden	Feelings expressed

Staffing and team readiness

The staff members need to be keen and prepared to take on the responsibility of student clinical education. If they feel poorly prepared, the process may fail, time will be wasted and students (and staff) could be damaged. The team of staff needs to have the opportunity to discuss their views about clinical education, competing demands in the workplace, appropriateness of the caseload and their confidence in providing supervision (Box 4.2).

Resources available

There are a number of practical physical and resource issues which can impact on the effectiveness of a clinical placement. Very few clinicians would describe their workplace as being sufficient to meet all their needs even before they

> **Box 4.2   How have you planned to ensure that staff members have the competencies and capacity to undertake the important role of clinical educator? What is the evidence that you have done this?**
>
> For example:
>
> - Is clinical education identified in the staff member's position description?
> - Has the staff member had the opportunity to participate in education programmes to develop clinical education skills?
> - If the staff member is keen to be involved, but has not participated in any programmes, is supervisory support available? (This support may be from the same discipline or from an experienced supervisor from another discipline.)
> - Other evidence:

consider including a student (or two or three). It can be very difficult to have a student who needs to observe a clinical session sitting with you, the client and the carer in a room the size of a broom cupboard and with only three chairs available. It is therefore important to have considered the physical and resource requirements for each clinical experience (Box 4.3).

> **Box 4.3   How have you planned to optimise the physical setting and resource requirements for a placement? What is the evidence that you have done this?**
>
> For example:
>
> - Have you planned to have observation facilities so that observation either *by* the student or *of* the student is not too intrusive?
> - Is there a place where students can sit to work independently – a desk, a chair, a shared student office?
> - Are there certain days when space is at a premium and it would not be feasible to have another person present?
> - Will you need additional test materials, computer access, other clinical materials for the particular placement?
> - Other evidence:

Placement requirements and goals

It is important that you and the university share the same expectations for the placement. Most requests for clinical placement specify the type of client, the frequency of attendance, the learning goals and the number of students to be placed. You and your team need to consider what resources you have to offer, and then match these with the requirements of the placements requested (Box 4.4).

However, because placements are always at a premium, managers may be asked to rescue a student who has been let down by another clinic. As a good manager you will, of course, not be unduly swayed by the desire to help out if you are truly unable to meet the minimum requirements for the clinic. If

Box 4.4   Have you planned and negotiated to ensure that you will provide the core requirements for a placement? What is the evidence that you have done this?

For example:

- Have you identified the number and type of clients or activities you provide in which students can meaningfully be engaged?
- What level of student independence is required for successful involvement in the clinical education programme? (For instance, if you can only provide observation, it is not useful to offer final-year placements in which the student needs to demonstrate independence.)
- Have you confirmed with the university the appropriateness (or otherwise) of the clinical experience your agency can provide?
- Other evidence:

you have identified what you can and cannot offer, it will be easier to ensure you are not risking the student drowning in your attempt to perform a rescue.

Frequently there are competing demands for students from different universities. In some parts of Australia, university clinical education coordinators have established clinical consortia to attempt to streamline the placement of students from different academic programmes and this has eased the complexity of conflicting loyalties. Managers may think this is a good idea and encourage similar developments in their area.

Organisation

It is important for a manager to ensure that policies and procedures for clinical education experiences have been developed and are understood within the agency. The purposes of such policies should aim to ensure, inter alia, that roles and responsibilities are specified and legal and other contractual obligations are understood and followed (e.g. if a placement agreement exists between the agency and the university), that channels of communication are specified for all involved (at the agency and the university) and that all stages of the placement are planned (Box 4.5), including consideration of contingencies (e.g. if the client caseload changes or if a staff member becomes ill).

Box 4.5   How have you planned and organised in preparation for the clinical placement? What is the evidence that you have done this?

For example:

- Have you prepared and reviewed your policies and procedures relating to clinical education? Are staff members familiar with and in agreement with these policies and procedures?
- Is there an agreement in place clarifying legal and contractual agreements between the agency and the university?

continued over

- Have you clarified the role of the university should any difficulties arise during the placement?
- Do all staff members involved have copies of the university guidelines regarding the placement?
- Do the other staff members in the organisation know you will have students in their wards or departments?
- Do you have contingency plans, such as video case studies and other learning packages, for the inevitable "down-times"?
- Have you identified issues of potential concern or situations which may impact on the student's experience, such as areas or topics which would not be suitable or could act as distractions from the key learning objectives for the placement?
- Other evidence:

Orientation

Students report that their best clinical experiences start with the receipt of an orientation package (Box 4.6) before the commencement of the placement. This is true of long placements away from home, where issues like accommodation and local facilities are important. It is also true of short placements where it is vital that the student is as well briefed as possible to arrive at the clinic prepared for the materials, resources requirements and other local expectations. Obviously details about public transport, parking, lunch facilities and other daily requirements are also very important. The orientation and welcome at the commencement of the placement are covered below.

Box 4.6 **Have you planned how a student will learn about all the relevant local as well as clinical issues which will ensure a good start and shared understanding before the commencement of the clinic? What is the evidence you have done this?**

For example:
- Have you developed an orientation package and programme?
- Have you reviewed the effectiveness of the package and updated it?
- Other evidence:

IMPLEMENTATION

This section reviews the managerial functions undertaken by a nominated manager or clinical educator, if you are in a sole position, of the period whilst the student is on placement in your agency. Specifically, the first-day experience and the day-to-day managerial responsibilities are considered. Once the student has completed the placement it is also a managerial function to guide an evaluation phase of the placement experience for both the student and the supervisor(s).

The first day

The first-day experience for the student is an important time to manage. Students respond positively to a warm welcome which also includes the apparent organisation of practical matters such as desk space, facilities to lock away their personal valuables, an orientation to the physical layout of the department and an oral/written briefing about the procedures used in the department. Other first-day tasks may include implementing hospital security policies and the provision of authorised name badges.

As previously described, it is a function of the managerial role to facilitate an atmosphere/climate of anticipation, organisation and enthusiasm for the opportunities provided by the student for mutual learning (Box 4.7).

Box 4.7   Did the first-day experience of the student go as planned? What is the evidence?

For example:

- Were all necessary processes and procedures explained to the student?
- Did the student experience a warm welcome?
- Was a positive, learning-oriented impression formed by the student on the first day?
- Other evidence:

Day-to-day monitoring

The manager role assumes the task of monitoring the progress of the placement experience for both the clinical educator and the student. Opportunities for learning by the clinical educator around the education experience may be encouraged by the manager. Within this role there exists the opportunity for the manager to model a supportive approach to learning the skills of clinical education. Skills in setting "just right" challenges can be modelled by the manager in the expectation that these will inform the teaching–learning relationship of the clinical educator and student.

Specifically, the use of techniques such as critical incident analysis may be useful for either or both supervisor and student.

Critical incident analysis

The primary aim of the clinical education component of the curriculum which prepares allied health professionals for entry into their respective professions is to integrate theory with practice, i.e. to situate the academic knowledge, skills and attitudes inside a specific context and to draw the theory and the practical together. A critical incident analysis technique (Brookfield 1995, Fook et al 2000) is a useful method of facilitating the integration of the theory and exploring the dimensions of advanced practice. Critical incident analysis is most commonly used within a reflective practice framework of adult learning.

Critical incidents are not necessarily crisis occasions experienced by the student or the clinical educator. Any event that serves as a breakthrough for the learner can be regarded as a critical incident. Events that are part of everyday practice may be regarded as significant if they have provided an opportunity for an essential insight. The steps within a critical incident analysis (Brookfield 1995, Fook et al 2000) are outlined in Box 4.8.

Box 4.8

Critical incident analysis

1. Identify an incident from your (learner) experience that was critical. Allow some time for it to emerge.
2. Fully describe what happened, including:
   a. social context
   b. personal context
   c. organisational context
   d. reasons for selecting the particular incident.

The written description of the incident is from your (learner) perspective. It is a concrete description of the event rather than an analysis. It is written like a story, is often a couple of pages long and constitutes the raw data for later use.

3. Analysis of incident

This may occur with one other person or in a small group. It includes "asking, answering and discussing questions which articulate the theory, practice and assumptions which are implicit in the description" (Fook et al 2000, p. 227). Some questions that may be relevant are:

- What are the main themes or patterns that emerge from my description?
- How are my thoughts, feelings, actions, intentions and interpretation interconnected?
- What knowledge and assumptions are embedded in my account – are they relevant and appropriate in the situation?
- Are there gaps in my description – what perspectives are missing?
- Does the language I am using reflect something about the way I interpret the situation (adapted from Fook et al 2000, p. 227).

The use of the tool is consistent with a self-directed learner-focused approach to learning which places the supervisor/manager in the role of facilitator. Such an approach sits well with providing learners with opportunities to develop self-reflective skills to support life-long learning.

EVALUATION AND ONGOING REVIEW

At the conclusion of the placement an evaluation of the placement from the student and supervisor perspectives is part of the role of the manager. Placement experience evaluations usually cover a broad range of areas, including:

- the variety of client contact, including the opportunities provided for learning
- the organisation of the placement and its structure

- the teaching and supervision methods
- the usefulness of orientation materials
- the orientation experience itself
- the facilities/resources for students.

In implementing a formal evaluation process some issues need to be considered. These include:

- the timing of the evaluation
- the purpose of the data collection and how the data are to be used
- the methods used – for instance, can/should respondents be anonymous?

The provision of a standard evaluation form available for perusal by the student in the orientation folder at the start of the placement reflects an agency's ongoing commitment to quality and makes explicit the sections under review.

If feedback on the learner's perception of the supervision experience specifically is desirable, an evaluation task proposed by Brookfield (1995) and outlined below may be used. Brookfield argues:

> that seeing ourselves as our students see us makes us aware of those actions and assumptions that either confirm or challenge our power relationships … and help us to check whether students take from our practice the meaning that we intend (p. 30).

This activity may be undertaken with the manager and clinical educator or clinical educator and student. The questionnaire aims to give the person in the facilitator role some specific information about how the supervisory practice is perceived by the learner. The five questions Brookfield (1995) uses are:

1. At what moment (in the supervision session this week) did you feel most engaged with what was happening?
2. At what moment (in the supervision session this week) did you feel most distanced from what was happening?
3. What action that anyone (teacher or student or other) took in the supervision session this week did you find most affirming and helpful?
4. What action that anyone (teacher or student or other) took in the supervision session this week did you find most puzzling or confusing?
5. What about the supervision session this week surprised you the most (could be something about your own reactions, something someone did, or anything else).

(Brookfield S Becoming a critically reflective teacher. Copyright © 1995 Jossey–Bass, San Francisco. This material is used by permission of John Wiley & Sons, Inc.)

Such information provides valuable opportunities for clinical educator development. Further, the information provides a means of flagging potential problems, allows students to practise being reflective learners, builds trust and strengthens the case for diversity in clinical education methods – that is, the need to use a range of supervision techniques because "one size does not fit all".

CONCLUSION

This part of Chapter 4 has identified key functions of the manager role in the planning and evaluation phases of the clinical education experience. Specifically, the manager role has a central focus in developing and maintaining an organisational culture that is positively oriented and responsive toward learning. Such an environment is instantly recognisable by visitors and forms a lasting impression. Other planning tasks, such as staff/team readiness, resource availability, organisational policies and procedures and orientation duties, are also necessary within the role. In addition, the chapter provides an outline of some reflective techniques that, as mentioned earlier in the chapter, complete the application of the Kolb cycle of experiential learning.

REFERENCES

Brookfield S 1995 Becoming a critically reflective teacher. Jossey-Bass, San Francisco

Fook J, Ryan M, Hawkins L 2000 Professional expertise: practice, theory and education for working with uncertainty. Whiting & Birch, London

Higgs J 1992 Managing clinical education: the educator-manager and the self-directed learner. Physiotherapy 78(11):822–828

Higgs J 1993 Managing clinical education: the programme. Physiotherapy 79(4):239–246

Knowles M, Holton E, Swanson R 1980 The adult learner. Gulf Publishing, Houston

Knowles M, Holton E, Swanson R 1998 The adult learner, 5th edn. Butterworth-Heinemann, Woburn, MA

Kolb D 1984 Experiential learning: experience as source of learning and development. Prentice Hall, New Jersey

McLeod S, Romani J, Cohn E, Higgs J 1997 Models and roles in clinical education. In: McAllister L, Lincoln M, McLeod S, Maloney D (eds) Facilitating learning in clinical settings. Stanley Thornes, Cheltenham, p 252–295

Turney C, Cairns L, Eltis K et al 1982 Supervision development programmes: role handbook. Sydney University Press, Sydney

PART 3 Instructor, observer and provider of feedback

Jennifer Marriott and Kirstie Galbraith

The roles of instructor, observer and provider of feedback are closely related and interdependent, yet each demands a very different set of skills. This part aims to explore the key requirements of each role and offers suggestions and strategies for effective student learning.

INSTRUCTOR ROLE

Perhaps new clinical educators may view the role of instructor as one associated with teaching students important facets of their job. Based on their own past experience and without a knowledge of different supervisory styles (see Chapter 6), some clinical educators may assume that a didactic approach is required. Cheetham & Chivers (2001) define instruction as: "the inculcation of specific knowledge or skill-related principles to one or more individuals at the same time". However, if clinical education is to involve the student in the learning process, this demands the use of skills other than telling. These skills are expanded further by Turney et al (1982).

The clinical educator maybe involved in:

- Presenting
    - suggesting
    - modelling
    - explaining

- Questioning
  - lifting the level
  - pausing
  - probing
  - asking divergent questions

- Problem-solving
  - delineating the problem
  - identifying factors and gathering information
  - seeking solutions
  - applying and appraising solutions

- Conferencing
  - planning for the conference
  - guiding discussion
  - terminating the conference.

Such diversity of activities has been incorporated in the task of coaching, where one-to-one learning support is tailored to the needs of the individual (Cheetham & Chivers 2001).

Collins et al (cited in Cheetham & Chivers 2001) propose a model that includes the following six elements:

1. modelling: an expert demonstrates to the learner
2. coaching: the learner practises while the coach offers feedback
3. scaffolding: the instructor provides support that is gradually reduced as the learner becomes more proficient
4. articulation: the learner describes his or her problem-solving processes
5. reflection: the learner reflects on the comparison between individual problem-solving processes with those of a peer or more experienced practitioner
6. exploration: the learner moves to autonomous problem-solving.

Other important components of instruction include:

- Providing suitable conditions for self-directed learning
- Directing the learner's attention towards significant factors of a task
- Imparting the hidden secrets of mastery, rather than just the mechanics of a task
- Ensuring basic knowledge and skills are mastered before more complex tasks are undertaken (hierarchical learning).

Instruction must also take into account the expertise of the learner. Dreyfus & Dreyfus (cited in Cheetham & Chivers 2001) describe the transition from novice to expert as a gradual transition from a rigid adherence to taught rules and procedures, through to a largely intuitive mode of operation, which relies heavily on a deep, tacit understanding (see Chapter 5 part 1 for a more detailed discussion on novice–expert differences).

> ### EXERCISE
>
> Think of an example of effective instruction when you were the learner.
> Take a moment to write a few sentences describing the experience.
> What made this a good experience for you?

Brainstorming sessions undertaken with groups of clinical educators over a number of years have generated a remarkably consistent list of criteria describing a good instructor. This list includes: good listener, patient, negotiator, passionate, helper, affirming, supportive, unhurried, clear/constructive feedback, pitched at the right level, approachable, wise, knowledgeable, admits to not knowing everything, clear expectations, puts things in context, flexible, persistent, able to use different approaches to solve problems, relaxed, chunking information, asks students if they understand, asks questions, uses analogies/experience, helps student to problem-solve (not just providing the answer), enthusiastic and motivating, role model, realistic expectations, life experience, clear communication, confident, giving student opportunity to practise new skills, being accessible, allocating time for the student, accurate observer, giving feedback at an appropriate time/place, treating student as a peer, consistent, passionate, adaptable.

These criteria are consistent with research into the qualities of effective clinical teachers by Irby (1978) (Table 4.2).

> ### EXERCISE
>
> Think about the last time you were an instructor.
> Which of the above components did you do well?
> Which areas could be improved?

OBSERVER ROLE

Definition

The observer role in clinical education involves the active task of observing clinical performance and may include skills and behaviours, as well as communication and body language. Without this important role it is very difficult to provide feedback to the student.

When is the role of observer particularly important?

1. *New learner or new skill.* It is important for the supervisor to observe the new learner in order to develop trust and confidence in the student's ability and to identify the learner's existing skill level.
2. *Assessing competence.* Formal observations of set tasks are important in an ongoing assessment of competence as the learner moves from novice to expert.
3. *Providing feedback.* Personal observations of a student by the clinical educator are essential as the basis of appropriate feedback. First-hand

Table 4.2 Qualities of effective clinical teachers

Quality	Characteristics
1. Organisation and clarity	– explains clearly – presents material in an organised manner – summarises and emphasises what is important – communicates what is expected to be learnt
2. Group instruction skills	– establishes rapport – shows respect for and personal interest in students – emphasises problem-solving (the process, not just the content) – listens attentively – answers questions carefully and precisely – questions students in a non-threatening manner
3. Enthusiasm	– is dynamic and energetic – enjoys teaching – has an interesting style of presentation and stimulates interest in the subject
4. Knowledge	– discusses current developments and research – cites references – reveals broad reading and directs students to useful literature – discusses divergent points of view
5. Clinical supervision	– demonstrates clinical procedures – provides practice opportunities – offers professional support and encouragement – observes student performance frequently – identifies strengths and limitations objectively – provides feedback and positive reinforcement
6. Clinical competence	– objectively defines and synthesises patient problems – demonstrates skill in data interpretation – manages clinical problems – works effectively with a health care team – maintains a humanistic orientation and good rapport with the students
7. Modelling professional characteristics	– is self-critical – takes responsibility – recognises own limitations – shows respect for others and demonstrates sensitivity – has self-confidence

observations establish credibility and provide irrefutable evidence of the student ability or behaviour.

4. *Risky situations.* In situations where a mistake by the student may put the client at risk it is important that tasks are closely observed to protect the welfare of both parties.

Who can take on the role of observer?

The role of observer may be undertaken by a number of people depending on the situation:

1. *Clinical educator*. The clinical educator is the most common person to take on the role of observer. Observations may be used in both formative and summative assessment and to provide feedback.
2. *Student*. The student may observe a more experienced practitioner undertaking a task in order to learn the requirements of the task.
3. *Peers*. Other students may observe as part of peer review. This is useful as part of the teaching process, but needs to be undertaken carefully to avoid inappropriate feedback or competitiveness. The use of checklists as part of peer observation can be particularly useful to reinforce the processes involved in successful completion of the task.
4. *Others*. Other members of the student's profession who have obtained a higher level of competence in completing the set task may be asked to observe and provide feedback to the student. Clients may also take on the role of observer.

Prior to the period of observation, discussion between the clinical educator and the student may negotiate or clarify the specific tasks to be observed. It may be helpful to define objectives for the student. Again this will assist in providing feedback to the student at the end of the session. Aspects of performance being observed may include the student's:

- ability to perform a certain task
- ability to communicate and interact with the patient or with other health care professionals
- knowledge of a particular topic.

> **EXERCISE**
>
> Think about a time when you were in the observer role.
> Which aspects of this role did you find difficult?

What strategies could you use to overcome these difficulties (identified in above activity)?

1. *Notes taken whilst observing the learner*. Formal records may be more credible if they represent an accurate, objective record of what occurred; however they are time-consuming and may not be feasible in many situations.
2. *Checklists*. Checklists may save some time and are useful if it is important that certain elements of a task are undertaken or undertaken to a predetermined standard. Universities will often provide checklists to assist clinical educators in their observations and subsequent feedback.
3. *Audio*. Tape recordings of student–client interactions aid memory so that the student can hear both what was said and the tone/inflection used. These are objective records and allow students to comment on their own performance. Tape recordings can also be used for peer-observation and feedback sessions.

4. *Video*. Video recordings may be useful for providing feedback on particular tasks and behaviours. It may be difficult to reduce artificiality as both students and clients will be conscious that a video recording is being made and may modify their actions or language accordingly. Remember that consent from the patient must be obtained before audio or video taping.

FEEDBACK ROLE
Definition

Feedback is information given to indicate the level of competence that has been achieved in performance of a task. Feedback can therefore be positive or negative depending on whether the task was completed well or not. Although these terms are well accepted it may be preferable to consider feedback as either supportive or corrective (Latting 1992). It is usually more difficult to give corrective feedback than supportive feedback.

Based on the individual's performance in the workplace, either in completing individual tasks or overall, clinical educators are aware of the students' level of competence. The clinical educator is able to provide specific information to assist students to recognise the standard they have achieved in undertaking the task. This information may include positive reinforcement and praise for those tasks completed correctly or information about areas in which the student is not yet competent.

Effective feedback serves two major functions: it instructs by helping to clarify deviations between preferred and actual behaviour; and it motivates by increasing student desire to perform well (Latting 1992).

Types of feedback

The type of feedback utilised (Latting 1992, Best & Rose 1996) (Table 4.3) will depend on the facilities available, the task being appraised, the learning style of the recipient or the time available.

Characteristics of effective feedback

It is generally considered that feedback must be specific, accurate, objective, timely, usable, desired by the receiver and checked for understanding to be effective (Latting 1992, Brinko 1993).

Source of feedback

Information obtained from a number of sources

The use of several different sources of information will add credibility to the feedback that is being given. This applies to both positive and negative feedback. It has the tendency to de-personalise and reduce the subjectivity of the feedback, increasing its validity and reliability and making it more effective. It is recommended that the person giving the feedback has been involved in the observation of the student.

Table 4.3 Advantages and disadvantages of different types of feedback

Feedback	Advantages	Disadvantages
Written	Useful for ongoing consideration Forms permanent record to view for progress/assessment purposes	Does not allow for discussion, clarification or further elaboration
Verbal	Allows discussion and elaboration of points	Has to be scheduled Difficult for some supervisors to give negative feedback face to face
With audio/video assistance	Provides permanent record to check for, or verify, particular behaviours Allows more detailed analysis after a session when student can concentrate more without performance pressure	Subtle behaviours, e.g. facial expressions and small comments, may be missed Need to check for accuracy Can be biased if only a portion of the reality is recorded
Individual	Can discuss sensitive issues more easily Can focus on individual specific points	Time-consuming
Group	Time-efficient Allows for peer input	Difficult for some students to be genuine and reveal weaknesses with peers
Direct	Time-efficient in the short term Useful for novice students at times	Does not allow students independently to problem-solve Can set up a power game of expert who knows all the answers and novice who knows little
Indirect	Allows students to generate their own feedback and problem-solving skills Encourages student confidence in own ability to learn Gives students a chance to present their own interpretation of events rather than defending themselves against the supervisor	May be time-consuming for novice practitioners
Peer	Gives another perspective on performance May be accepted by student with less resistance	May not provide sufficiently broad frame of reference

The source of the information for the feedback must be perceived as credible, knowledgeable and well-intentioned

It is important the person receiving the feedback perceives the person giving the feedback as someone with an appropriate level of knowledge and expertise with which to make an accurate judgement on performance of the task. To be effective it is recommended that feedback be non-judgemental and that the student trusts the motives and intentions of the person giving the feedback. Critical feedback given in an attempt to control or to rationalise unfair decisions will lead to resentment by the recipient.

Modify feedback according to the recipient's level of experience or education

Effective feedback takes into consideration the level of training students have attained and the amount of experience they have had in undertaking the task at hand.

Method of providing feedback

Feedback may be more effective if it is given using a variety of methods

The method of providing feedback may depend on the recipient's preferred learning style. Different methods of providing feedback will be more informative, meaningful and relevant than other methods to different individuals. Visual learners may prefer video feedback, aural learners may prefer verbal feedback, others may prefer written feedback. The method of providing feedback may depend on the task being assessed. In some situations use of more than one method of providing feedback may be beneficial.

Content of feedback

Feedback information must be accurate and irrefutable

Feedback information should be factual and clear. The recipient is more likely to be receptive if information is seen as being accurate and unbiased. It is important to the feedback process that the recipient listens carefully to the feedback and is given an opportunity to clarify content they are unsure about.

Feedback should contain specific data

Recipients prefer specific information rather than vague generalisations. Feedback that refers to specific tasks or areas is more likely to result in improved performance than a general comment on performance.

Feedback should be focused on the behaviour rather than the person

Focusing on changeable behaviours rather than personal characteristics minimises a student's defence response and optimises opportunity for change.

Feedback should be descriptive rather than evaluative

Feedback information that describes rather than evaluates reduces defensiveness. Attributing poor performance to a particular cause should be avoided where possible as it may be based on false interpretations of the cause. It is important that the emphasis of the feedback is on skill-building rather than fault-finding.

Timing of feedback

Feedback is more effective when it is given as soon as possible after completion of the task

In general, the longer the delay in providing feedback, the less effective it will be, as recollections of the event may be faulty and may differ. Immediate feedback may not always be possible and it may need to be delayed to a more appropriate time and/or place.

Give negative/corrective feedback privately

Corrective feedback given publicly may cause the recipient to be defensive and also has a negative effect on others.

Feedback is more effective when it is a routine part of the process

The frequency of receiving feedback influences the effectiveness of the feedback that is received. Several instances of feedback may be required to change behaviour. Feedback should therefore be frequent enough to benefit the recipient but not excessive. Too frequent feedback may lead the recipient to depend on external cues for behavioural change rather than self-reflection.

The feedback process is more effective when the recipient engages in it voluntarily

Actively seeking feedback is an indication that the recipient is motivated to improve performance. Feedback to those who do not voluntarily seek feedback can still be effective if it is seen as part of the routine process or a professional expectation.

Giving feedback

Be sensitive to the recipient's self-esteem

Individuals low in self-esteem rely more on feedback from external sources. Those with high self-esteem may not recall negative information as clearly as positive information and may respond less to negative information than those with low esteem.

Include a moderate amount of positive feedback with a limited amount of negative feedback

Emphasise desired rather than undesired behaviours. In general, positive feedback is more accurately perceived and recalled than negative feedback. Feedback conversations are more effective when they begin and end with positive information. The negative information is more likely to be accepted as valid.

Feedback must be relevant and meaningful to the recipient

To be relevant and meaningful it is recommended that feedback be timely, and relate specifically to behaviours of the recipient, conveyed in language that is understandable to the recipient.

Allow for response and interaction

Be prepared for the recipient to respond in a defensive or embarrassed manner. Make certain that the recipient has understood the intent of the feedback and resist the temptation to retaliate. Invite a response as the recipient may suggest a course of corrective action that will lead to a more positive outcome. Invite the recipient to provide feedback to you on your performance.

Relate the feedback to goals defined by the recipient or to rewards that result from positive performance

Problem identification and goal setting by the recipient produces internal motivation and a desire for feedback.

Use the first person (student name, I) or a question when giving feedback

Statements made in the second person (you) may seem more accusatory and may not be received as well. Turning the information into a question has the effect of softening the effect and making it seem less critical. The answer may then lead to a discussion that may provide the opportunity for presenting alternatives.

Choose appropriate language

Because negative information is very difficult to hear it is important that the language used to convey it is chosen very carefully and the use of inflammatory language is avoided. Beware of voice tone and body language as these can be seen as threatening and aggressive.

EXERCISE

Integrating the roles of instructor, observer and provider of feedback

Best & Rose (1996) detail a useful development exercise in teaching learning and assessment. This activity involves learning a new skill that incorporates all three roles – instructing, observing and providing feedback. It requires a minimum of three people:

– an observer (O)
– an instructor/teacher (T)
– a learner (L).

1. The T selects a skill at which he/she is proficient. The L must be a novice in this activity. Suitable activities may be: card tricks, origami, highland dancing, foreign-language phrases, nappy-folding, musical instrument-playing, yo-yo tricks, etc.
2. The T and L establish criteria for successful completion of the task
3. The T teaches the L the task
4. The L performs the task
5. The O observes the process from stages 2 to 4
6. The T writes a self-evaluation of his/her teaching and the L's performance, and gives both of these to the O
7. The L writes a self-evaluation of the learning or performance and an evaluation of T's teaching and gives both of these to O
8. The T gives verbal feedback to the L about the L's performance
9. The L gives verbal feedback to the T about the T's teaching
10. The O comments on the match between the written evaluations and the verbal feedback
11. The three participants talk about what they felt was successful and what they would change if they were repeating the exercise. Some questions to address are:
    – How well did the self-evaluations match the verbal feedback?
    – Did the O notice things that the T and L did not?
    – Did the T accurately hear L's feedback?
    – What might have affected recall?
    – What methods do you currently use to instruct and give feedback?
    – Was there anything in the exercise that you might use to modify your current methods of supervisory practice?
    – What was it like to be aware that you would be receiving feedback? Did this awareness affect your performance?

REFERENCES

Best D, Rose M 1996 Quality supervision. Theory and practice for clinical supervisors. W B Saunders, London

Brinko K 1993 The practice of giving feedback to improve teaching. What is effective? Journal of Higher Education 64:574–593

Cheetham G, Chivers G 2001 Part 1: How professionals learn – the theory. Journal of European Industrial Training 25:250–269

Irby D 1978 Clinical teacher effectiveness in medicine. Journal of Medical Education 53:808–815

Latting J 1992 Giving corrective feedback: a decisional analysis. Social Work 37:424–430

Turney C, Cairns L, Eltis K et al 1982 Supervision development programmes: role handbook. Sydney University Press, Sydney

PART 4 Counsellor role
Michael McGartland

INTRODUCTION: WHETHER TO COUNSEL

In contrast to some of the other supervision roles, the role of counsellor has attracted a diverse array of responses in the past. There are those supervisors who see the role of counsellor as a necessary and integral part of the supervision process, while others see it as something quite separate from supervision – perhaps to be carried out by a psychologist. As with all wide-ranging points of view, there are no doubt many more supervisors who fall somewhere along the continuum between these two positions and who perhaps change their views about their role as counsellor from time to time. There seem to be a number of reasons to explain the range of views.

Concerns that counselling and psychotherapy do not work and are unscientific

From the 1950s to the 1980s there was much debate about the effectiveness of counselling. However, in more recent years the evidence is clearly in and "the efficacy of psychotherapy is now firmly established and is no longer the subject of debate" (Wampold 2001, p. 59). For those receiving counselling the average person is better off than 80% of those untreated, and the improvements are sustained (Asay & Lambert 1999). It is likely that these results are comparable to other disciplines in the health and medical sciences. As for being scientific, theoretically based and evidence-based practice is advocated and in widespread use. In addition, many approaches to counselling also pay attention to the art of the practice, as well as the relationship between the counsellor and the client.

The definition of counselling is not clear

The debate in this area does not pose a problem for those whose career is in counselling. However, the lack of a readily available, uniform definition of counselling in the literature and the apparent similarity of the practice to everyday activities may be confusing to those who use counselling skills in their work. Counselling is a systematic approach to help another deal with a

Figure 4.2 Counselling sits on a continuum of interpersonal interaction between interviewing and psychotherapy

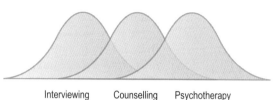

Interviewing   Counselling   Psychotherapy

difficulty or sort out a problem. Writing for a general medical practitioner audience, Davies (2003, p. 53) describes counselling with some clarity:

> *The aim is for the person to cope as well as possible with the stressor. The problem is not treated as an illness. The person is not treated as being 'sick' but rather as a coping adult. The theory of counselling is that through facilitating the expression of feelings about the stressor in the context of a good therapeutic alliance, the person will be able to clarify and understand his or her problems better and solve them rationally to the best of his or her ability. ... Counselling begins by understanding and clarifying the problem.*

Counselling can be viewed as sitting on a continuum of interpersonal interaction between interviewing and psychotherapy (Fig. 4.2). Interviewing is the process of finding out information from another and can be quite brief in duration. Interviews are conducted by many people in a range of occupations and are often part of a larger process, such as selecting a school for a child, or finding a new job. In contrast, psychotherapy can be a lengthy process, usually measured in months, where a professional psychotherapist enters into a specific relationship with another person (couple, family or group) to deal with particular and sometimes complex psychological problems. While approaches to counselling can vary quite considerably, there are a basic set of attitudes and behaviour that are accepted to be beneficial by most practitioners. While only some professionals concentrate their practice on counselling and psychotherapy, many health professionals use counselling skills in their day-to-day work both with patients and as supervisors.

Appropriate boundaries

The third reason why there may be reservations over embracing the counselling role is that there can be a concern over appropriate boundaries. Not all supervisors may be comfortable about finding out personal information about a student's (and potential colleague's) personal life, and there may be concerns that knowing this information may influence future working relationships. In addition, there may be concern that adopting a counselling role may be in conflict with other roles, for example as an assessor.

Fear in the role of supervisor

The fourth reason for the range of views could be our own fear as supervisors. We may fear that we could harm the student; that perhaps encouraging students to explore and express their concerns and feelings may lead them to feel worse. Perhaps this issue can be clarified by considering a somewhat extreme example from everyday life. Many people, concerned that a depressed friend may be suicidal, are often unwilling to ask about this possibility for fear that they may put the idea into the distressed friend's head. Educational campaigns about suicide by mental health professionals usually contain reassurance that the person, if seriously depressed, is likely to have already thought of suicide. Some direct talk about thoughts and plans can be beneficial.

This is related to the second possible component of our fears as supervisors – the fear of the expression of emotions, particularly the so-called negative ones of sadness, depression, anxiety and anger. The full-time counsellor lives in the realm of emotions and expects to deal with them in the course of a consultation. Others, however, can be concerned by the expression of emotions, particularly if they are expressed strongly. One of the premises of counselling is that acceptance and exploration of emotions can be beneficial. In some ways there is the belief in the value of a holistic approach rather than favouring the Cartesian mind–body split, where practitioners would only deal with the mind or the body. Thus it can be helpful for supervisors in professions that can focus more on bodies to remember that thoughts and feelings can be explored in the same way as behaviour.

These considerations of whether to counsel need to be considered against our pastoral responsibility for those whom we supervise.

WHEN WOULD WE CONSIDER ENGAGING WITH THE STUDENT IN OUR COUNSELLING ROLE?

As a background to this question it should be remembered that psychological and relationship problems are common. For young adults who make up many of those whom we will supervise, they can be at an age in life when there is considerable change, e.g. moving out from home, choosing a career, establishing intimate relationships. In addition they can be under considerable financial pressure. In any year in Australia about 20% of the population meet the accepted clinical criteria for anxiety disorders, depression and substance abuse disorders (Meadows & Singh 2001). Young adults are well represented in this group.

Times to consider counselling the student include:

- When the student's work performance is deteriorating or poor. We can then have a responsibility to address the cause at some level. Sometimes the cause is how the students are feeling about themselves and their work, and sometimes it has to do with factors external to the placement. It can also have to do with interpersonal issues on the placement.
- If the student is obviously having trouble coping with life or is unwell the supervisor may then wish to raise the issue gently.
- If the student approaches the supervisor for assistance then it is necessary to respond somehow.

It is argued here that the question is not whether to engage in counselling with the student but that we as supervisors are already engaged in a helpful relationship with the student. The decision is how we are going to engage with the student. We are engaged in this counselling role like it or not, even if it is just to the point of recognising that there is an issue and perhaps referring on.

- These days we are all expected to be skilled interpersonally and at least to some degree be able to interact with others such as clients/patients in a therapeutic way. To support this, virtually all undergraduate medical and health science courses (as well as those in many other disciplines) include some education and training on interpersonal and counselling skills.
- Where necessary, the decision to be made is not whether to refer but at what point to refer (if at all). Even where we do refer on, we are likely to be engaged with the student about the issue and/or its effects at some level
- As with the other roles in supervision we need to perform this role well and to whatever level is appropriate.
- Of course, in engaging in this role we need to counsel within our own limitations and skill levels.

HELPFUL ATTITUDES AND BEHAVIOUR

Understanding the issues

As mentioned earlier, counselling begins with understanding the issues. For this to happen the supervisor has to set the scene on a variety of levels.

As with the other supervision roles it is helpful to have clarified the *structural* issues such as the relationship between the student, supervisor, agency and university, clarification of expectations and roles within the supervisory relationship and some understanding of privacy, confidentiality and its limitations.

A quiet *setting* as free as possible from distractions is desirable. Similarly, it is preferable to have a period of time set aside of, say, half an hour. More time can be arranged as required. Students usually appreciate that there are other demands on supervisors' time and are happy to make another time to continue. The period between discussions can be valuable to allow the student time to reflect and possibly work on the issue.

It can be helpful to remind ourselves that people are both *fragile* and *robust* and we need to strike the right balance when working with them.

The supervisor must have the *disposition* to help.

It is helpful if supervisors understand that it is not their *role* to resolve the particular issue. Their role is to help the student understand the issue better, perhaps understand how it may be influencing the student's work, and possibly to consider some of the courses of action available to move towards a resolution.

Similarly it is preferable if the supervisor does *not accept responsibility* for solving the problem. Sometimes we as supervisors can enter into some sort of tacit agreement with students that they can unburden the problem on to us, and that we will solve it and hand them back a neat and elegant solution. It is often not possible to sort out someone else's (sometimes complex) problem this way. This arrangement often leads to students being disappointed and the supervisors having a residual feeling of burden for the unresolved problem. Two ways to tell if this dynamic is in progress is firstly when supervisors are engaged in "20 questions" – they take over responsibility for running the interaction as though they are working to some agenda (in a similar way to conducting a diagnostic interview). The second scenario is when the supervisor is suggesting solutions one after the other, e.g. "Have you tried this?" In this situation the suggestions are usually met with a "yes, but … " response. Occasionally we can be tempted to jump in with solutions having only listened to the student for a few sentences. Although few writers say it explicitly, an interaction like this risks being insulting. It implies that the issue troubling the student is so simple that one can grasp it in less than a minute, and that the student is not intelligent enough to have already thought of the obvious solutions. Both of these situations above tend to end in silence. The supervisor has taken the lead in the interaction and eventually has nowhere to go. Except in extreme circumstances responsibility for solving the student's problem rests with the student; we can only offer assistance.

It is also helpful if the supervisor is aware of particular categories of *risk*. One is that young people have high rates of anxiety disorders, clinical depression, eating disorders and substance use disorders. While the student may be well aware of these if they become evident during placement, some gentle direction to receive professional assistance would be appropriate. If the student is depressed it is also possible that the student may be concerned with and disclose thoughts of suicide. In this instance it is important that supervisors are clear about the limits to confidentiality. Contemporary practice is that if we are concerned that there is a serious risk of suicide we should contact an appropriate person, even if the student is unwilling to give permission. People to contact include the student's family, the student's general practitioner, the university counselling service, the local psychiatric emergency service, ambulance and/or police. While this is a rare situation for clinical supervisors to be in, it is helpful to have thought through the issues beforehand so that we are clear about the courses of action open to us.

It can be important to remember that the *process* can be as important as the outcome. Times of difficulty and crisis can also be opportunities to learn how to do things differently. Learning how to solve a problem can be as important as finding the solution. Sometimes the development of a rapport between the supervisor and student can be an aid to the development of an excellent trusting working relationship in the future. The student-focused care evidenced when the counsellor role is working well is also an excellent role model for students when they are working with clients and with students themselves one day.

It is also important to be able to tolerate the expression of *emotion*. It is not uncommon for people in difficulty to be angry or sad or to cry. We don't have to stop them but just to accept the flow of emotions. Similarly we may need to be able to tolerate *ambiguity*. Sometimes people's worlds are not entirely rational and they can entertain some quite contradictory thoughts and feelings. Often these are not problematic either. O'Hanlon (2003) has written that many issues are not "or" but can be "and"; that is, that we do not necessarily have to be cut and dried in our interactions with the world, we can embrace ambiguity. An example is that a female student in a difficult romantic relationship may capture her predicament by saying that she wants to remain in the relationship *and* she wants to leave it.

Respect and empathy

Once the preliminaries are established, what to do can be guided by the two underlying principles of respect and empathy. In turn, these are made up of:

Adopting a *non-judgemental* position. Our role as counsellor is to assist students to sort out their own issues, not tell them that they were right or wrong. Judgement tends to limit trust and exploration.

You need to *listen well* to try and understand, in a rich sense, what it is like to be this other person. In doing this you listen not just to what is said but to the non-verbal components of the communication, as well as to what is not said. Being listened to very well can be therapeutic in itself. Sometimes that is all that is required.

Part of listening very well is to *feed back* your understanding to the students. This helps them to feel understood and offers a means to clarify any misunderstandings.

Some reflection of *what we bring* to the interaction can be very helpful. We may have a desire to be very gentle and look after this person or perhaps we find the person to be difficult and want to keep our distance. This can be helpful in telling us either about our habitual style of interacting and/or giving us some very helpful information about the student with whom we are interacting. Maybe others feel the same way and it gives us an insight into one habitual way that the student relates to others.

In this component of the counselling it is usually *unhelpful to offer advice*. Similarly, if the student is telling a story about an interaction with another person it is usually unhelpful to take the other person's perspective. The aim is to inhabit the student's shoes and see the world from the student's perspective.

Clarifying questions to help you understand the student and the story being told are helpful. However, one must be on guard not to use questions as a means of giving advice. "How did you feel when that happened?" is an example of a clarifying question. "Don't you think that you should talk to her" is really advice-giving dressed up as a question. Remember the aim of all our counselling interactions is to help us and the student understand the student, not tell the student what to do.

Sometimes if the story being told is vague, it can be helpful to be *concrete* and specific. For example, you could ask: "when was the last time that your mind went blank?"

When listening to the story it is important to be listening to the student's *strengths* as well as difficulties. Sometimes it is helpful to remind someone of the strengths and abilities that you have observed, e.g. "I have observed you in other settings and I have noticed that you have well-developed research skills for investigating alternatives".

It can also be helpful for students to be aware of resources available to assist themselves. We can provide resource details but sometimes, depending on the issue, it can be beneficial for students to play an active role in researching these.

Moving towards resolution

Often just listening well to the student is all that is required to assist the student to start to deal positively with the issue. Sometimes some assistance towards action can be helpful. Again the emphasis is on a respectful approach, recognising that the student is capable of making decisions and taking action in the student's own life. A problem-solving approach can be helpful.

How has the student resolved similar problems in the past? Sometimes thinking of very broad categories of similarity to the current issue can be helpful, e.g. interpersonal issues, times when you have felt stuck, times when you have been ambivalent.

Students can be asked how they think they will move forward. If they don't know, the supervisor could either work through a problem-solving approach (e.g. Hawton & Kirk 1989, D'Zurilla & Nezu 2001) with the student (possibly in another session) or could show a problem-solving procedure to the student and let the student work through the process in the student's own time. The usual problem-solving steps are as follows:

- Clearly identify one problem. If there are a number of problems it may be necessary to prioritise. If possible starting with an easier problem makes learning the process easier.
- List all the alternative solutions open to them. While it's OK for the supervisor to make a suggestion or two in the process, it should be student-driven as much as possible. In keeping with the principles of brainstorming the alternatives are not evaluated at this point in time. The emphasis is on generating a range of creative alternatives.
- For each alternative the advantages and disadvantages are listed. The best solution is then selected. Note that this may not be the perfect solution; a perfect solution may not be available.
- The steps needed and resources required to implement the preferred solution are then identified.
- The solution and plan of action are then reviewed to ensure that they are sensible.
- The plan is then carried out.

The process is reviewed with the student to consider what worked well and what may need modification. In this stage students can be encouraged to congratulate themselves for having started to deal with a tricky solution. These days too little attention is paid to celebrating our achievements. Celebrations can assist in consolidating the learning.

THE NEXT STEP – REFERRING ON

At some stage the supervisor may wish to refer the student on. This time may vary from supervisor to supervisor and from situation to situation. Of course, if the student has a clear course of action mapped out to address the problem then you may not need to do anything. Students can be encouraged to identify resources available to them.

When to refer

- When it is not or no longer within your role as supervisor
- When you feel out of your depth
- When you do not have adequate time to devote to the situation
- When the student needs specialist assistance.

In referring it is important to let the student know that you are not abandoning them but that you are unable or unwilling to continue dealing with the issue and that you are suggesting a more appropriate next step. It may be appropriate to ask the student to let you know how things turn out.

Where to refer

These days it is expected that supervisors would have at least a basic knowledge of the services available to their students. Some of the standard places that students can be referred to include:

- student/placement/course coordinator at the university
- university student counselling service
- the student's general medical practitioner
- the counselling service of the student's local community health service
- a clinical or counselling psychologist in private practice
- a reputable telephone counselling service, such as Lifeline
- the local psychiatric emergency service (often located at major teaching hospitals).

Lists of specific resources should be available from the university staff member organising the student's placement, and from staff such as social workers and psychologists at the placement agency.

LOOKING AFTER OURSELVES

In the process of supervision we have to deal with many tricky (as well as potentially rewarding) situations. It can be very helpful for us as supervisors to have our own supports in place. Professional counsellors for example not only are expected to have regular supervision, they eagerly seek it out.

MAJOR APPROACHES TO COUNSELLING

It can be helpful to know the major approaches adopted in counselling both for when you refer someone on for counselling and for informing the way you practise the counselling component of your role as supervisor. While there are many approaches to counselling the major ones are:

- psychodynamic therapy
- behaviour therapy and cognitive-behaviour therapy (CBT)
- the humanistic approach
- family/systems approaches
- narrative therapy.

Descriptions of the details of these approaches can be found in Patterson (1989), Corsini & Wedding (2000), Dryden (2002), Davies (2003) and McLeod (2003).

In summary, this part of Chapter 4 has argued that the question is not whether to counsel but when to counsel and when to refer. Counselling is a seamless part of the interpersonal component of our supervisory relationship with a student. When students would benefit from assistance with some work-related or personal issue in their lives it is the job of the supervisor to decide how much to help. The specific incident of breaching confidentiality when someone's life may be in danger was mentioned. While there are differences between different schools of counselling there are some common factors seen as being fundamental for good human relationships. The most basic of these are empathy and respect. Within this role it is helpful for supervisors to be aware of services to be able to refer students should the need arise. Finally, it is noted that the interpersonal aspects of supervision can be trying and it is recommended that supervisors put in place support mechanisms to support them in their work.

CHECKLISTS

The following questions may be helpful to ask of ourselves.

1. Does the student need counselling?
- Does the student respond to feedback positively and improve performance in following sessions?
- Does the student show an awareness of the client's needs and have a willingness and capability to respond appropriately to these needs?
- Is the student punctual for clinic, appropriately dressed and able to maintain social interactions with you and other agency staff?
- Does the student show motivation to learn in the clinic?

2. Are we the ones to counsel or should we refer?
- What is it that might be troubling the student?
- Are you ready to put aside your hypotheses and hear the student's view?
- Can sufficient privacy be provided?
- Can adequate time be made available to allow for an uninterrupted conversation?
- Are you the student's assessor and how would the student's self-disclosure affect your assessment?
- Are adequate resources available if the situation goes beyond your expertise?
- Are you aware of your own motives for wanting to counsel the student?
- Does the student present with issues troubling him/her that parallel your own personal difficulties? If so, how will you be able to put your own situation aside and not personalise the student's situation?

REFERENCES

Asay T P, Lambert M J 1999 The empirical case for the common factors in therapy: quantitative findings. In: Hubble M A, Duncan B L, Miller S D (eds) The heart and soul of change: what works in therapy. American Psychological Association, Washington, p 23–55

Corsini R B, Wedding D (eds) 2000 Current psychotherapies, 6th edn. Peacock, Itasca, IL

Davies J 2003 A manual of mental health care in general practice. Commonwealth Department of Health and Ageing, Canberra

Dryden W (ed) 2002 Individual therapy: a handbook, 4th edn. Sage, London

D'Zurilla T, Nezu A M 2001 Problem-solving therapies. In: Dobson K S (ed) Handbook of cognitive-behavioral therapies, 2nd edn. Guilford, New York, p 211–245

Hawton K, Kirk J 1989 Problem solving. In: Hawton K, Salkovskis P M, Kirk J, Clark D M (eds) Cognitive behaviour therapy for psychiatric problems: a practical guide. Oxford University Press, Oxford, p 406–426

McLeod J 2003 An introduction to counseling, 3rd edn. Open University Press, Buckingham

Meadows G, Singh B (eds) 2001 Mental health in Australia: collaborative community practice. Oxford University Press, Melbourne

O'Hanlon B 2003 A guide to inclusive therapy. Norton, New York

Patterson C H 1989 Theories of counseling and psychotherapy, 4th edn. Harper Collins, New York

Wampold B E 2001 The great psychotherapy debate: models, methods and findings. Lawrence Erlbaum Associates, Mahwah, New Jersey

PART 5 Assessor role

Helen McBurney

INTRODUCTION: ASSESSMENT IN CLINICAL SETTINGS

Assessment requirements can have major impacts on both the assessor and the student and on their relationship with each other from the outset of a clinical placement. These impacts may be positive or negative depending on the situation and the individuals. Assessment in a clinical setting is usually more complex for both the assessor and the learner than a written examination. Who is the assessor, what is being assessed, the importance of all components to the total assessment, and how this is amalgamated into an assessment outcome or decision need to be clearly understood.

Why assess in clinical settings?

Assessments of actual practice are thought to provide a better reflection of routine performance than any assessment undertaken under test conditions. However, Norcini (2003) suggests that, whilst the assumption underlying this view is sensible, it is still unproven. To have any sense of relevance for the individual being assessed it is important that the reason for the assessment is understood and that the format of the assessment is able to address relevant criteria.

Cox (1988) provides eight reasons to assess: (1) certification; (2) promotion; (3) selection; (4) appointment; (5) ranking; (6) prediction; (7) diagnosis; and (8) analysis.

Each of these reasons places the assessor in a slightly different role and may alter the focus or criteria used for the assessment. The first six require a judgement about performance or ability to act at a defined level. In some of these instances this includes a comparison with others. Points seven and eight require a coaching role, as a colleague, teacher or mentor. They address issues such as strengths and weaknesses and how to improve. These have an important place in developing clinical practice behaviours.

There are two major reasons for formal clinical practice assessment during the progression from new student to graduate health professional. These involve defining competency at specific points in a course and the final certification of competency for entry-level practice.

Defining competency levels

Assessment is used in clinical settings to decide competency at specific tasks and readiness to move to the next level of development or appointment. Competencies may be set at differing levels across the progress of a student from entry level to graduation. Achievement of these competencies may be used to define progress throughout the student's professional development. In early formative stages, competencies might have increasing levels of complexity and may include: application of knowledge, component skills of clinical performance as separate tasks, performance of specific tasks with a patient or client, finally reaching clinical performance and embracing the habitual practice of responsible professional clinical practice.

Judging entry to practice

Entry into practice is frequently assessed on the final stage of competency – the student has attained an entry level of performance in clinical practice skills and can demonstrate this as usual behaviour. Clinical assessments have to contend with case specificity – the variance in actual patients and in performance that occurs over a number of different patients. Case specificity suggests that clinical performance with one patient and his/her problem does not reliably predict performance with subsequent patients or problems (Smee 2003).

Aspects of assessment

Yaphe & Street (2003) provide evidence that examiners use three main steps in the assessment of a student. These three steps may be likened to the research process of hypothesis generation, hypothesis testing and findings. In their study, 26 examiners of medical practitioners were found to form an initial impression of the level of a student's performance very early in the assessment process (a hypothesis). The initial impression (or hypothesis) was tested by an exploratory process in the clinical encounter in order to define more precisely the level of achievement. This testing then confirmed a final mark.

Within this process examiners were able to articulate attributes that enhanced or detracted from the student's performance. Despite examiner training, it was found that some of these features related to personal attributes of the student rather than to application of knowledge or demonstration of behaviours and skills identified as important in the training programme.

Defining terms

There are three terms commonly referred to in the literature on assessment and each is very applicable in the clinical practice setting.

Continuous

In the clinical context, continuous assessment is an ongoing process of judgement across the time span of a clinical experience. Bond & Spurritt (1999) assert that this may also be considered by students as continuous harassment!

Formative

Formative assessment usually takes place during a course. It usually involves a structured session for feedback and should be designed to help students understand how they are progressing. It may also include re-evaluation of learning needs and strategies and might not contribute to the final mark.

Summative

Summative assessment comes at the end of a specified course or time and involves a final assessment or judgement.

Separating feedback and assessment

In many clinical situations the clinical educator may also have an assessor role. Both students and assessors need to understand clearly the difference between feedback and assessment. Feedback may provide constructive criticism and suggestions for improving performance. Assessment is the judgement of performance in relation to criteria or standards.

Patients as providers of feedback and contributors to assessment

Patients are rarely invited to participate in assessment of students; however, Spencer (2003) observes they are frequently able to contribute useful feedback to both the student and assessor from their perspective of a clinical interaction and can have a powerful influence on clinical assessment.

Questions for assessors

Is the assessment reliable? Does the assessment consistently measure what it is supposed to measure? Is this consistency apparent both within and between students and within and between different examiners?

Improved reliability can be achieved by standardising patients (using patients with the same problem and a comparable level of function and ability to participate) or the use of a simulated patient (an individual trained to play the role of patient, with all candidates being assessed on their interaction with the same "patient"). Well-understood examination criteria and standardisation of examiner behaviour can also each have a major effect on improving reliability.

Is the assessment valid? Do the assessment procedures actually measure what they are supposed to measure? At the most basic level the answer to this question should describe the links between the objectives of the curriculum and the content and criteria for the assessment.

DEMONSTRATING PROFESSIONAL COMPETENCE

Clinical performance and competency can be assessed at differing levels of complexity and responsibility. Norcini (2003) cites the framework proposed by George Miller in 1990 for the assessment of clinical competence. This suggests the lowest level of clinical competence is knowledge (knows facts), followed by competence (knows how to do), performance (shows how or demonstrates as an isolated activity or for assessment purposes) and action (does as an integral part of everyday practice). This framework could be applied at the level of a specific task or for the management of a full and complex caseload. Within this framework, action is not based on artificial tests but on what actually occurs in practice. This highest level of clinical competence is seen to be best assessed by gathering information about performance in everyday practice.

Attitudes

Professional competence is not only defined by actions in relation to knowledge and technical skill ability but also by the display of appropriate attitudes to the clinical situation and individuals, be they staff, clients or carers. The development of professional attitudes within the health professions is a complex process to which all individuals bring their own beliefs and values. Attitudes that are important in the clinical context might include the ability to respect others' rights and opinions, to learn, accept feedback and work in a team. Behaviours that indicate the desired attitudes are established and demonstrated in the clinical setting and become a part of effective patient–therapist interactions. Attitudes then become an important part of the demonstration and assessment of clinical competency.

Safety

Professional competence also carries the requirement of due consideration of safety. Safety in the clinical environment includes the patient and staff, and may also include visitors or others, as well as equipment and procedural aspects. This is rarely discussed in the literature on assessment; however it is an important underlying concept in efficacy of treatment. It is possible to do little and be very safe but ineffective, to do as much as possible in a risk-taking manner, or to do all that is possible with due consideration for the safety of all concerned. Safety in clinical practice is an important part of the demonstration of an appropriate level of knowledge and skill.

Assessment processes

Setting clinical problems relevant and important to the curriculum

In order for the assessment to be relevant it is imperative that clinical problems relevant and important to the curriculum are assessed using criteria that are both appropriate for the level of the students in the course and allow students to demonstrate their understanding of the issues and ability to work with the patient.

Setting criteria or standards and making these known to both students and assessors

Knowing the purpose for which an assessment will be used helps in the design of the assessment task. In many instances students will concentrate their learning on what they believe is to be assessed. Assessment can then drive learning. Optimal student performance is enhanced by understanding the purpose of the assessment and the criteria to be used.

Applying criteria

It is rare that an entire cohort of health professional students in a course will be assessed in the clinical context by one examiner. It is far more likely that a number of examiners and a number of clinical settings might be involved in the same assessment process. It then becomes important that all examiners have similar standards and expectations of performance in relation to each of the assessment criteria so that the assessment is equitable for all students. In practice this might involve examiners meeting to set criteria and discuss standards. A review and discussion of previously taped student clinical interactions with performances at differing levels can be valuable as a part of the assessment standardisation process.

Ongoing performance assessment

Assessment skills are like many other clinical practices. The more they are used and refined, the more reliable they become. This would suggest that all examiners should participate in assessment processes as regularly as possible and that one-off sessions as an examiner are less desirable from the perspective of the student. There is some evidence that the development of expertise in a particular aspect of clinical practice does not improve assessment capacity in this area. Yaphe & Street (2003) express concern that examiners of higher academic rank were more severe in their assessments of medical student performance. Perhaps with the development of expertise, clinicians become further removed from the performance level that can reasonably be expected of a student.

Assessment types

Oral

The use of oral examinations in a clinical setting will provide some evidence of students' level of knowledge and how it might be applied in a specific clinical setting. It might also give some indication of students' level of communication skills with the examiner; however it will not examine students' communication with patients, their level of skill at clinical tasks or their ability to communicate with other staff. Performance anxiety can be heightened to such an extent that it impedes performance in oral examination procedures and thus lessens the validity of the assessment.

Practical skill

Practical skills may be examined using a model, a simulated patient or an actual patient. The level of complexity of the task will depend on what is being assessed. Do the criteria emphasise technical skills or is communication included? A model may allow demonstration of technical skill but it is difficult to demonstrate communication skills when there are no responses. Do all patients have the same capacity to communicate with the student? The advantage of a simulated patient is that all students are assessed in their interaction with an individual trained to give appropriate responses.

An objective structured clinical examination (OSCE) is a series of defined clinical tasks around which all students rotate (Newble 1988). This approach allows a wide variety of tasks to be assessed within the practical limitations imposed by the setting and number of students. It is easier to construct tasks to assess technical skills or interpretation of test results than to construct tasks that validly assess interpersonal and attitudinal components of clinical practice and competence; however the use of a simulated patient and input from this person to these aspects of the assessment can be useful.

Clinical performance

The assessment of actual clinical performance is the most difficult for both the student and the examiner. Not all patients are the same in terms of complexity of case or ability to communicate. Feeling unwell can make the patient less amenable to participation. Nervousness about an examination situation can impede both the student and the examiner. A continuous clinical assessment process offers the opportunity for evaluation over a longer time span and in a variety of clinical situations. It is more likely to reflect usual practice, but can have the student feeling under scrutiny at all times. The caseload available at the time might also limit the range of skills that the student is able to demonstrate. The assessor can also feel some conflict between the role of teacher or mentor and the assessment task.

Logbook

A logbook may be a useful method of documentation as a part of clinical assessment. It might include: a record of exposure to various clinical tasks, self-reflection of clinical performance, formal recording of clinical educator observation sessions or recording of changes in learning experiences and goals. All of these may contribute to the assessment of a clinical placement. Gordon (2003) reports the use of a portfolio to assess the personal and professional development of medical students.

Self-reflection

There is some evidence that students are well able to assess accurately their own performance at a task (Best & Rose 1996). Fitzgerald et al (2003) demonstrated this in a study of self-assessment with medical students. However, the medical students were shown to be less reliable when the task was altered from performance in written examinations to clinically oriented assessment. This is not unexpected given the inherent increase in variability of the task in a clinical performance.

Project

A project usually provides the opportunity for work on a specific area of clinical practice and can provide the opportunity for in-depth exposure to a specific question or part of the curriculum. The student also needs to be able to draw on principles for practice that may be gleaned from such a project, so that learning from this project can be applied to other areas of clinical practice.

Case study

A case study provides for in-depth discussion of the details of an individual's problems and also for the application of broader discussion of principles depending on the opportunities offered by each case. A case specifically developed for the purpose may be able to cover a wide portion of the learning needs; a case selected for specific interest may cover a narrower area of curriculum in depth. An actual case selected from the student's workload will have different opportunities than those provided by a paper case. In deciding if a case should be used we need to return to the question of the purpose of the assessment and the curriculum being assessed.

The possibilities of assessment in relation to clinical practice are many and it is more likely that a rounded picture of the clinical abilities of a student will be reflected if more than one form of assessment is utilised. This brings us to the question of how different forms of assessment should be weighted to provide an overall decision.

A further two aspects of assessment should also be considered in this discussion.

Judging by norms

Assessment by the criteria of what is normal achievement for the level of the student within a course may help with the development of pass/fail criteria, but is not necessarily the best or most appropriate assessment of clinical performance. The use of normal achievement goals does not encourage individual students to extend themselves to achieve their potential; rather it encourages the achievement of what might be considered a satisfactory standard by all.

Demonstrating achievement of goals

This is one way of assessing performance of specific tasks to a specific level, but may indicate only that the required standard has been met on one occasion and does not necessarily demonstrate usual clinical practice.

Challenges in clinical assessment

Clinical assessment in the health sciences is frequently a major component of overall assessment, particularly in later years of a programme. The outcome can have a major impact on the students and their later career opportunities and decisions.

Remaining fair and objective

The use of clear standards and criteria will greatly enhance the ability of an assessor to provide a reliable and valid assessment of performance. It is in the interests of all concerned that personal reactions to any student do not influence the assessment of performance. Cross-cultural differences may adversely affect assessment (Yaphe & Street 2003). Senior examiners have also been found to be more severe in their assessments.

Reliability and sampling

Performance that is sampled across a range of clinical situations and problems is more likely to provide information about usual performance than is a one-off examination. Hamdy et al (2003) found that the reliability of a clinical assessment was increased when four patient encounters were observed.

Equivalence in patient difficulty and performance assessment

Patients with the same condition may vary in complexity depending on the severity of their condition, any comorbidities and their ability to understand and comply with clinician recommendations. This can increase the complexity of decisions about students' clinical performance.

Providing constructive feedback as an adjunct to assessment

Asking students how they think they have performed and using their reflections allows the assessor to see their performance from their perspective and use this as a starting point for feedback. Providing feedback based on observed behaviour, in a practical, timely and concrete manner, assists students in their ongoing self-reflection and development, as well as giving students an understanding of the elements of their performance that have contributed to the assessment. Identifying specific areas where performance was good and areas where performance could be improved helps students to understand their learning and their ongoing needs.

Assessing the struggling student

If serious concerns are identified there is an obligation to identify these clearly to students. However, identification alone is insufficient and the addition of constructive strategies to address the problems will make the experience far more valuable for the student, particularly within formative assessment where there is time to address issues within the existing placement.

The failing student

Failing a student is a difficult and anxiety-producing situation for both the assessor and the student. If the assessor is also the clinical educator then there is frequently a level of distress and potentially some feeling of having failed in the educative role. Best & Rose (1996) remind us that: "You don't fail the student ... the student fails the assessment." In a well-developed assessment system with clear expectations and criteria, adequate feedback for the student and opportunities for improvement, the student should have had every opportunity to achieve the required standard.

Maintaining the dual supervisor and assessor role

Where assessment is to be provided by the clinical educator at the end of a clinical placement there is a need for the assessor to judge the performance in an impartial manner, separate from his/her personal reaction to the student. This can be emotionally demanding on both the student and the assessor. Again, clear criteria and an objective impartial approach to the assessment task will help both student and assessor.

DEVELOPING AS AN ASSESSOR

Assessment skills can be developed in the same manner as other clinical practice skills and the assessor can benefit from using a number of adult learning techniques in the same way as a student in the clinic. Reflective practice techniques can be utilised to review performance as an examiner. The ability to self-evaluate critically and use this to improve performance is as important to the assessor as it is to the student.

In the same way as for any learned behaviour or skill, regular use, review and further training can enhance the ability to apply techniques. The reliability of clinical assessments is likely to improve with exposure to different students and with regular exercise of these decision-making skills, regular re-evaluation of assessment practice and of current professional standards. Actually participating in clinical practice at the same level as the student also reminds an assessor of the complexities of the tasks being undertaken and can help to keep the assessor grounded.

It should be apparent from the above comments on development as an assessor that self-evaluation processes learned and implemented as students can have a major contribution to life-long learning in clinical practice after graduation and the achievement of professional autonomy. Indeed, skills in self-evaluation and reflection can be utilised to assist learning and development in other life settings and experiences.

In all clinical assessments it is important to the development of students that the assessment provides assistance to their learning. Whatever the clinical assessment, there is a need for feedback to assist the student to learn from the situation. In some instances there may also be a need for an independent debriefing of the student and/or the assessor.

Assessments that focus on the learner are most likely to yield practitioners able to evaluate their own performance critically in whatever context they may practise. Making assessment a positive experience that achieves this outcome is a challenge to all students and educators.

REFERENCES

Best D, Rose M 1996 Quality supervision: theory and practice for clinical supervisors. W B Saunders, London

Bond H, Spurritt D 1999 Challenges of assessment. In: Higgs J, Edwards H (eds) Educating beginning practitioners: challenges for health professional education. Butterworth-Heinemann, Oxford, p 228–235

Cox K 1988 How to assess performance. In: Cox K, Ewan C (eds) The medical teacher, 2nd edn. Churchill Livingstone, Edinburgh, p 180–188

Fitzgerald J, White C, Gruppen L 2003 A longitudinal study of self assessment accuracy. Medical Education 37:645–649

Gordon J 2003 Assessing students' personal and professional development using portfolios and interviews. Medical Education 37:335–340

Hamdy H, Prasad K, Williams R et al 2003 Reliability and validity of the direct observation clinical encounter examination. Medical Education 37:205–212

Newble D 1988 How to plan and run structured clinical examinations. In: Cox K, Ewan C (eds) The medical teacher, 2nd edn. Churchill Livingstone, Edinburgh, p 175–179

Norcini J 2003 Work based assessment. British Medical Journal 326:753–755

Smee S 2003 Skill based assessment. British Medical Journal 326:703–706

Spencer J 2003 Learning and teaching in the clinical environment. British Medical Journal 326:591–594

Yaphe J, Street S 2003 How do examiners decide? A qualitative study in the process of decision making. Medical Education 37:764–771

SECTION 2

Teaching and learning

SECTION CONTENTS

Chapter 5

Domains of teaching and learning

CHAPTER CONTENTS

PART 1 Understanding clinical knowledge and developing clinical expertise

Helen Edwards, Dawn Best and Miranda Rose

INTRODUCTION

The aims of this chapter are:

- to assist clinicians to understand the development and acquisition of clinical knowledge in students and health care professionals
- to explore the relationship between practical and theoretical knowledge
- to encourage research which articulates the rich tacit knowledge of experienced clinicians.

Before you start reading the body of this chapter, please read this short dialogue. Pam, a speech pathologist, is being interviewed about James, a patient she has seen recently. The dialogue explores what clinical knowledge and expertise Pam needed to know in order to achieve a successful outcome with James.

Interviewer: *Tell me about the patient you have chosen to talk about.*

Pam: *Let me give you some background. James is a 65-year-old male with motor neurone disease (MND). He was trying to walk and fell. Because of the MND his arms don't work, so when he fell he hit the ground and shattered his jaw. I knew he had been admitted to Ward D which is an evaluation, management and palliative unit and not in the active rehab stream.*

Interviewer: *What did you think at this stage – after referral but before you had met James?*

Pam: *My first thoughts were around MND. "How awful ... it's a shocker". Short terminal disease. "Expect big swallowing problems." Assume James will need counselling.*

I was expecting difficulties with feeding, chewing and swallowing and also probably with communication.

Interviewer: *Where do your strong feelings about MND come from?*

Pam: *I thought it was appalling when I first learned about it at university. I learned about it in a theory lecture. It hooked into a visceral response. It's progressive and fatal. Patients don't get better but they stay fairly cognitively intact. I've seen a number of patients with MND. I've read about it. I've thought about the ethics, I've discussed theory with experts. I've explored diagnostic possibilities – video-fluoroscopy. My clinical observations have taught me that there are big social implications. Does the patient have social contacts and who is involved?*

In this case there was a son involved who wanted his father to be "normal". He didn't want his father to be a sick person. I got an angry call from the nurses on the ward saying the son was feeding his father a pie, even though he'd been told his Dad would find it easier if his food was minced.

Interviewer: *Why did the nurses ring you?*

Pam: *I had worked with the nurses to help them to note problems and let me know. The patient had been referred to me by the nurses. They didn't want to feed him because they were afraid he would choke and they'd be responsible.*

Interviewer: *How are you working with James?*

Pam: *I'm trying to do what he wants. My philosophy is to do everything to increase the quality of his life. With MND patients I try to work with their preferred activity – self-determination. Clinically I have to accept I can't "fix things". I'm not going to effect a recovery.*

Interviewer: *When did you know that?*

Pam: *Instantly, as soon as I got the phone call and it was from Ward D I knew it wasn't rehab. I expected there would be swallowing problems, probably dysarthria. In that setting you know other clinicians will have been involved and you don't want to have to subject him to unnecessary extra assessment. I hoped someone good had been with him to deal with social and emotional issues.*

Interviewer: *Do you always have an emotional reaction with MND?*

Pam: *Always. I think: "Oh hell, this is so hard." Yet I know I am professionally confident, know what I'm doing in the area. Intellectually I'm comfortable. I started thinking about what the patient wanted, what his food preferences might be and how the family was. I did a diagnostic procedure with his swallowing, observed him and what he could do. I came up with some options*

Interviewer: *And are you happy with the outcome?*

Pam: *Yes. Yes, I'm happy. James has surpassed expectations. I've got the staff prepared to consider humanistic care, to look at future planning short of palliative care. It's been a positive outcome for James and for Ward D.*

EXERCISE

What sources of clinical knowledge did Pam draw on? How did she acquire them?

Before you read the rest of this chapter you might like to reflect on how you develop clinical knowledge. Think about a patient or client you have seen recently where you had to stretch yourself beyond your routine practice but where you also achieved a satisfactory outcome.

– Who was the patient/client and what was the condition?
– Why were you seeing him/her?
– When did you notice that this was not a "routine" case?
– What clues did you pick up? How did you know they were significant?
– How did you proceed? What were you thinking?
– What did you do? Why did you do this? How did you know what to do?
– Did you relate the case to something that you'd done previously, to something you had read, to what other people might have done?
– What theoretical knowledge did you draw on?
– Did you consider the individual, the wider social setting?
– What was the outcome for the patient/client?
– What was the outcome for you?
– What do you know now that you didn't know before?
– Where does this fit on your repertoire of clinical knowledge?
– How do you feel about the achievement and the outcome?

This chapter will now explore how clinical knowledge develops and how clinicians can assist students to develop clinical knowledge.

VIEWS OF KNOWLEDGE

The traditional view of learning in clinical settings was a process of "applying theory to practice". For many years health science and medical curricula were structured with theoretical or preclinical components followed by clinical or applied components. The process of learning for both students and practising clinicians was seen as applying theory to practice. Theoretical knowledge, "knowing that", was the favoured knowledge in academic and university settings. Practical knowledge, "knowing how", was less highly valued and little understood. For readers interested in this area, Higgs & Titchen (2000) provide a very accessible account of the different ways we have come to understand knowledge. Gradually, we have come to realise that the reality of acquiring clinical knowledge is far more complex than applying theory to practice. A variety of scholars and theories can help us better understand and appreciate clinical knowledge and the complexity of clinical practice.

Let us begin by thinking about types of knowledge and ways of knowing. Back in the 1950s Polanyi (1958) differentiated two very different types of knowledge. One, explicit written knowledge, is in the public sphere and accessible to all via texts and courses. This is the stuff of academia. The second type is tacit knowledge. Tacit knowledge resides inside individuals, is not codified, spoken about or formally recorded. Much expertise in clinical professions takes the form of tacit knowledge and as such is not easily accessible to students.

Another related way of thinking about knowledge is to distinguish between *knowing that* (book knowledge) and *knowing how* (practice knowledge). The philosopher Heidegger (1962) challenged the traditional view of the relationship between the two types of knowledge. The received wisdom was that knowing that (theory) preceded knowing how (practice). Heidegger postulated that the relationship in fact was reversed, that knowing how preceded knowing that. Knowing how is the practical stuff of everyday life as well as the skilled practice of professionals. It can be seen in many contexts from market places (measuring and calculating), to work sites (using tools, creating artifacts) to health care facilities (treating patients, using instruments). Knowing how, suggests Heidegger, has a number of characteristics. Importantly, people are actively engaged – they are doing. Further, they are setting out to accomplish a specific purpose. People can reflect on their activity and actions. Activities are repeated and are changed as a result of experience. Activities have a "rich referential context" – people are surrounded by products, outcomes, places, actions and people to which their knowing how relates. To a naïve observer, knowing how looks easy. It is practical, engaged, non-reflective, smooth and unproblematic – take, for example, a skilled health professional carrying out a complex but routine task.

A speech pathologist, Jill, works with a man, Bob, who is unable to produce speech following a stroke. Jill attempts to facilitate speech production by asking Bob to become aware of how individual speech sounds are made, where the tongue, teeth and lips are positioned, whether the voice is on or off, what the speech sounds look like when Jill produces them, and how it feels to make the sounds. Jill uses many kinds of cues and considerable knowledge of how speech is produced to structure the activities in such a way that maximises the chances of Bob making the sounds. Jill does this utilising a complex hierarchy from least to most support, aiming to have Bob produce the sounds with the minimum of her assistance/maximum independence. In doing this Jill is manipulating approximately 20 variables in her mind as she decides how to work with Bob. To the casual onlooker it appears as an easy, smooth and almost relaxing/peaceful activity.

But what happens when something goes wrong, or doesn't turn out quite as expected? Then, suggests Heidegger, people begin to engage in analytical and elemental thinking, to engage in present-at-hand thinking:

- I need to change that for this client
- What do the textbooks say?
- Perhaps I shouldn't have ...
- Why is this happening?

The practitioner begins critical reflection, develops hypotheses, begins to study properties, wonders what would happen if things were done another way. Through this process, suggests Heidegger, knowing how moves towards knowing that – theory develops *from* practice.

Knowing how or practice knowledge has long been acknowledged as the key component of working in clinical settings. Yet we are only just beginning to research and explore the phenomenon. It is a difficult task because so much of practice knowledge is tacit knowledge and so much of research involves a positivist quantitative paradigm that is inappropriate for exploring tacit knowledge. Fortunately, however, there is a growing body of qualitative research that examines clinical knowing.

NOVICE TO EXPERT

Patricia Benner, from the University of California, was a pioneer in looking at clinical practice, in particular the development of expertise and the characteristics of experts. Using a qualitative framework including observation and interview, Benner observed a range of nurses working in clinical settings – from nurses new to practice through to nurses acknowledged by their colleagues as outstanding practitioners. From this work she described a hierarchy of practice in clinical nursing that she encapsulated in the title of her book – *From Novice to Expert: Excellence and power in clinical nursing* (Benner 1984). Benner's five stages of development are novice, advanced beginner, competent, proficient and expert. The book contains beautiful insightful descriptions of each stage and the model has been adopted by others in exploring their profession and developing curricula. Let us examine each stage in a little more depth.

1. *Novice attributes*: The novice clinical practitioner has no experience of the situation and thus works with what Benner terms the attributes of the situation. Novices work on objective measurable parameters (e.g. weight, blood pressure) that can be recognised without previous experience of the situation. Novices tend to be rule-governed and inflexible and have limited behaviour that they can use in clinical settings. They have little understanding of the contextual meaning of learned textbook terms.

Does this describe some of the undergraduate students you have seen in clinical placements?

2. *Advanced-beginner aspects*: Advanced beginners demonstrate what Benner describes as marginally acceptable performance. They work on the aspects of a clinical situation and have enough real-life experience to note the recurring meaningful situational components. Working with aspects of a situation requires prior experience in the actual situations to

recognise key areas. The example Benner gives is assessing clients' readiness to learn. Aspects of a clinical situation may be made explicit, even developed into guidelines, but aspects cannot be made completely objective. This contrasts with the attributes of the novice stage where attributes can be observed, quantified and measured. Benner suggests graduating students are at the stage of advanced beginner. Advanced beginners still need support in the clinical setting.

The last three stages, competent, proficient and expert, are developed through clinical practice

3. *Competent – planning*: The characteristic of competent practitioners is the capacity for planning. Competent practitioners see actions in terms of long-range goals or plans. They have a feeling of mastery and ability to cope with and manage the many contingencies of the clinical setting. Note that students in clinical settings do not yet have the experience to function at this level. Nor does the short length of time students generally stay in clinical settings allow this longer-term perspective.

4. *Proficient – perceives wholes*: Proficient practitioners perceive wholes. Perspectives present themselves – they are not thought out. Proficient practitioners learn from experience what typical events to expect in a given situation and how plans need to be modified in response to those events. They are able to recognise when the expected normal does not materialise. They are very aware of the nuances of a situation.

5. *Expert – intuitive grasp*: Expert practitioners have an intuitive grasp of each situation. They zero in on the accurate region of the problem without wasteful consideration of the range of unfruitful, alternative diagnoses and solutions. They have well-developed perceptual acuity and recognition ability. Note, though, that a clinician can be expert in one situation, for example, acute care and novice in another, for example, community-based care.

Benner went on to analyse what is at the heart of expert nurses' abilities. Building on work that had been carried out on experts in other diverse areas – pilots and chess players – she highlighted *pattern recognition* as being a key skill and ability. Experts recognise patterns without being able to state all the particulars. They can recognise de novo something that is similar to something else without having preset criteria.

A second characteristic of experts in clinical practice is *skilled know-how*. Experts have developed a multitude of areas where they display skilled know-how, e.g. inserting a drip, manipulating a patient's spine, making a plaster cast, transferring a heavy, non-ambulant patient, positioning a patient with multiple fractures for X-ray, reading a video-fluoroscopy film. Skilled know-how is an example of embodied intelligence – it encompasses both knowing how and tacit knowledge.

The third characteristic of an expert nurse clinician that Benner identified is *common-sense understanding*. Experts using common-sense-understanding have the ability to grasp the worlds and concerns of patients and clients. They use that understanding to make good assessments. They recognise subtle changes and can hone in on the accurate region of the problem. Again, this is not a formal system that can be quantified.

Finally, there is *sense of salience*. Experts know and realise what is important – things stand out for them. This is in contrast to novices who are faced with a barrage of information that goes unnoticed or is difficult to organise into priorities.

EXPERT PRACTICE IN PHYSICAL THERAPY

In reporting this research, the five steps from novice to expert and the characteristics of expert practice, Benner provided much-needed insight into and valuing of clinical practice. What she said made sense to practitioners and people began to explore the novice to expert process and expert practice in their own clinical professions. An excellent example of this development is the volume *Expertise in Physical Therapy* by Jensen et al, published in 1999.

Jensen and her colleagues were responsible for an impressive 10-year qualitative study using a grounded-theory approach that explored the nature of expertise in physical therapy practice in the USA in all branches of the profession. From their analysis of observational and interview data, they developed a theoretical model for expert practice in physical therapy that identified *knowledge, clinical reasoning, movement* and *virtue* as the key components of expertise.

In the area of knowledge, expert physical therapists:

> *held a deep understanding of their clinical specialty and continually worked toward enlarging their scope of knowledge pertinent to their practices. They were engaged in learning as they transformed their knowledge base through reflection – that is, thinking critically about practice*

> (Jensen et al 1999, p. 182).

Experts' knowledge had two characteristics – it was multidimensional and it was focused on the patient.

The second component of expert physical therapy practice was clinical reasoning. The authors characterised clinical reasoning as contextual collaboration – collaboration between therapists and patients or with patients and their families. Having identified a problem and understood the context, experts engaged in collaborative problem-solving with the patient and the family.

The third component identified as part of expert physical therapy practice was movement. The facilitation of movement is the core of physical therapy practice. It is the focus of activity, the area where skills are developed.

The final area of expertise identified by Jensen et al (1999) was virtue or caring commitment. Experts demonstrated consistent and strong moral commitment:

> *They all set high standards and aimed at doing their best for patients and maintaining professional competence. Clinical practice for these therapists was exciting and provided them with the opportunity to continue learning through reflection*

> (Jensen et al 1999, p. 191).

Experts were morally committed to their patients, and this often translated into an advocacy role for patients or serving on local and professional groups.

In teasing out the elements of clinical expertise, the authors identify some of the differences between novices and experts. They see a fundamental difference in the way novices and experts bring knowledge to problems. For experts, the patient is the primary focus, the primary source of knowledge, even though the experts are at the same time accessing their multidimensional existing knowledge. Experts have a deep level of propositional knowledge combined with a strong procedural and practice knowledge.

The clinical reasoning processes of experts were very practical and client-focused. Experts were proficient in knowing when and how to carry out tasks like data collection, and when to take risks. They were comfortable with ambiguity and uncertainty. In all of this, they used metacognition – monitoring and controlling their own thinking processes and problem-solving strategies. Jensen et al (1999) point out that clinical reasoning is not an analytical, deductive or rational process as is sometimes portrayed in the literature.

EXERCISE

Different professions have different understandings and approaches. You may like to consider what the characteristics of expertise are for your profession.

ACTION AND NARRATIVE – CLINICAL REASONING IN OCCUPATIONAL THERAPY

The profession of occupational therapy has been researched by Fleming & Mattingly (2000). They explored clinical reasoning in occupational therapy and other professions, building on ground-breaking ethnographic work they had completed over the previous decade. Fleming & Mattingly believed that the medical problem-solving model that emphasises hypothetical deductive reasoning was too narrow to cover the ways that health professionals interacted with their clients. Thus, they developed an approach that better reflected the social dimensions of expert clinical reasoning and the ways health professionals actually practise. They claimed: "in order to be truly therapeutic clinicians must understand their patients and the ways in which they make meaning in lives that are changed by illness and injury" (Fleming & Mattingly 2000, p. 61). Strategies used by clinicians include narrative reasoning and active judgement.

Narrative reasoning is a form of meaning-making – the process we use to understand social life. Clinicians use narrative reasoning to understand concrete events and to relate them to desire and motive. When clinicians reason narratively, clinical problems and treatment activities are organised as an unfolding drama with a cast of characters and examination of motives. Narrative reasoning involves a search for motives and how they lead to critical key actions. Fleming & Mattingly give the example of an occupational therapist deciding when and how to use a splint and demonstrate how narrative reasoning is manifest in expert practice.

One can make a splint, for example, without needing to have tremendous skills in interpreting the meaning of splint wearing for one's client.

> *However, one cannot make a good decision about when to give a client a splint, or figure out how to get that client to wear it, without developing a capacity to assess the beliefs, values and concerns of that client*
>
> (Fleming & Mattingly 2000, p. 57).

Action and judgement on action are core elements of health professional practice. In the therapeutic interaction, both the patient/client and the therapist are required to act and make judgements on that action. This action and judgement do not necessarily occur in a fixed, linear sequence of think–act–reflect. Rather, thought and action occur in rapid dynamic relation to one another (Fleming & Mattingly 2000, p. 54). Health care professionals use imagination and action to make professional judgements; they use observations and interpretations; they build up patient/client capacity and confidence over time. They take action while treating patients and gain information as they undertake treatment. Action is both the concrete event and the reasoning strategy. Clinicians learn if and how their treatment strategies worked. In this way, clinicians build up a wealth of personal/professional expertise. And due to the way in which it was developed, much of this expertise is what Polanyi (1966) called tacit knowledge.

The question then arises as to how as teachers we can facilitate the development of action, judgement and narrative reasoning.

Another typology – propositional knowledge, professional craft knowledge and personal knowledge

In an illuminating and integrative chapter on knowledge and reasoning, Higgs & Titchen (2000) build on much of the preceding work. They propose that clinicians need to develop and use three types of knowledge: propositional knowledge, professional craft knowledge and personal knowledge.

Propositional knowledge is a type of knowing that. It is:

> *the public, objective knowledge of the field and knowledge of the external world. It encompasses book knowledge and the presentation of the abstract, logical and formal relationships between concepts or constructs, and formal statements concerning interactional and causal relationships between events*
>
> (Higgs & Titchen 2000, p. 27).

It deals with empirically established facts.

Professional craft knowledge is the actual competencies required of professionals in the field. It is knowing how, and it has lower status, especially in the rarified world of academia. It is hard to codify and make explicit, but it is the essential basis of everyday functioning as a health professional.

Higgs & Titchen's third type of knowledge is *personal knowledge*, which they define as the:

> *unique frame of reference and knowledge of self which is central to the individual's sense of self. It is the result of the individual's personal experiences and reflection on those experiences*
>
> (Higgs & Titchen 2000, p. 28).

Personal knowledge assists health care professionals and students to understand complex human desires for dignity, independence and support. It helps them appreciate the needs and frames of reference of clients. Personal knowledge allows people to cope with pain, frailty and human endeavour and is essential in learning to deal with ethical dilemmas in the clinical situation.

Higgs & Titchen's (2000) work emphasises the complexity that is clinical knowing and adds the additional emphasis on the importance of personal knowing. Being aware of such complexities will help clinical educators to have realistic expectations of students in their clinical settings.

Understanding students' stage of development of knowledge

Much of the discussion on clinical knowing thus far has focused on a progression towards expert practice in the health professions. But there are many ways of looking at development of knowledge that have been developed outside the health professions. Some can be applied to and provide useful insight into students in clinics. One such development is the Biggs & Collis (1982) SOLO (structure of observed learning outcomes) taxonomy. In a doctoral thesis presented to Hong Kong Polytechnic University in 2003, Kit Sinclair applied this SOLO taxonomy to occupational therapy student behaviour in clinics and suggested it might be a useful tool for grading

Table 5.1 Using the SOLO taxonomy to grade student progress (reproduced with permission from Sinclair 2003; adapted from Garrett & Schkade 1995)

SOLO stage	Cognitive behaviour	Professional skills
Unistructural	Falls back on "student role" to avoid action, decision-making or problem-solving, when working with clients Addresses only one issue at a time	Takes inappropriate position in relation to the client (e.g. across the room, behind the client). Avoids interaction
Multistructural	Keeps client "busy" but may not follow treatment plan; treatment goals show poor organisation or relation to theory base; addresses many issues at once without coordination	Manipulates task materials haphazardly, resulting in incomplete or inaccurate instructions to client; uses lecture or scolding to attempt to bring about change in client's behaviour or skills and cooperation
Relational	Consciously relates treatment with assessment and goals; chooses relevant activities, but does not think beyond	Endeavours to coordinate tasks to provide integrated instruction for client, using appropriate interaction with client toward expected goals
Extended in abstract	Develops treatment goals related to functional improvement; chooses activity for treatment purpose based on treatment plan and activity analysis	Accurately demonstrates tasks in smooth unhurried movements Uses combination of therapeutic process and use of self to elicit improved function

students' progress (Sinclair 2003). Her summary table is reproduced in Table 5.1. You may recognise some of your students in the descriptions.

Another framework useful in reflecting on the state of students' knowledge is provided by Bloom (1956) and described by Shepard & Jensen (1997). Bloom suggested a six-level taxonomy from lower-order (knowledge) to higher-order (evaluation) cognitive processing, representing the stages students go though in acquiring knowledge. The descriptor verbs (actions) associated with each of the six levels are of great practical assistance (Fig. 5.1). Clinical educators could reflect on the type of cognitive activities they are expecting of their students in terms of these actions and check that their expectations are consistent with the students' expected levels of development for a particular stage of the clinical placement.

Further, clinical educators might suggest activities to students, taking into consideration the developmental increments outlined by the taxonomy. For example, a student new to your clinical context and with little prior

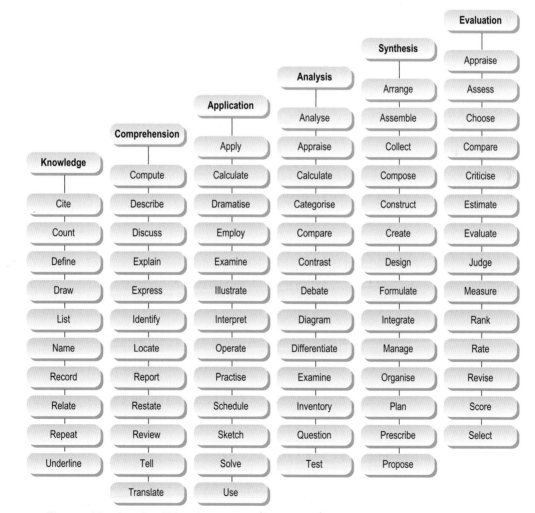

Figure 5.1   The cognitive domain of Bloom's taxonomy (Bloom 1956)

experience in the clinical population may be at the point of consolidating basic theoretical knowledge (knowing that) and thus be able to "cite, count, define and list (knowledge stage)" information about the clinical population rather than "analyse, appraise, compare and contrast (analysis stage)". You might encourage the student to explain and restate information about this clinical population as a developmental increment toward the later analysis, synthesis, and evaluation activities. We have utilised the taxonomy in our clinical education programmes in speech pathology at La Trobe University by encouraging students to use the descriptors as an aid to the self-evaluation of their progress towards clinical competence (McAllister et al 1995).

IMPLICATIONS FOR CLINICAL TEACHERS

We conclude this section on developing clinical expertise by highlighting the implications for clinical educators.

First, be clear that learning in clinical settings and developing clinical knowledge is *not* simply application of theory to practice. It is far more complex, and works on many fronts and modalities. Students require time to *develop* their clinical knowledge. The process includes social maturation, building up experience and thus a web of perspectives, having enough experiences to see patterns, developing the capacity to reflect and to understand core self. Articulating the knowledge you use in your professional practice and how you apply it will enhance students' understanding of the depth, complexity and subtlety of clinical practice.

When we develop clinical education programmes we need to include:

- hands-on clinical experience
- opportunity to develop experiential knowledge
- capacity and opportunity for reflection before, during and after any event
- acknowledgement of emotional aspects of learning in clinics
- realistic expectations for students with the particular level of experience
- adequate time to enable knowledge to develop.

We need to establish trust in the learning environment, to have faith that the journey and the process that the students are undergoing will end with the desired outcome. To prepare students for ongoing practice we must:

- model the processes
- articulate knowledge sources (speaking aloud, story-telling)
- observe, listen, question
- give feedback on performance
- more than that, we must take responsibility to inform new research projects that can describe expert practice in our professional area
- and, of course, we must continue to develop our own practice.

REFERENCES

Benner P 1984 From novice to expert: excellence and power in clinical nursing practice. Addison Wesley, Menlo Park, California

Biggs J, Collis K 1982 Evaluating the quality of learning; the SOLO taxonomy (structure of observed learning outcomes). Academic Press, New York

Bloom B (ed) 1956 Taxonomy of educational objectives. Handbook 1: The cognitive domain. David McKay, New York

Fleming M, Mattingly C 2000 Action and narrative: two dynamics of clinical reasoning. In: Higgs J, Jones M (eds) Clinical reasoning in the health professions, 2nd edn. Butterworth-Heinemann, Oxford, p 54–61

Garrett S T A, Schkade J K 1995 Occupational adaptation model of professional development as applied to level II fieldwork. American Journal of Occupational Therapy 49(2):122

Heidegger M 1962 Being and time. Harper and Row, New York

Higgs J, Titchen A 2000 Knowledge and reasoning. In: Higgs J, Jones M (eds) Clinical reasoning in the health professions, 2nd edn. Butterworth-Heinemann, Oxford, p 23–32

Jensen G, Gwyer J, Hack L, Shepherd K 1999 Expertise in physical therapy practice. Butterworth-Heinemann, Boston

McAllister L et al 1995 Developing competency based skills for speech pathology students: indicators of emerging competency. Queensland University, Brisbane

Polanyi M 1958 Personal knowledge. Routledge and Kegan Paul, London

Polanyi M 1966 The tacit dimension. Routledge and Kegan Paul, London

Shepard K, Jensen G 1997 Handbook of teaching for physical therapists. Butterworth-Heinemann, Boston

Sinclair K 2003 A model for the development of clinical reasoning in occupational therapy. PhD thesis presented to Hong Kong Polytechnic University

PART 2 Manual skills

Margaret C. Hodge and Matthew Oates

INTRODUCTION

Most health science practitioners use manual skills every day, to a lesser or greater degree. Any task that involves work done by hand or uses human energy or power is a manual task, and skill is required to perform that task correctly, efficiently and safely. Manual skills used by health practitioners range in difficulty from those required to perform a relatively straightforward task, such as adding a page to a medical record, to those used in a complex and sometimes dangerous task, like the manufacture of a limb prosthesis.

All manual tasks require the purposeful performance of motion using motor structures of the body. In simple terms, the brain and motor neural pathways provide controlling signals to muscles, which act on body segments to bring about purposeful movement. Some manual tasks need precise, fine motor control; other tasks call for the application of more gross movement or strength. Sensory mechanisms provide the brain with information used to select or modify the movement. An important aspect of gaining a new motor skill is learning how best to apply sensory information received.

Because manual skills are integral to our roles as health practitioners, much clinical education, supervision or mentoring is directed towards the development of manual skill competency in the learner. Skill training usually begins within university practical classes. University educators aim for the learner to have grasped basic skills before engaging in manual skill performance in a clinical facility. This controlled setting allows the learner to focus on applying theory and practising manual techniques, at a slow pace that is appropriate for a learner, without the added complexities of a clinical environment. A disadvantage of the separation between the practical class and real practice is that students may have difficulty transferring their learning into the clinical setting. The clinical educator plays a vital role in assisting the student to build on skills previously learned. An understanding of how we learn manual or motor skills can assist educators in this role.

MODELS OF LEARNING MANUAL SKILLS

Various models of learning manual skills exist. Presented in Table 5.2 are two contrasting models that have been applied to clinical tasks.

The model described by Payton (1986) is traditional, in that it begins with understanding of the skill, progresses through supervised practice in a learning environment with feedback and arrives at real-life applications and teaching of others. This model has similarities to those described by others (Marteniuk 1979, Turnbull 1982, Benner 1984), which involve early cognitive processing, a period of task repetition and, eventually, automation in a fluent manner.

Sanson-Fisher and colleagues (2002) presented an experimental model that reflects more recent developments in teaching and learning theory. The students involved were asked to learn clinical skills through a systematic clinical appraisal and learning (SCAL) strategy. Students initially conducted independent clinical tasks with a patient and documented their findings. They then observed the clinical tutor completing the same tasks and compared their own findings to those of the clinician. On the basis of disagreements between their own performance and that of the tutor, students established their own learning objectives, which were then discussed with the tutor. Sanson-Fisher et al concluded that the SCAL appeared to offer advantages in the development of independent decision-making. This self-directed approach to learning, with no formal demonstration or practice phases, clearly placed physical examination manual tasks within the context of patient treatment and was equally effective in physical examination skill development as the traditional model.

Of course, models of learning are not necessarily mutually exclusive. A novice practitioner could use a self-directed or problem-based approach to learning manual skills, which gradually provides sufficient experience to

Table 5.2 Examples of clinical learning models. This table lists two models of clinical skill acquisition that are very different from each other. The Payton model summarises a fairly traditional view of learning; the Sanson-Fisher offers a self-directed approach

Payton 1986	Sanson–Fisher et al 2002
Define and illustrate the skill	Independently perform the task and form own judgements
Identify the skill when it is performed by someone else	Observe an experienced clinician performing the task
Demonstrate the skill	Determine level of agreement between self and tutor
Practise the skill with feedback	Establish own learning goals based on disagreements
Use the skill in a real situation	Receive feedback from tutor
Teach someone else the skill	

develop sophisticated pattern recognition strategies and perform tasks in an automatic fashion.

Before focusing on implications for clinical educators, we should note that motor skills are used in all facets of human life and are taught in many fields. Sport involves the development of quite bizarre motor skills that have little direct application away from the arena, purely for enjoyment or fitness. Musicians develop precise motor skills that enable them to produce not only sounds in a sequence, but to modulate those sounds to convey mood or emotion. Motor skills used by dancers also convey emotion, but through performance of the movement itself. Manual skills are vital in trades and industry, and are used by surgeons and by parents. Models of teaching motor skills in all these fields have traditionally paralleled that of Payton, involving explanation, demonstration, practice and completion. Development of proficiency in clinical manual skills used by health practitioners is another example of motor learning, and it is not surprising that learning follows a similar path. Clinical educators may find it useful to explore teaching literature associated with other fields. Many health practitioners are expert in teaching motor tasks to their patients, but can forget that clinical manual skills require the same type of learning.

IMPLICATIONS FOR CLINICAL EDUCATORS

As clinical educators of health science students, it is important to recognise the importance of both the motor and cognitive components of skill development. Because both elements are integrated, for the purpose of this text, we have described the process of manual skill development as consisting of:

- skill and context definitions
- demonstration of the skill
- student practice of the skill
- provision of feedback
- facilitation of skill transfer.

Each of these components will be explored individually.

Skill and context definitions

Beyond the basic performance of clinical manual skills there is an essential requirement of the health care student to understand what the skill is, when it should be applied and, in the case of patient assessment, how the findings arising from the performance of the skill should be interpreted. In order to facilitate learning of the skill, the student needs to be able to place the skill in the context of patient treatment or professional practice and have an understanding of the skill to be learnt. Furthermore, the student can be made aware of any alternative contexts in which the application of the particular skill is desirable.

To demonstrate this, let us consider the podiatrist's use of a scalpel as an example. It would be very easy simply to demonstrate the correct technique for loading a scalpel handle with a scalpel blade and then to demonstrate the correct technique for holding and using the scalpel. Students could practise this over and over again until they were comfortable with this skill. Beyond the attainment of this manual skill, an understanding of when and why a scalpel should be used (or not used) is vital. The student must know that this skill can be used to improve patient comfort and mobility by removing unwanted callus or other painful skin lesions such as corns or warts.

In the case of a diabetic foot ulcer, the removal of dead tissue with a scalpel can assist in the healing of such a wound. Moreover, depending on what the scalpel is being used for, the way in which it is held or manoeuvred may change. Similarly, there are different blade sizes that are available and these may be indicated in particular circumstances. Scalpels are sharp instruments able to cause serious injury if not used appropriately and therefore discussion of any relevant safety issues and informed consent is also mandatory.

So, using this example, one can begin to appreciate that the teaching of manual skills alone is insufficient in facilitating student understanding of competence in manual skill performance. The student is required to:

1. Have an overall understanding of the skill to be learnt. Example: loading a scalpel handle with a scalpel blade and using the scalpel.
2. Place the skill in context of patient management and professional practice. Example: the scalpel can be used to manage safely and effectively various skin lesions (callus, corns, warts) and subsequently improve patient comfort, mobility and independence. This is a unique service that podiatrists provide to their patients.
3. Be aware of alternative contexts in which the skill can be used. Example: the skill of scalpel use can be also be applied to assist in wound healing by removing dead or necrotic tissue from a chronic wound.
4. Be aware of safety considerations and any contraindications to the use of the skill. Example: care needs to be taken as the scalpel is very sharp and able to cause injury.

Marteniuk (1979) and Turnbull (1982) suggested that skill acquisition can be divided into three phases, the first of which they described as a cognitive phase where the student must have an idea of the overall skill to be learnt. By working through this initial defining process, we hope that students are, at a cognitive level, comfortable with the purpose of and justification for learning the skill, are aware of safety considerations, and that subsequently their ability to acquire this skill is enhanced.

Demonstration of the skill

Following conceptualisation of the purpose and context for learning a new skill, it makes sense that the skill is demonstrated to the student by an experienced and competent person. There are different ways of demonstrating a skill or task and the method chosen may vary depending on the nature of the skill. While traditional techniques have focused on demonstrating the skill in logical and sequential steps, modern approaches to skill demonstration include such things as the use of internal commentary and the incorporation of real-life scenarios as key features of the demonstration (Murdoch Eaton & Cottrell 1999, Studdy et al 1994).

Mackway-Jones & Walker (1999, as cited in Fraser 2003, p. 541) described four stages in the teaching of skills using a commentary:

1. The instructor demonstrates the skill silently at normal speed while the learner observes.
2. The instructor repeats the skills in a number of small steps with dialogue. At this stage questions are clarified.
3. The instructor repeats the skills, with the learner providing the dialogue.
4. The learner performs the skills with commentary.

Perceived advantages of this approach are repetition of the demonstration and the absence of distraction that could occur if the demonstrator used dialogue in the initial stage.

Studdy et al (1994) described a similar process but suggested that the skill be demonstrated as part of a realistic scenario, to support learning of the skill in the context in which it is defined. In the variation by Murdoch Eaton & Cottrell (1999), called the silent run-through, after stage 2, the learners work in pairs and perform the skill on each other while providing an audible commentary, then repeat the practice while silently running the commentary through their minds. The authors concluded that, although this technique did not appear to improve clinical problem-solving skills, the breaking down of complex manual tasks into smaller, digestible components and using a silent commentary appeared to be an effective way of teaching complex clinical skills.

Alternatively, a stepped approach may be adopted in which only part of the task is demonstrated and practised at a time. Once competency in each part has been achieved, the sections are put together to perform the complete task. Using our earlier example of scalpel technique, the first component of the task would be to open the scalpel blade packet and hold the scalpel blade and handle correctly in preparation for loading the handle with the blade. After the student has practised and is comfortable with this, the skill of loading the blade on to the handle would be demonstrated and practised, followed by demonstration of correct debridement technique, followed by unloading and disposal of the scalpel blade. Then, ideally, the student should be able to put these smaller tasks together and perform the entire skill of scalpel debridement from start to finish.

This part-practice approach may be of particular benefit where a complex clinical process consisting of a number of steps is to be learned. However, this technique is dependent on the skill being able to be broken down into smaller tasks that can be practised independently. Commentary techniques outlined above have been identified as useful in breaking down a complex task to facilitate learning.

Intricately woven with demonstration of a manual skill is the obvious need for the student to practise the skill, in order to achieve not only manual competence, but to allow the student to develop long-term retention of the skill.

Student practice of the skill

Students need to practise a manual skill repeatedly in order to gain competence. Researchers have demonstrated that repeated practice of a motor skill creates neural linkages, which enable swift and accurate response when the need for a practised action is anticipated (Elsner et al 2002, Drost et al 2004). A classic model of skill acquisition, applied to a clinical setting by Benner in 1984, relies on repetition of experience to advance from a novice state to that of expert. Repeated practice of a skill allows the practitioner to accumulate sufficient experience of similar encounters eventually to be able to recognise patterns in patient responses. This pattern recognition technique is a feature of proficient and expert practice, produces fast and almost intuitive decisions and cannot develop without repeated experience.

Although the need for repeated experience is widely accepted in motor learning, there is some conflict amongst researchers as to the timing and planning of opportunities to practise skills. As mentioned in the previous section, practice of small segments of a complex task until competence in each segment skill is achieved, before undertaking the whole task, is one approach to practice. It is believed that part-practice allows students to focus attention on one component at a time, avoiding the stress that may accompany having to perform all steps sequentially (Oldmeadow 1996).

Schmidt (1991, as cited in Best & Rose 1996, p. 54) acknowledged improvement in performance when tasks were grouped together in a logical and ordered sequence, but argued that retention of the skill was improved by random allocation of task order. Schmidt suggested that once the student can perform tasks, the order in which tasks are presented should be rotated and interspersed with other activities so as to avoid repetition by rote. Such a scenario is more closely analogous to clinical practice, in which patient pathologies present in a random fashion. The student would need first to identify what task was required before performing it, thus practising decision-making. This is where practice with real patients, such as occurs on a clinical placement, can be of great benefit. As patients with differing pathologies present to these clinics, they provide a random allocation of tasks for the student to perform, and a variety in cultural and social influences which impact on health care.

A clinical educator's planning and organisation of practice sessions will largely depend on the nature of the skill and whether the focus is on smooth performance of the skill or on long-term retention. It is worth noting that, when we are planning and organising practice of skills, we must consider the implications of errors in student performance. Allowing students to practise using real patients requires careful consideration if errors in the performance of certain skills may place patients at risk of injury.

Provision of feedback

None would argue against the importance of providing feedback to students about their performance. Bilodeau (1966, as cited in Kidulski & Rice 2003, p. 329) suggested that "Feedback is one of the key influential variables in the acquisition of motor skills, second only to practice." The general principles for feedback are discussed earlier (Chapter 4, part 3). It is often difficult for clinical educators to balance the demands of increasing workloads with the need to provide students with regular, constructive and thoughtful feedback.

The research about feedback with respect to motor skill development considers a number of factors related to the provision of feedback on performance, including:

- type of feedback
- timing relative to performance of the skill or task
- frequency of feedback provision.

The influence of these factors on the learner's acquisition or retention of manual skills is discussed below.

Feedback may be broadly classified into two types, intrinsic and extrinsic (or augmented). Intrinsic feedback is that which is generated from performance of the skill itself while extrinsic feedback is offered by sources other than the task, such as that given by a clinical educator (Kidulski & Rice 2003).

Intrinsic feedback is particularly useful in skill acquisition, as the learner receives sensory information during task performance. Because intrinsic feedback is provided directly by the task to the learner, clinical educators have little influence over its provision. An educator may, however, direct the learner's attention to key sensations. Intrinsic feedback can be facilitated by biofeedback that enhances sensory input. An auditory beep may reinforce correct instrument placement, for example (Zheng 2002).

Kilduski & Rice (2003) investigated the effects of two types of augmented or extrinsic feedback – qualitative and quantitative knowledge of results – on motor skill acquisition and retention. Qualitative knowledge of results referred to verbal encouragement while quantitative knowledge of results was in the form of an error score. Participants were randomly allocated to one of four conditions: (1) those who received qualitative verbal encouragement only; (2) those who received just the quantitative error score; (3) those who received both qualitative and quantitative knowledge of results; and (4) those who received no feedback on performance of the motor task. The results of this study suggest that qualitative feedback alone or in conjunction with quantitative feedback improves skill acquisition but not retention (Kidulsky & Rice 2003).

Knowledge of performance, another example of extrinsic feedback, provides students with information about the patterns of movement they use when learning a skill. This type of feedback is considered important for learning the skill and may be provided using a variety of techniques, including videotape replays, kinematic feedback, biofeedback and kinetic feedback (Schmidt & Lee 1999).

The literature in relation to the timing of feedback indicates that extrinsic feedback given during performance of the manual skill hinders performance while that given after completion of the task enhances manual skill learning (Annett 1959, Newell 1976). Best & Rose (1996) suggested that the complexity of the task should guide the timing of feedback provision. They recommended that feedback be offered after a prolonged delay in order to enhance retention of simple manual skills, while feedback be provided very soon after completion of more complex skills.

Retention of a skill can be improved if summarised knowledge of results is provided following a number of consecutive trials, as long as this is delayed in the acquisition phase (Schmidt & Lee 1999). It is important to note that, while retention improves with this delayed summarised feedback, there may be detrimental effects on motor performance (Schmidt & Lee 1999). Best & Rose (1996) suggested that frequent feedback improves performance of manual skills but may hinder long-term retention of the skill as the learner becomes dependent on this frequent feedback.

As clinical educators, our understanding of these issues related to feedback provision may help us provide our students with an opportunity to enhance their acquisition and retention of manual clinical skills.

Facilitation of skill transfer

To become proficient and independent practitioners, students must be able to transfer manual skills from one environment to another. This includes skills they learned and practised in the controlled environment of the university practical class, and skills developed in the clinical environment. Whittle & Murdoch Eaton (2001) demonstrated that a group of medical students clearly understood the importance of having good transferable skills, including manual skills. Such understanding is necessary for learners to be motivated to develop skills transfer and it is hoped that all heath science students are aware of this need.

The clinical placement provides the primary opportunity for health science students to begin the process of skills transfer. An educator can encourage students to recall and consider skills learned elsewhere and can promote opportunities for them to make decisions about alternative application of their skills. To do this, however, educators must accept that a student may use techniques that are different from their own preferred method, but are equally effective. When this occurs, an astute educator can learn a new technique from the student, while providing an opportunity for the student to advance through Payton's learning model by teaching the skill.

A final point to note is that motor skill proficiency is affected by changes in environment or equipment used to perform the skill. This may partly explain an educator's observation that a student has difficulty with a task that was satisfactorily completed in the university practical programme or in another clinic. Therefore, it is helpful to allow a student to become familiar with equipment in your facility before a task begins. This may simply involve allocating time for the student to examine and practise with the equipment, or a demonstration may be needed. Safety orientation is mandatory if the equipment has the potential to cause harm to the student or patient.

Gradual reduction in supervision

Seeing a student improve in ability to apply manual skills appropriately in real-life professional practice is one of the most rewarding aspects of clinical education. The challenge in achievement of this reward is that the clinical educator must learn to stop teaching.

One of the hallmarks of an effective manager is to nurture the professional development of staff, so that staff members may be promoted to roles of increased responsibility. Similarly, as clinical educators we must be willing slowly to withdraw our assistance (or control), and allow our students to become increasingly responsible for the selection and implementation of their manual skills. In the health sciences this means that we need to give our students the opportunity to work autonomously with patients attending our clinics. The pace of this transition should be considered in light of each student's competency, and even those who are reasonably proficient in their manual skills should be encouraged to seek advice when they encounter unfamiliar or uncertain situations.

The aim of many university health science programmes is to develop competent entry-level practitioners. Graduates of health sciences still have much to learn and it would be unwise to assume that new graduates, or novice practitioners, do not require some level of supervision. Ideally, we expect that after a year or two of work, the novice practitioner would function more independently but would still require mentoring. Payton (1986) suggested that the final stage of manual skill development may be that of being able to teach the skill to someone else. The Benner model culminates in intuitive performance of tasks at an expert level and may occur after five or so years (Benner 1984). Clinical education is an important stage along the process towards independent practice, but is not the final step.

Future developments in manual skill education

Manual skill education will continue to be a vital and necessary component of our education and practice as health care professionals. However, we live in a litigious climate where increasing claims against health care professionals have affected the cost and availability of professional insurance. The future use of real-life patients in the clinical setting, for the purpose of student skill development, may become increasingly obsolete in response to these issues.

Future developments in manual skill education may focus on offering simulated experiences that allow students to pursue development of manual clinical skills through alternative environments such as simulated patients or virtual-reality teaching.

Some professions are already using these alternatives to teach practical skills and allow students to practise these. For example, teaching aids such as manikins, instructors using role play or even the use of animals or cadavers have been used to varying success in the medical and health science professions (Fraser 2003). Sophisticated computerised systems are being developed that allow examination of a completely virtual patient (Caudell et al 2003). Although the authors cited distance education as the primary application, the system would allow any student to practise physical examination skills without using a human patient. It is likely that such developments will change the way in which some clinical manual skills are taught in the future. Each simulator has its own advantages and limitations but nonetheless, given the nature of the skill to be taught, these alternatives may be acceptable. To be so, learners must enact skills transfer to real clinical practice, and transfer will probably be under the guidance of clinical educators or mentors.

CONCLUSION

In this section we have outlined a number of ways in which a clinical educator can facilitate the development of manual skills by a learner. Teaching of manual skills may involve simple descriptions, demonstrations and practice or more sophisticated educational techniques such as internal commentaries. If you would like to know more about motor learning, the reference list at the end of the section offers a starting point for further reading.

EXERCISE

Which of the models of learning outlined in Table 5.2 most closely matches your experience in teaching clinical manual skills? Do you routinely demonstrate a task first or do you let the student try? Imagine using the opposite approach when working with your next learner practitioner. How would you feel about it? What would the risks be? What advantages might you encounter? Try to identify a clinical manual task in which the alternative model would work.

REFERENCES

Annett J 1959 Learning at pressure under conditions of immediate and delayed knowledge of results. Quarterly Journal of Experimental Psychology 11:3–15

Benner P 1984 From novice to expert: excellence and power in clinical nursing practice. Addison-Wesley, Menlo Park, p 13–34

Best D, Rose M 1996 Quality supervision: theory and practice for clinical supervisors. W B Saunders, London, p 53–56

Caudell T P, Summers K L, Holten J T et al 2003 Virtual patient simulator for distributed collaborative medical education. Anatomical Record 270B(1):23–29. Online. Available: http://www3.interscience.wiley.com/cgi-bin/fulltext/102524540/PDFSTART 15 May 2004

Drost U C, Rieger M, Brass M et al 2004 Action-effect coupling in pianists. Psychological Research. Online. Available: http://springerlink.metapress.com/app/home/contribution.asp?wasp=agxyplrutrdt1xvrlh87&referrer=parent&backto=issue,7,28;journal,1,27;linking publicationresults,1:101575,1 16 May 2004

Elsner B, Hommel B, Mentschel C et al 2002 Linking actions and their perceivable consequences in the human brain. Neuroimage 17(1):364–372

Fraser J 2003 Teaching practical procedures in general practice: a primer for supervisors of medical students and registrars. Australian Family Physician 32(7):540–543

Kidulski N C, Rice M S 2003 Qualitative and quantitative knowledge of results: effects on motor learning. American Journal of Occupational Therapy 57(3):329–336

Marteniuk R G 1979 Motor performance and learning: consideration and rehabilitation. Physiotherapy Canada 31:187–202

Murdoch Eaton D, Cottrell D 1999 Structure teaching methods enhance skill acquisition but not problem-solving abilities: an evaluation of the "silent run through". Medical Education 33:19–23

Newell K M 1976 Knowledge of results and motor learning. Exercise and Sports Sciences Reviews 4:195–228

Oldmeadow L 1996 Developing clinical competence: a mastery pathway. Australian Physiotherapy 42(1):37–44

Payton O 1986 Psychosocial aspects of clinical practice. Churchill Livingstone, New York, p 21

Sanson-Fisher R W, Rolfe I E, Jones P et al 2002 Trialling a new way to learn clinical skills: systematic clinical appraisal and learning. Medical Education 36(11):1028–1034

Schmidt R A, Lee T D 1999 Motor control and learning: a behavioral emphasis, 3rd edn. Human Kinetics, Champaign, IL, p 323–408

Studdy S J, Nicol M J, Fox-Hiley A 1994 Teaching and learning clinical skills, part 2 – development of a teaching model and schedule of skills development. Nurse Education Today 14:186–193

Turnbull G 1982 Some learning theory implications in neurological physiotherapy. Physiotherapy 68:38–41

Whittle S R, Murdoch Eaton D G 2001 Attitudes towards transferable skills in medical undergraduates. Medical Education 35:148–153

Zheng Y 2002 Operation manual of TUPS (tissue ultrasound palpation system). Jockey Club Rehabilitation Engineering Centre, Hong Kong Polytechnic University, p 10

PART 3 Attitudes

Dawn Best and Megan Davidson

INTRODUCTION

The domains of learning listed by Shepard & Jensen (1997) provide a framework for health science education that focuses on classifying learning outcomes in the following five domains:

1. cognitive
2. skills
3. attitudes
4. psychomotor
5. spiritual.

The preceding two sections have discussed knowledge and skill development, which includes the psychomotor area. This part will explore the development of attitudes – an area that many clinical educators find challenging. It is certainly more difficult to define and more problematic than knowledge and skills to assess. There is some debate about whether the spiritual domain should be included within health science education at all. In some professional areas of practice such as palliative care where it is acknowledged as an important and integral component of practice, it is included within the affective domain. It is also acknowledged that, although there are practice differences between professions, individual academic and clinical teachers have great variation in personal comfort in acknowledging the spiritual domain (Shepard & Jensen 1997). Although the classification into the domains of learning is a useful guide for planning, orientation, feedback and assessment, it is important to recognise that each domain is integrally linked. Moral and ethical development could be included in the affective domain but is not included here since this topic is expanded in Chapter 10.

This part aims to:

- provide an explanatory framework for the development of professional attitudes in health science students
- acknowledge the process of professional socialisation
- explore relevant literature on personal biases and stereotyping
- increase awareness of personal biases and professional attitudes
- provide clinical educators with strategies for facilitating the development of effective professional attitudes in students.

Although there is general agreement on the specific areas that belong to professional behaviour, there is considerable variation between the actual behaviours considered as appropriate in the individual placements. The climate of the placement will determine the level of formality expected in interdisciplinary communication and the appropriate channels for information. Few orientation programmes provide details of the specific professional behaviours that are expected in the individual clinical facility. Fitting in to the department is very much left to the student to get it right. Consequently students are often criticised for sitting on the beds, being too familiar with clients, being too formal with patients, being too pushy or too passive according to the specific expectations of the group. There is a marked difference between appropriate professional behaviour in acute care facilities and rehabilitation centres, between metropolitan and city placements or even between individual placements. Student clinical assessments often require supervising clinicians to make judgements on ethical and professional attitudes without clearly defining the behaviour for the specific placement environment.

DEFINING ATTITUDES

Attitudes have been defined as:

- Internal states that modify choices of personal actions towards objects, persons or events (Gagne 1977, p. 49)
- Evaluations of ideas, events, objects or people (Sdorow & Rickabaugh 2002, p. 487).

The attitudinal domain is rarely considered when students enthusiastically arrive at clinical placements, fit in smoothly and make good progress. However, when the student has problems with professional behaviour then it can present considerable challenges for all.

Attitudes have emotional, cognitive and behavioural components (Sdorow & Rickabaugh 2002). As clinical educators we can observe the expressions and behaviours of the student and listen to what is said to each other and to clients and then use these as a guide for any judgement of the student's attitude.

The following sequence for affective development places lower-level attitudes on a continuum that progresses to more organised behaviours, which develop as the attitudes become more internalised into a way of viewing the world. This inherently creates a problem for us as clinical teachers since it asks that we increase our awareness of those very behaviours that are often unconsciously integrated into our professional and personal lives.

The five-stage affective developmental sequence (Krathwohl et al 1984) is outlined below:

1. *Receiving*. The lowest level of learning outcome ranges from an awareness of existence of a phenomenon to selective attention on the part of the learner.
2. *Responding*. This level refers to active participation of the student in response to awareness of the phenomenon.
3. *Valuing*. Valuing is based on the internalisation of a set of specific values, which are characterised by consistent behaviour.
4. *Organisation*. This category is typified by the synthesis of different values to form a system of values, which form the basis for a philosophy of life.

5. *Characterisation of a value*. Once the learner has developed a value system that is demonstrated by controlled behaviour for a sufficient length of time, persistent and predictable lifestyle characteristics are developed.

The sequence provides a framework for understanding learning in the affective domain with some appropriate teaching strategies to optimise student learning in this important area. It certainly justifies the need for explicit orientation to the desired behaviours expected in each clinical environment.

Once we have become socialised into our profession, these attitudes and values are so much part of our own behaviour that we may not be aware of them. Briefing a new learner to the specific behaviours of a task when our own behaviours are unconscious becomes a challenge. We may forget to brief at all or have difficulty identifying the specific behaviours associated with the task.

An interesting illustration of the model is provided by a qualitative study of physiotherapy student perceptions of their learning following a semester of clinical experience (Best 1992). All students were in the third year of a four-year undergraduate programme but their responses indicated the following very different perceptions of themselves in relation to their enrolment. The responses included:

1. Being a university student

   I have enough trouble coming to terms with the fact that I am a university student at all, let alone a third year physiotherapy student. I feel a long way off from the physiotherapist I want to be ... I realise the depth of skill involved is greater than I had previously appreciated.

2. Being a university student enrolled in physiotherapy

   Until now physiotherapy was just a university course that I would be studying for 4 years. I didn't think about it as a profession for life until I completed the clinics.

3. Accepting a professional identity

   Six months ago I considered myself to be a Uni student studying physiotherapy. Today I am a physiotherapist in training.

4. Integrating personal life with professional identity

   As the course races by I see myself more and more as a physiotherapist and this carries over a lot more into everyday life.

It is obvious that the attitude the student has to becoming a health care clinician will influence learning knowledge and skills in both academic and clinical settings. However, it is important to remember that the opportunity to work in the clinical environment for a period of time appears to be the catalyst for the change in identity.

PROFESSIONAL SOCIALISATION

Much of the learning associated with attitudes and values is concerned with the process of professional socialisation, which sometimes remains a hidden curriculum.

All professions have specific traits, which unite members with a common identity and shared attitudes and values. This process of professional socialisation requires both learning and the internalising of behaviour patterns, customs, feelings, morals and values of the group. Jensen et al (1999), in a 10-year qualitative study of US expert physical therapists from a range of different areas of practice, identified common professional values which the authors called virtues. These included a strong commitment to others and a passion for excellence as well as compassion, empathy and patient-centred problem-solving.

Ramsden (1985), in considering the socialisation process of the new graduate physiotherapist with the profession, states that the full-time responsibility of professional practice includes:

- identification with a peer group
- clarification of the role by the explicit and implicit behavioural norms of the group
- opportunity for constant rehearsal of the role
- responsibility for patient care.

Experience in the clinical environment provides students with these opportunities which as busy clinicians we may overlook.

Professional socialisation builds on other socialisation processes from childhood and adolescence. Attitudes related to gender and culture are established very early in childhood and will impact on later professional attitudes and behaviour. It must be acknowledged that professional socialisation is a continuous process as over time professional knowledge and clinical workplaces and culture change (Cant & Higgs 1999). Let's look at your own expectations of students.

1. Using the list below, construct a description of the student you would most like to have as your next student, and a description of the student you would least like. Write down why you would most/least like the students you have described.
   - Age: 20, 25, 30, 35, 45
   - Gender: male, female
   - Ethnicity: Anglo-Celtic, Indian, Greek, Jewish, Vietnamese
   - Weight: underweight, normal weight, overweight, obese
   - Religion: atheist, Jewish, Christian, Muslim, Hindu
   - Health: No health problems, diabetes, anxiety disorder, chronic low-back pain, depressive disorder
   - Interests: Football, cinema, tennis, bush-walking, fashion.
2. Consider:
   - How similar to you is your preferred student?
   - How unlike you is your least preferred student?
   - What impact might this have on your clinical education responsibilities?

Cognitive bias

Cognitive biases are systematic errors that arise from the limited information-processing capacity of the human sensory system. When we consider that the central nervous system can utilise about 50 bits of information per second, yet the human ear can receive 10,000 and the eye 4 million bits per second (Stewart et al 1979), cognitive strategies that reduce and order this information are vital.

What is cognitively processed depends largely on what is expected, or what is most salient in a particular situation. This selectivity of perception, although part of normal cognitive processes, can result in biased or erroneous perceptions of people and situations. Some cognitive biases that have been widely studied and that are likely to operate in student–clinical educator interactions as well as student–patient and clinical educator–patient interactions are outlined in this section.

Stereotyping

A stereotype is "a set of beliefs about the personal attributes of a group of people" (Ashmore & Del Boca 1981).

Stereotypes are a constellation of beliefs, ideas, associations and emotions and can contain positive and negative elements. Many social stereotypes are acquired from a young age, and you cannot "not know" the stereotypes transmitted by your culture. Write down the stereotypical attributes of the following groups:

- teenagers, the elderly
- men, women
- the unemployed, the middle class, the rich
- Irish, Jews, Chinese, English, French, Indian, American, Arabs, Australians
- doctors, lawyers, used-car salesmen, accountants, nurses, politicians, teachers.

Stereotypes allow one to generate an expectation of the likely characteristics of individuals, based on their membership of a group. A person's gender, age, ethnicity or appearance activates stereotypes that may influence person perception, interpersonal processes and judgements of performance and competency.

People generally hold less positive stereotypes about groups of which they are not a member (out-groups) and more positive stereotypes of their own or in-group (Stroebe & Insko 1989). Positive information about an in-group and negative information about an out-group is more likely to be recalled (Stephan 1989).

Halo effect

The halo effect occurs when one attribute of a person influences judgements about unrelated attributes. In performance evaluation, a general feeling about a person may bias ratings of performance consistently in a positive or negative direction (Sdorow & Rickabaugh 2002).

Self-fulfilling prophecy (self-confirming bias)

A feature of cognitive processing is the tendency for self-confirmation. We will tend to pay attention to, process and recall information that is congruent

Figure 5.2   Comparison of intentional and automatic processes

with our prior expectancies. As Hamilton (1981) put it, "I wouldn't have seen it if I hadn't believed it."

Although cognitive biases are automatic, they can be modified and inhibited by conscious, intentional processes (Devine 1989). Intentional processes require more time and effort than automatic processes (Fig. 5.2) and this has obvious implications in a workplace where the clinical educator is cognitively busy balancing the competing demands of patients, students and managers.

LINKING RESEARCH FINDINGS TO CLINICAL EDUCATION

The following section provides details of some relevant research findings on professional attitudes of both clinicians and students. Although the attitudes of patients will also impact on student learning, no studies were found which addressed this aspect.

Clinical educator attitudes – to student, patient

Health professionals are not immune from cognitive biases such as the positive halo effect of physical attractiveness (Nordholm 1980) and negative halo effect of a visible disability (Gething 1992a). Some studies have shown relatively neutral attitudes of health professions toward the elderly (Lookinland & Anson 1995, Slevin 1991) while others have reported negative and ageist attitudes (Kearney et al 2000, Gething et al 2002). Health professionals' attitudes toward disabled people seem to be relatively positive (Gething 1992b, 1993, White & Olson 1998). The study by White & Olson found that occupational therapists had more positive attitudes than physiotherapists or nurses toward people with disabilities.

A clinical educator's perceptions of student competency may unconsciously be negatively or positively influenced by stereotypes. Haskins et al (1997) demonstrated that, when presented with videotapes of white, Hispanic, Asian and black physiotherapy students reciting identical scripts, physiotherapists rated the black student consistently lower than the other students.

Student attitudes – to own/other professions, patients

Streed & Stoecker (1991) asked physiotherapy and occupational therapy students to rate both professions on a range of attributes. Both groups rated their own profession more positively than the other profession.

Tunstall-Pedoe et al (2003) found that medical, radiography, physiotherapy and nursing students had stereotyped views of their own and the other professions when they began their university course and that those stereotypes were stronger after a first-year interprofessional programme. The strongest stereotypes were held by students whose parents were health professionals. Work by Hind et al (2003) with medical, nursing, dietetic, pharmacy and physiotherapy students showed that students at the start of their professional training identified strongly with their own professional group and held largely positive attitudes toward their own and other professional groups.

Studies suggest that students' attitudes toward the elderly are either neutral (Kaempfer et al 2002) or positive (Brown et al 1992, Tovin et al 2002, Menz et al 2003) and their attitudes toward people with disabilities are relatively positive (Gething 1992b).

REFLECTIVE TASKS

Increasing personal awareness

- Think about your own practice and list the beliefs on which your own professional practice is based.
- Your list will reflect your employment and personal experiences.
- Perhaps it includes attitudes related to a specific concept, e.g. rehabilitation, health, disability.
- Perhaps it includes some beliefs related to professional ethics, e.g. confidentiality and client autonomy.
- Perhaps it includes attitudes towards a particular population, e.g. people with physical or mental disability, people with particular diagnoses, elderly people, the terminally ill and dying, and other health science professionals.
- It is probably also influenced by personal experiences or individual contact with family, friends or acquaintances.
- As you look at your list, can you remember how you learnt these attitudes?

Clarifying departmental expectations of students

We have adapted the following activity suggested by Davis (1991) in our preparation course for clinical educators. She advised that all members of the department – porters, cleaners, assistants, clinicians, secretaries and the department head – be included. Brainstorm the components of professional behaviour that are accepted by the group within the department as a preliminary exercise to the student orientation. It is also recommended that time be spent deciding what constitutes satisfactory and unsatisfactory performance.

Owning personal biases and modifying practice to account for them

If we are concerned with the development of professional attitudes then we need to be explicitly aware of those we are concerned with and the behaviours that reflect them. Re-read the research findings and identify any biases you have which may impact on your student or client interactions. Once we are aware of our biases we can modify our behaviours so that they do not impact on our student and practice responsibilities.

ENCOURAGING DEVELOPMENT OF EFFECTIVE STUDENT PROFESSIONAL ATTITUDES

Role modelling

Student attitudes are, at least in part, influenced by the attitudes of their clinical educators. Wilhite & Johnson (1976) reported that nursing students' attitudes toward the elderly improved during an eight-week course, and the amount of change was associated with the educators' attitude. Remember that we are role models for students. They are watching all we do and are likely to follow our behaviour. Also keep in mind that, although we may all aspire to ideal professional behaviour all of the time, it is an unrealistic goal to achieve in all the complex health care situations we are faced with today.

Davis (1975) challenges us to identify our not-OK behaviours. In modelling our ability to reflect on our own professional behaviour, in developing awareness of what we are doing or saying and adjusting our practice to account for any inconsistencies, we provide students with realistic expectations for their own practice as well as clear guidelines for what we believe is important in professional behaviour.

Education

An increase in knowledge, particularly where myths or misconceptions are replaced by accurate knowledge, has been shown to be associated with an increase in positive and/or a decrease in negative attitudes. Negative attitudes toward people with a severe mental illness have been shown to be ameliorated by education that challenges common myths about mental illness (Corrigan et al 2001).

Thompson et al (2003) measured an increase in positive attitudes in nursing students toward disability over their final year and Brown et al (1992) showed a favourable shift in physical therapy students' attitudes toward the elderly following educational and clinical experiences.

Personal contact

Wooliscroft et al (1984) reported improvement in medical students' attitudes toward the elderly during contact with elderly people in a variety of health care facilities and Adelman et al (1992) reported improved student attitudes after contact with healthy elderly people. Exposure to elderly patients in nursing homes does not appear to result in more negative attitudes amongst medical (Fields et al 1992) or nursing students (Langland et al 1986). Close contact with disabled people was associated with a more positive attitude among physiotherapists (Gething 1993) and contact with people suffering from a mental illness produced significantly more positive attitudes in college students (Corrigan et al 2001).

Remember to include the affective domain in all of your clinical educator roles

During orientation provide students with a clear definition of the component behaviours expected in the specific clinical placement. For example: "Although the clinic starts at 8.30 am, in this clinic we expect you to arrive at least five minutes before the starting time."

Observe student performance and listen for clues of developing professional attitudes

Provide feedback to students on their behaviours that relate to their ability to meet these guidelines. Remember to give positive feedback to students when they comply with these behaviours, as well as letting them know when they infringe them. It is always helpful to focus on the behaviour. For example, rather than describing a student as "rude", it will be more helpful to use a sentence such as: "You seemed to ignore the parents of the child and did not refer to her by name."

Assess student behaviour that reflects the attitudes, values and beliefs that are essential to professional practice in your workplace. Remember that this involves two stages: defining what to assess as well as judging the extent they are met.

REFERENCES

Adelman R D, Fields S D, Jutagir R 1992 Geriatric education. Part II: the effect of a well elderly program on medical student attitudes toward geriatric patients. Journal of the American Geriatrics Society 40(9):970–973

Ashmore R D, Del Boca F K 1981 Conceptual approaches to stereotypes and stereotyping. In: Hamilton D L (ed) Cognitive processes in stereotyping and intergroup behaviour. Erlbaum, Hillsdale, NJ, p 1–35

Best D 1992 Perceptions of learning in clinical placements: a study of third year physiotherapy students. M Ed thesis La Trobe University, Melbourne

Brown D S, Gardner D L, Perritt L, Kelly D G 1992 Improvement in attitudes toward the elderly following traditional and geriatric mock clinics for physical therapy students. Physical Therapy 72(4):251–257

Cant R, Higgs J (1999) Professional socialisation. In: Higgs J, Edwards E (eds) Educating beginning practitioners. Butterworth-Heinemann, Oxford, p 46–51

Corrigan P W, River L P, Lundin R K et al 2001 Three strategies for changing attributions about severe mental illness. Schizophrenia Bulletin 27(2):187–195

Davis C 1975 Clinical education awareness of our "not-OK" behaviour. Physical Therapy 55:505–506

Davis C 1991 Evaluating student clinical performance in the affective domain. In: Proceedings of the 11th International Conference of World Confederation for Physical Therapy, WCPT, London

Devine P G 1989 Stereotypes and prejudice: their automatic and controlled components. Journal of Personality and Social Psychology 56:5–18

Fields S D, Jutagir R, Adelman R D et al 1992 Geriatric education. Part I: efficacy of a mandatory clinical rotation for fourth year medical students. Journal of the American Geriatrics Society 40(9):964–969

Gagne R 1977 The conditions of learning. Holt Rinehart & Winston, New York

Gething L 1992a Judgements by health professionals of personal characteristics of people with a visible physical disability. Social Science and Medicine 34:809–815

Gething L 1992b Nurse practitioners' and students' attitudes towards people with disabilities. Australian Journal of Advanced Nursing 9(3):25–30

Gething L 1993 Attitudes toward people with disabilities of physiotherapists and members of the general population. Australian Journal of Physiotherapy 39(4):291–296

Gething L, Fethney J, McKee K et al 2002 Knowledge, stereotyping and attitudes toward self ageing. Australasian Journal on Ageing 21(2):74–79

Hamilton D L 1981 Illusory correlations as a basis for stereotyping. In: Hamilton D L (ed) Cognitive processes in stereotyping and intergroup behaviour. Erlbaum, Hillsdale, NJ, p 115–144

Haskins A R, Rose-St Prix C, Elbaum L 1997 Covert bias in evaluation of physical therapist students' clinical performance. Physical Therapy 77(2):155–163

Hind M, Norman I, Cooper S et al 2003 Interprofessional perceptions of health care students. Journal of Interprofessional Care 17(1):21–34

Jensen G. Gwyer, G. Hack, L et al 1999 Expertise in physical therapy practice. Butterworth-Heinemann, Boston

Kaempfer D, Wellman N S, Himburg S P 2002 Dietetics students' low knowledge, attitudes, and work preferences toward older adults indicate need for improved education about ageing. Journal of the American Dietetic Association 102(2):197–202

Kearney N, Miller M, Paul J et al 2000 Oncology healthcare professionals' attitudes toward elderly people. Annals of Oncology 11(5):599–601

Krathwohl D, Bloom B, Masia B 1984 Taxonomy of educational objectives. David McKay, New York

Langland R M, Raithel J A, Benjamin G et al 1986 Change in basic nursing students' attitudes toward the elderly after a nursing home experience. Journal of Nursing Education 25(1):31–33

Lookinland S, Anson K 1995 Perpetuation of ageist attitudes among present and future health care personnel: implications for elder care. Journal of Advanced Nursing 25(1):47–56

Menz H B, Stewart F A, Oates M J 2003 Knowledge of aging and attitudes toward older people. A survey of Australian podiatric medical students. Journal of the American Podiatric Medical Association 93(1):11–17

Nordholm L A 1980 Beautiful patients are good patients: evidence for the physical attractiveness stereotype in first impressions of patients. Social Science and Medicine 14A:81–84

Ramsden 1985 Bases for clinical decision making: perceptions of the patient, the clinician's role and responsibility. In: Wolf S (ed) Clinical decision making in physical therapy. Davis, Philadelphia

Sdorow L M, Rickabaugh C A 2002 Psychology, 5th edn. McGraw Hill, Boston

Shepard K, Jensen G 1997 Preparation for teaching in academic settings. In: Shepard K, Jensen G (eds) Handbook of teaching for physical therapists. Butterworth-Heinemann, Oxford

Slevin O D'A 1991 Ageist attitudes among young adults: implications for a caring profession. Journal of Advanced Nursing 16(10):1197–1205

Stephan W G 1989 A cognitive approach to stereotyping. In: Bar-Tal D, Graumann C F, Kruglanski A W, Stroebe W (eds) Stereotyping and prejudice: changing conceptions. Springer-Verlag, New York, p 37–57

Stewart R A, Powel G E, Chetwynd S J 1979 Person perception and stereotyping. Saxon House, Westmead, Hants

Streed C P, Stoecker J L 1991 Stereotyping between physical therapy students and occupational students. Physical Therapy 71(1):16–20

Stroebe W, Insko C A 1989 Stereotype, prejudice, and discrimination: changing conceptions in theory and research. In: Bar-Tal D, Graumann C F, Kruglanski A W, Stroebe W (eds) Stereotyping and prejudice: changing conceptions. Springer-Verlag, New York, p 3–34

Thompson T L, Emrich K, Moore G 2003 The effect of curriculum on the attitudes of nursing students toward disability. Rehabilitation Nursing 28(1):27–30

Tovin M M, Nelms T, Taylor L F 2002 The experience of nursing home care: a strong influence on physical therapist students' work intentions. Journal of Physical Therapy Education 16(1):11–19

Tunstall-Pedoe S, Rink E, Hilton S 2003 Student attitudes to undergraduate interprofessional education. Journal of Interprofessional Care 17(2):161–172

White M J, Olson R S 1998 Attitudes toward people with disabilities: a comparison of rehabilitation nurses, occupational therapists, and physical therapists. Rehabilitation Nursing 23(3):126–231

Wilhite M J, Johnson D M 1976 Changes in nursing students' stereotypic attitudes toward old people. Nursing Research 25(6):430–432

Wooliscroft J O, Calhoun J G, Maximum B R, Wolf F M 1984 Medical education in facilities for the elderly. Impact on medical students, facility staff, and residents. JAMA 252:3382–3385

Chapter 6

Learning about learning

Dawn Best, Miranda Rose and Helen Edwards

This chapter aims to provide a theoretical framework for clinical educators and mentors that will introduce key educational terminology and concepts in order to:

- provide some guidance about how to optimise learning in a specific situation or with an individual learner
- explain and understand your own experience as a learner and an educator
- suggest strategies for planning and managing some of the complex issues which are linked to clinical and professional education
- assist you to predict outcomes of what may happen in a given situation
- increase your confidence in the important role of being a clinical educator
- stimulate your interest to explore a topic in depth in your own further reading and research.

The chapter includes:

- an introduction to experiential learning as a framework to assisting in the development of an understanding of learning in the clinical environment

- a brief review of some of the literature from psychology, education, social anthropology and workplace action research relevant to learning in the clinical environment
- discussion of a systems model of the teaching and learning process to explore some of the variables related to the individual learner, clinical educator, and learning context.

Learning is a complex topic and there is an enormous amount of literature available. Although there are many theories that contribute to an understanding of the learning processes in the clinical environment there is currently no one theory that answers all our questions. Hence, this is a demanding section. You may have to be in the mood for it! You may have to read bits of it more than once. Remember that it sometimes takes time to get used to new theory and concepts. We expect this of our students all the time.

Initially, learning in clinics may seem deceptively simple. Our health science students enrol in programmes in academic institutions and then, depending on the curriculum structure, spend time in the clinical environment to develop skills in professional practice with the help of you, the clinical educator. However, there is more to it. One of the most exciting things for the authors, as we begin to write this chapter collaboratively, is the potential for a clearer understanding. We have all been involved in clinical education for over 20 years. We have been clinicians, teachers, researchers and students. We have worked in academic settings and practice settings. We come from very different professional backgrounds. We have found theories that clarified our practice and even developed some theories from our practice. Although a simple theory for clinical learning is still elusive, it is our hope that this chapter helps you in the development of one that "works" for you in your context.

LEARNING PROFESSIONAL PRACTICE

One of the challenges of writing a book for professionals from different health care professions from different countries is the lack of a shared understanding of simple words. There is an additional problem when "learning" is both the outcome of the process as well as the process itself. Another of the reasons for the complexity relates to the nature of professional knowledge that is explored in Chapter 5.

In clinical education, our students are actually involved in a variety of distinct but related activities. Students are:

- learning practice, i.e. learning to operate within a tradition
- learning from practice, i.e. learning by watching and maybe copying
- learning by practice, i.e. learning by the opportunity for repetition of the action
- learning through practice, i.e. learning about principles through specific actions (Fish & Twinn 1997, p. 80).

There is a lot of activity going on so we will begin by looking at experiential learning.

EXPERIENTIAL LEARNING

It would seem appropriate to introduce a theoretical understanding of clinical education in the experience and actions of the clinical environment. Experiential learning has been defined as:

- the process whereby knowledge is created through the transformation of experience
- a continuous process which integrates experience, perceptions, cognition and behaviour (Kolb 1984)
- an active process of exploration and discovery, often leading to unexpected outcomes (Boud et al 1985).

Boud & Pascoe (1988) describe the following three critical criteria for experiential learning:

1. How close is the learning environment to the real environment? Clinical placements present the student with real-life experience, but experience per se does not lead to learning. It is the quality of the experience that is vital to learning, as well as the context in which the experience is located.
2. What level of involvement is required in the learning activity? Experiential learning involves the full attention of the individual student – the intellect, body, emotion and interpersonal response.
3. How much control does the learner have over the learning experience? Learners need to have some control over their learning experience if their learning is to be personally relevant and based on previous experience and prior knowledge. This implies a need for some degree of negotiation with the clinical educator. The extent to which this negotiation actually occurs varies enormously in the clinical environment.

All clinical placements present real-world experience. Although some environments such as university-based clinics are organised primarily to provide students with clinical experience, the majority of placements are concerned primarily with health care delivery. Boud & Pascoe (1988) make an important distinction between the clinical environment and the degree of learner autonomy and involvement of self that the situation allows. Facilitating and controlling these additional characteristics in the clinical environment depend on you – the clinical educator. The majority of us have little preparation for our education role and little time to devote to learning objectives such as fostering student autonomy and involvement of self. This is further complicated by the reality that in many clinical placements students are shared between more than one educator.

There is also a difference between information assimilation, or academic learning, and experiential learning (Coleman 1976). Information assimilation requires a shared understanding of language to transmit information and organise it into general principles before it can be actively applied. In experiential learning the learning process is reversed so that information is generated from action without requiring language. We may talk about a clinical example in great detail in theoretical sessions but until the student has experienced this we cannot be sure that we share an understanding. As educators we may have to help students connect their clinical experience to theoretical concepts or to recognise a theoretical construct in the clinic.

In the clinics we sometimes see students who have difficulty remembering theory, or others who are unable to apply what they have learnt at the university. It is easy to label such students as lacking in knowledge and blame them or their university for their deficits. An understanding of the differences between experiential and theoretical learning allows us to be less hasty in our judgement and provides us with some indications of how to help students make the transition between these two very different types of learning. Coleman states that both types of learning have characteristic properties (Table 6.1).

The key ideas about experiential learning were summarised by Boud et al (1993) as:

- experience is the foundation and stimulus for learning
- learners actively construct their experience
- learning is a holistic process
- learning is socially and culturally constructed
- learning is influenced by the socio-emotional context in which it occurs.

REVIEWING EDUCATIONAL THEORIES FROM PSYCHOLOGY

This section highlights and reviews some relevant learning theories from psychology that have clear implications for learning professional practice. Although it is likely that much of the following section is included in the curriculum of health professional courses, in our experience as workshop facilitators for health care clinical educators, it appears that, sometimes, new insights emerge when these theories are revisited and applied to the learning of students or junior colleagues in the health care environment.

Table 6.1 Strengths and weaknesses of academic and experiential learning

Positives	Negatives
Academic learning (information assimilation)	
More time-efficient	Ambiguities of language, e.g. What is really meant by muscle tone?
Uses the experience of others	Difficulty in retaining the learning (memory loss)
Extrinsic motivation	Requires the translation of abstract principles to concrete situations
Experiential learning	
Intrinsic motivation	Time-consuming
Knowledge is easily remembered	Difficulty in translating experience to general principles
Holistic experience	Difficulty in verbalising experience

Behavioural psychology

Considerable research activity at the beginning of the last century focused on experimenting with the behaviour of animals. This work established that events external to the organism affected its behaviour. A stimulus was presented which created a response. This could be manipulated by positive and negative rewards. Do you remember the findings of Pavlov with a bell and his salivating dogs, and Skinner and his rats in mazes and pecking pigeons? But does this research apply to learning in clinical environment? The obvious answer is yes. However, we may be less likely to apply this theory to our clinical education practice even if it is firmly embedded in our clinical practice. Welcoming the novice, smiling and using a name are powerful reinforcers and motivators while frowns, negative comments and punishing behaviours have a profound influence. Behaviouralism is strongly entrenched in our teaching and learning in the form of:

- learning behavioural objectives
- in the individual check sheets of acceptable behaviours used in clinical examinations
- in objective structured clinical examinations (OSCE)
- in computer-based learning packages and notions about the effects of reinforcement of learning
- in our grading system and prize allocation.

If we were to make behavioural theory more explicit as a theory of use for our practice we would:

- acknowledge the power of feedback in learning
- remember the importance of positive feedback and how it sustains effort and motivation
- check that, as clinical educators, professional supervisors or mentors, we are not inadvertently reinforcing ineffective behaviours
- remember that task repetition is essential in changing individual behaviour at this unconscious level.

Cognitive psychology

Research in the last 50 years in cognitive psychology has focused on a very different domain in the exploration of how humans think. Here the focus is on the individual's search for meaning and the study of thought processes. Theories developed in this area now provide an understanding of the development of schema, the organisation of long-term memory, influences on memory storage and retrieval, problem-solving and transfer of concepts, concept formation and decision-making (Regehr & Norman, 1996). This work created the foundation for studies in information processing which has studied expert systems and clinical reasoning and was further explored in Chapter 5 part one.

Gestalt psychology

Contributions from the field of gestalt psychology provide us with an understanding of how the stimuli, especially the visual images in our environment, are linked to perceptions in our search for meaning. Based on the German word meaning "configuration", this research showed how we organise visual cues to make sense to us. Studies in figure ground perceptions found that individuals appeared to interpret sensory cues on their past experiences. As clinicians we attend more to some visual or auditory cues than others. We look for a big picture that takes into account our ability to recognise similarities from our past experiences.

The practice expertise of expert clinicians is based on this ability to recognise a variety of patient cues and organise them into a cohesive pattern so that client diagnosis and management decisions appear to emerge from an almost unconscious level. This pattern recognition ability develops over time from the experience and reflective analysis and has already been discussed in the Knowledge (Chapter 5 part 1) and Attitudes (Chapter 5 part three) chapters. If the student has not attended to nicotine-stained fingernails on the patient's hands and has not heard the coughing which intersperses the patient's verbal responses to assessment questions, then attention is less likely to be given to the effect of chronic airways disease in the student's clinical reasoning process.

Humanistic psychology

A group of psychologists working in the United States of America in the middle of last century provided us with additional useful concepts that further highlight the need to focus on the individual learner.

Carl Rogers' early work in psychological counselling became the basis for educational theories that recognised that experiential learning involves emotional as well as cognitive aspects of the learner. Individual learner thoughts and feelings are focused in a search for meaning which is focused in what is learnt, how it is learnt and evaluated (Rogers 1969, p. 5). The recognition of the importance of learner autonomy fundamentally changed the traditional role of the teacher to a facilitator of learning. Rogers' view that significant learning is most influenced by the personal learner–teacher relationship identified the following 10 principles of learning (Rogers 1969, p. 157–163):

1. All humans have a natural potential for learning.
2. Effective learning occurs when the learning is perceived as relevant to the learner.
3. Learning which involves a change in self-concept is threatening and tends to be resisted.
4. Learning which is threatening to the self is facilitated in a supporting and encouraging environment.
5. Opportunities for learning which fundamentally changes the self can only occur when threats to the learner are minimalised.
6. Significant learning occurs through doing.
7. Learning is facilitated when the learner is responsible for the learning process.
8. The most lasting and sustaining learning involves feelings as well as intellect.

9. Interdependence, creativity and self-reliance are all facilitated with self-evaluation and when external evaluation is of secondary importance.

10. The most socially useful learning in the modern world is the learning of the process of learning, a continuing openness to experience and incorporation into one's self of the process of change.

These principles, developed over 30 years ago for classroom teachers, remain consistent with current educational philosophy in our acceptance of concepts such as adult learning, life-long learning, student autonomy or student-focused learning.

Abraham Maslow was another humanistic psychologist whose concepts are particularly useful to clinical educators. When prompted, most health science students and clinicians remember the pyramid model developed by Maslow to describe a hierarchy of human needs (Maslow 1970). This triangle places basic physiological needs such as sleep, food and water as the foundation for all other higher needs. Safety needs are located on the next level, followed by the need to belong and then for self-esteem. Self-actualisation is placed above all these other needs. It is important to remember that it is only when these more basic motivations are addressed that the learner is able to attend to the more important task of learning. Consider how this model might apply to your own learning experiences. Perhaps you may remember how difficult any learning was when you were sleep-deprived, when the room was too hot, when you were thirsty or very threatened by what you would be asked to do next. You may have observed the difficulty the anxious student has answering questions and undertaking higher-level cognitive tasks. Further examples of appropriate application for medical educators are provided by Hutchinson (2003).

Although earlier behavioural psychologists identified that human perception is an individual response, the humanistic psychologists highlighted the importance of the individual's development of a sense of self and the critical conditions that contribute to facilitating individual growth towards achieving the highest potential.

To summarise, application of these theories from humanistic psychology suggests that as clinical educators we will:

- focus on the development of a supporting learning environment
- accept that the role of clinical educator is linked to an ability to facilitate learning in our students effectively
- encourage our students to be autonomous learners
- remember the impact of anxiety and stress on learning.

APPLYING A SYSTEMS APPROACH TO LEARNING

A very different way of thinking about learning is provided by systems theory. Clinical education has been identified as an open system (Higgs 1993). This is defined as an assembly of components connected in an organised way where each component is affected by both being in the system and by influencing other components (Carter et al 1984). Higgs (1993) suggests that the complexity of clinical education is clearly described by viewing the

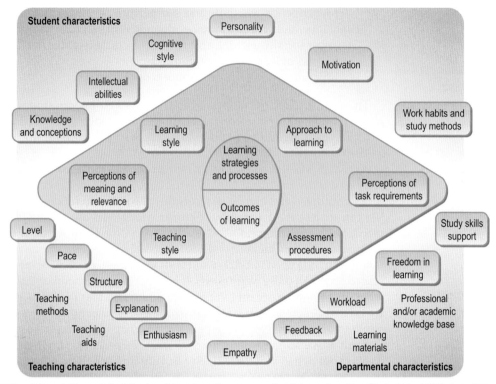

Figure 6.1   A heuristic model of the teaching–learning process in higher education (Entwistle 1987, Entwistle et al 1988; reproduced with permission from Rose & Best 1996)

individual learner, clinical educator and learning programme as subsystems contributing to a much larger entity. It also seems logical that the system will be more efficient when there is congruence between individual components. Think about your own experience in clinical education when things have not run smoothly and see if a lack of congruence between the subsystems can be identified in your own example.

Entwistle (1987) and Entwistle et al (1988) present a systems model of the teaching–learning process that clearly demonstrates its complexity and the number of variables involved. This model (Fig. 6.1) acknowledges the central interaction between the student's learning strategies and processes and the specific learning outcomes. It emphasises:

- relationship between student approaches to learning
- perceptions of the task
- understanding of relevance and meaning
- assessment procedures
- learning and teaching styles.

It sets these against the three different perspectives of the learner, the teacher and the context in which the learning takes place. The next section will provide a brief explanation of some of the topics located within the centre of the model:

- learning style
- teaching style (supervisory styles)
- approaches to learning.

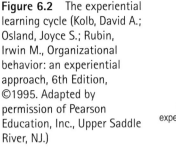

Figure 6.2 The experiential learning cycle (Kolb, David A.; Osland, Joyce S.; Rubin, Irwin M., Organizational behavior: an experiential approach, 6th Edition, ©1995. Adapted by permission of Pearson Education, Inc., Upper Saddle River, NJ.)

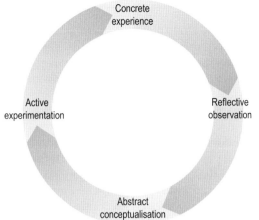

Learning style

Kolb et al (1974) and Kolb (1984) identified four very different activities that make up the learning process. Successful learning involves all these activities. However, Kolb recognised we all have an individual preference for one or two of the activities. Some of us are happier doing tasks (active experimentation) while others prefer to read theories (abstract conceptualisation) in order to receive information. Some prefer to reflect and observe (reflective observation) and others feel the need to modify their actions in the light of the information (active experimentation).

Kolb's learning cycle (Fig. 6.2) is represented by a circular model that moves from experiencing to observing and reflecting, to explaining and then to applying. It allows movement in the reverse direction and accepts that learning can begin at any point of the cycle. Learning style is seen as a preference for an activity and not as a fixed prerequisite for learning. Hence, this theory helps us to understand the impact individual differences have on learning and behaviour without labelling difficulties as personality conflicts. We might judge a student who is slow to interact with a client as lacking motivation and uninterested when in fact the student's preference would be to observe a client session first. Or conversely, the student who looks bored when watching a clinician may prefer to do a task before watching.

Learners who have a preference for action may be perceived as having an advantage in the clinical environment, especially if this preference is shared with their clinical educator. However, if the clinical educator's preference is to observe and reflect, or read the literature first, then such behaviour may be labelled hasty, unprepared or even unsafe. A knowledge of our own individual learning preference as well as the preferences of our learners provides a framework for the discussion of individual differences in order to plan for flexible learning opportunities. An early version of the Kolb learning-style inventory is available in Kolb et al (1974). Alternatively, a similar learning-style questionnaire has been developed by Honey & Mumford (2003).

Teacher styles/supervisory styles

Another area to explore in clinical education and other supervisory roles is supervisory styles. Supervisory styles concern the sometimes habitual patterns of behaviour we adopt when we are in educative or supervisory situations. To assist you in analysing what styles you may be using, the following is a brief overview of the styles that have been discussed in the literature. At the end of this chapter we suggest some exercises to help you identify and analyse your own preferred style(s) and some ways to make these more effective. The majority of information concerning supervisory styles comes from the area of organisational psychology and the preferred terms of the time when this information emerged were supervisor and supervisee. We could easily substitute clinical educator and student or mentor and mentee for these terms. In this following section, we have utilised the terms as they appeared in the literature.

Farmer & Farmer (1989) recognised that clinical education is a complex and dynamic process. They developed a conceptual framework to represent better the complex nature of supervisory behaviours called *styles*. They identified four key styles. We have listed the major goals of each style, the leadership styles associated with them, who makes the decisions, their relative emphases and uses:

Training
- to teach skills and knowledge
- directive
- supervisor makes decisions
- goals and tasks are set by supervisor
- emphasis on work, little overt concern for relationships.

Uses: crisis intervention, marginal students.

Monitoring
- to teach skills and knowledge with some attention to affective development
- supervisor makes decisions
- administrative
- supervisors sometimes gets supervisees' ideas and opinions in problem management
- supervision tends to operate on intuition and chance, supervisor has great freedom.

Uses: supervisees with low decision-making responsibilities such as aides.

Advising
- to facilitate affective development through genuine communication
- supervisor and student make decisions together
- consultative
- supervisor gets and tries supervisees' ideas and opinions
- emphasis on listening, accepting, trusting, advising and encouraging.

Uses: peer supervision, supervisees capable of moderate decision-making.

Transacting
- to facilitate affective and cognitive development through genuine communication
- decisions are negotiated
- collaborative
- supervisor always elicits supervisees' ideas
- goals and tasks are established jointly.

Uses: for advanced students capable of independent decision-making.

Each of the subtypes demonstrates a different focus on the various major constituents in the supervisory process – people, relationships, tasks and products.

Some examples of how supervisees with differing levels of clinical development might view a supervisor's style are well described by Hersey & Blanchard (1982). We have adapted their table and included it here (Table 6.2). Hersey & Blanchard refer to task behaviour and relationship behaviour as the two key dimensions of which a supervisor must be aware in supervision.

1. *Task behaviour*. Where supervisors focus on organising and defining the roles of the student, explaining what activities each is to do, and when, where and how tasks are to be accomplished.
2. *Relationship behaviour*. Where supervisors maintain personal relationships between themselves and students by opening up channels of communication, providing support and "psychological strokes" (Hersey & Blanchard 1982).

They point out that it is the relative degree of familiarity and experience that supervisees have had with a particular situation or task that determines how those supervisees will feel about the style of supervision they are being offered, e.g., a "telling" style will most likely be seen as effective by a novice or inexperienced student but highly ineffective by a student approaching competence or independence (Table 6.2).

For readers interested in ways to determine a particular student's "situational maturity" and therefore what supervisory style might be the most effective, Mawdsley & Scudder (1989) have developed their "integrative task-maturity model of supervision." This model builds on the work of Hersey & Blanchard. It is aimed at assisting the supervisor to gain an understanding of the situational maturity level of their student through the use of the Wisconsin procedure of appraisal of clinical competence (W-PACC). The supervisor can then select a particular style of supervision to meet best the needs of a particular student.

Approaches to learning

Biggs (1989) defines a learning approach as an interaction between the motivation for learning and different strategies for learning. Student perception of the learning task and the learning outcome will be influenced by the

Table 6.2   Differing views of supervisor styles

Basic styles	Effective	Ineffective
1. *Telling* – High task and low relationship (Style 1*)		
	Seen as having well-defined methods for accomplishing goals that are helpful to the students	Seen as imposing methods on others. Sometimes seen as unpleasant, and only interested in short-run output
2. *Selling* – High task and high relationship (Style 4*)		
	Seen as satisfying the needs of the student for setting goals and organising work, but also providing high levels of socio-emotional support	Seen as initiating more structure than is needed by the student and often appears not to be genuine in interpersonal relationships
3. *Participating* – High relationship and low task (Style 3*)		
	Seen as having implicit trust in people and as being primarily concerned with facilitating their goal accomplishment	Seen as primarily interested in harmony. Sometimes seen as unwilling to accomplish tasks if it risks disrupting a relationship or losing a *good person* image
4. *Delegating* – Low relationship and low task (Style 2*)		
	Seen as appropriately delegating to students decisions about how the work should be done and providing little socio-emotional support where little is needed by the student	Seen as providing little structure or socio-emotional support when needed by students

* Broadly equivalent to the Styles of Farmer & Farmer (1989).

approach to learning a student adopts. The learning approach adopted by a student in a clinical placement will influence the experience of the student in the placement. On the other hand, experience in the placement may facilitate a change in learning approach.

Considerable research on approaches to learning has been carried in the last 20 years. Marton & Säljö (1984) made the distinction between two different approaches to learning – *surface* and *deep*.

Deep learning is adopted by students who:

- search for personal meaning and understanding
- integrate aspects of the task into a whole
- relate new ideas to personal experience
- relate evidence to conclusions
- are interested in learning for learning's sake (intrinsic motivation).

Surface learning is adopted by students who:

- focus on memorisation and reproduction of the task
- view the specific aspects as discrete and unrelated details
- rely on teachers to define learning tasks
- are interested in qualification (extrinsic motivation).

A third approach is known as *versatile* or *strategic* (Entwistle 1987; Newble & Entwistle 1986; Ramsden 1984, 1988). Students with this approach:

- select the most appropriate approach for a given task in order to achieve high grades
- are highly organised
- investigate exam criteria and marking weightings
- rely on previous examination papers to predict questions.

The significant effect that clinical environment has on the student's approach to learning warrants special consideration. Coles (1989, 1990) observed that even medical students who were using a deep approach to learning and receiving high grades in the early years of their medical course had difficulty in transferring and using this learning in their clinics. On investigation he found that a significant number of medical students in their third year appeared to have altered their approach to the revision of their theory as a result of their clinical experiences during the year. In this programme the assessment of theory was scheduled following the clinical experience.

These students reported an increase in their motivation to learning, a recognition of the relevance of what they were studying and an ability to connect isolated topics. Coles (1989) called this new approach to learning *elaboration* and hypothesised that it occurred as a response to the learning requisition of the clinical placements. Students who adopted this elaborated approach to learning felt more confident that they would be able to retain what they were learning, and retrieve and use it in the future. Coles (1989) makes the observation that "elaboration does not happen proactively from abstract to concrete but retroactively from concrete to abstract". Students in the early years of the course with no clinical experience to relate to the information were unable to see the relevance of, or make generalisations with, the theory.

Coles (1990) adapted the earlier work on surface–deep learning approaches to student learning in the clinical environment. He devised the following four learning approaches:

1. *Restricted approach.* These students have a low self-image, feel overloaded by work, lack motivation for learning and consider dropping out of the course. They see little relevance in the material they are taught, which they try to memorise, and then tend to forget. They are disorganised and perform poorly in assessments.
2. *Adequate approach.* These students are better organised and have more self-confidence than the group using the restricted approach. Understanding the meaning of the material taught is the focus for learning but its relevance is not always apparent. Although these students perform better in examination than the first group, they have difficulty remembering and applying knowledge in the clinical setting. Motivation for learning is also external and relates to the achievement of high grades. This group often interprets B and C grades as failure. Students who use this approach may also consider withdrawing from the course.
3. *Clinical approach.* These students are more optimistic than students in either of the first two groups and report surprise at suddenly enjoying their learning as a result of their clinical involvement. They find that their clinical

experiences help them to understand the relevance and the meaning of theory. Students using this approach obtain satisfactory examination results, although they often have gaps in their knowledge and voice concern about perceptions that their revision appears non-rational.

4. *Elaborated approach.* This group is distinguished from the others as they approach their learning in a very different way. Their motivation for learning is intrinsic rather than focused on passing examinations. They are able to draw on their extensive knowledge in clinical situations and achieve the highest examination scores. However these students are concerned that to them their learning does not appear to be rational and organised.

STUDENT, TEACHING AND DEPARTMENTAL CHARACTERISTICS

The following section moves outside the centre of Entwistle's model (Fig. 6.1) and addresses student, teaching and departmental characteristics that affect teaching and learning.

Student characteristics

The learner attributes identified as relevant to learning in academic settings also apply to the students who arrive in your clinical workplaces. However, if you think about your own clinical and teaching experience, there are other individual student differences that could also be identified. Write a list of the student differences that you have identified as having an impact on learning in clinics. You may like to check it against the following list expanded from the Entwistle model.

Learner attributes:

- age
- learner's prior experience
- learner goals
- life situation
- level of competence
- level of maturity
- perceptions of task and role
- cultural background
- knowledge base
- learning preference
- cognitive style
- physical size
- health status.

Further work on learner differences has been provided by researchers investigating preferences for the various sensory modalities utilised in learning activities: visual, tactile, auditory and kinaesthetic. Generally, these preferences for sensory information are termed *modality learning styles*, although sometimes, somewhat confusingly, simply termed learning styles. The inference from these studies into sensory preferences is that instruction offered in a non-preferred sense will be less effective than a preferred sense. A study of school-aged children in the USA who self-rated their sensory preferences in learning found 20–30% of children were predominantly auditory learners, 40% visual, and 30–40% a combination of visual/tactile/kinaesthetic (Dunn & Dunn 1993).

A further study by Park (2000) investigated the sensory learning preferences of 709 high-school students of various ethnic backgrounds (Hmong, Vietnamese, Cambodian, Lao and Anglo-American) with less than 7 years of residency in the United States of America. Park found significant ethnic group differences in preferred sensory learning modality, with the Hmong and Vietnamese students showing the strongest preferences for visual learning and for tactile learning. However, recently the construct of modality preferences in learners has come under severe criticism (Klein 2003) in terms of the notion that learners can reliably be classified as one type or another. Klein points out the limitations of the classification methods used (self-report polar questionnaires) and the poor correlations between questionnaire results and actual observed learner activity. A more useful concept may be simply the notion of *preference*, taking into account that most learning activities involve multiple perceptual modalities and that most individuals report preferences for multiple or mixed modalities rather than simply one.

Teacher (clinical educator) characteristics

The teaching characteristics in the Entwistle model include some variables related directly to the teacher, and others that relate to the teaching methods used and the structure, pace and level at which the information is presented. Teacher characteristics include the degree of enthusiasm and the level of commitment for the teaching task. It is important to recognise that in the same way we all have a preferred learning style, teachers have a preferred teaching style. There are additional teacher characteristics that impact on learning in the clinical environment. One of the most critical of these is the level of expertise of the clinical educator. Novice–expert differences in practice are described in detail in Chapter 5 part one. It is important to acknowledge that the level of expertise of the teacher in no way influences the potential learning outcome.

Department characteristics

Department characteristics include study skills support, freedom in learning, the workload, feedback, learning materials and professional and/or academic knowledge base. When we apply this model to the clinical environment we must also include the geographic layout of the facility and the space available for students.

Limitations of the Entwistle model for clinical education settings

The Entwistle model provides a comprehensive model for learning in academic settings as well as learning in the clinical environment. However, there are some limitations in its application to clinical education when this spans both education and health systems and the output usually involves effective patient care as well as student learning. Hence, one of the limitations of the Entwistle model is the omission of the patient or client perspective in the learning outcome. This surely is one of the strengths of the clinical environment. An additional problem is that it fails to capture the complex challenge of transporting knowledge and skills between academic and clinical settings, or even between multiple clinical settings. For a greater understanding in these issues we need to look at the more recent research into workplace learning.

SOCIAL AND ANTHROPOLOGICAL CONTRIBUTIONS TO LEARNING

Social learning theory provides a very different perspective of learning. It moves away from a focus on the individual learner to explore work setting and work practices, and the relationship between the person and the environment. The research covers a wide variety of very different professions and tasks, with little contribution from health science. However, the findings are interesting and very relevant to clinical education, as well as professional supervision and mentoring.

Learning is described as a social, collective rather than an individual psychological phenomenon (Lave 1996). Anthropological studies of apprentices have raised awareness of the transformation of both the work practices and individual workers when novices and experts have the opportunity to work closely together. Learning is seen as a process of changing understanding in and through practice by participation in everyday activities (Lave 1996). We may be initially uncomfortable and perhaps see apprenticeship studies as a retrograde step when our professions proudly espouse a move away from this model. However, tied to this rejection is an assumption of an apprenticeship that encouraged rule-bound behaviour and which certainly did not encourage evidence-based practice and high-level cognitive skills (Best & Edwards 2001). The revived interest is based on very different assumptions. Termed cognitive apprenticeship, it is described as guided participation in social and cultural activities with guides or companions who support and stretch understanding (Rogoff 1990). This guided participation identifies:

- a movement from tasks of low accountability to others demanding highly accountable work activities
- access to knowledge that would not be learnt by discovery alone
- guidance from more experienced workers
- indirect guidance from others in the social and physical environment (Billet 2001).

The lessons for us as clinical educators from this perspective are consistent with research findings from education and psychology. Billet (2001) provides a summary of the key components for successful learning outcomes:

- positive relations between learners and guides (clinical educators/mentors) with a shared responsibility for collaboration
- clear goals and expectations and joint involvement of learners and guides
- regular contact between learners and guides
- thorough preparation of the guides (clinical educators, mentors) and briefing of the learners of the expectations, roles, responsibilities and potential benefits of their participation in the workplace.

This more recent vocational education research highlights the importance of the workplace community and the effect of the individual, and conversely the effect the individual has, on the workplace. Topics such as the transference or boundary crossing of knowledge and skills between schools and workplaces identify the importance of collaboration between workplaces (Tuomi-Grohn & Englestrom 2003). Even more exciting is the acknowledgement that this collaboration has the potential to transform both the learners and the practice.

New learners in the workplace need to develop a sense of the game and an understanding of the local culture; they need to acquire the words, grammar and actions that demonstrate they fit into the workplace. Once this is established they then earn the right to question the practice of the workplace (Bleakley 2002). The implications for us all as clinical educators and mentors are obvious. Bleakley interprets Englestrom's learning cycle to medical practice. This cycle moves from context of learning to cognition and on to contradiction. Questions from the novice that challenge the habitual practice of experts have the potential to raise awareness and stimulate new cognition that transforms practice and hence leads to changes in the context:

> *All forms of knowledge involve the construction of knowledge and skills understood as transformations rather than as the mere application or use of something that has been acquired elsewhere*

> (Tuomi-Grohn & Englestrom 2003, p. 3).

CONSTRUCTIVISM

There has been increasing interest over the last couple of decades in constructivism. Constructivism is a philosophy of learning that can be applied to any level of learning, from kindergarten to university (http://www.funderstanding.com/constructivism.cfm). Its central tenet is the idea that learners construct knowledge for themselves. Learners individually (and socially) construct meaning as they learn. This is achieved by reflecting on experiences. Individual learners generate their own "rules" and "mental models" which they use to make sense of their experiences. There are several guiding principles of constructivism:

- Learning is an active process, a search for meaning. Therefore, learning must start with the issues around which students are actively trying to construct meaning.
- Learning is a social activity associated with connection to other human beings, e.g. peers, teachers.
- Meaning requires understanding wholes as well as parts. Parts must be understood in the context of wholes. For this reason, constructivist learning focuses on primary concepts, not isolated facts.
- In order to teach well we need to understand the mental models that students use to perceive the world and the assumptions they make to support those models.
- The purpose of learning is for individuals to construct their own meaning, not just memorise the "right" answers. Assessment needs to be part of the learning process and provide students with information on the quality of their learning.

■ It takes time to learn. Learning is not instantaneous. For significant learning, learners need to revisit ideas, ponder them, try them out, play with them and use them.

■ Motivation is essential for learning.

Constructivism calls for a curriculum that is related to learners' prior knowledge and emphasises hands-on problem-solving. Teachers focus on making connections between facts and fostering new understanding in students. They rely heavily on open-ended questions and promote dialogue among students. Although developed for school education, clearly constructivism has direct application to learning in clinical settings. It provides an overall approach that can incorporate many other theories and approaches, such as experiential learning, reflection and problem-based learning. It allows clinicians to tailor educational experiences to suit their clinical setting and provides opportunity for students to integrate their learning. Above all, it puts responsibility on students to make sense of what is happening in clinics and encourages them to develop a deeper understanding of clinical expertise.

Problem-based learning

One approach to curriculum construction and educational delivery that is entirely consistent with constructivist ideals is problem-based learning (PBL). PBL is a method of teaching and learning that emphasises student-centred learning primarily in small groups of 8–14 students (for a recent meta-analysis of the effects of PBL, see Dochy et al 2003). Students work in small groups and together discuss and solve real-life clinical "problems" or cases. The cases provide the context and motivation for learning. Students' prior knowledge is activated by working through the cases and elaboration of knowledge is achieved through student-centred discussion.

Self-directed learning is emphasised, which further increases the motivation to learn. PBL curriculum weeks are often structured with a PBL case tutorial at the start of the week, followed by students having time to seek information independently about the issues they identified as being unresolved in the first tutorial. Following the seeking of information and perhaps attending lectures or practical classes provided by the teaching staff, the students return to a second PBL case tutorial toward the end of the week. At the second case tutorial the students review and share their newly acquired knowledge and evaluate solutions to the clinical problem at hand. Through these activities students acquire knowledge in integrated and clinically meaningful networks.

PBL has been championed as being an excellent educational method for the preparation of health science practitioners and is now widely utilised across the world. However, the ultimate PBL is, of course, clinical practicum, and this was well described by Davis & Harden (1998) in their discussion of the continuum of teaching and learning activities. Table 6.3 presents Davis & Harden's ideas concerning the changes in teacher and learner roles from didactic to PBL, but more importantly in the cognitive processes that students utilise in different educational experiences. The notion of a continuum may assist clinical educators to place the activities of clinical education within an overall framework of educational activity.

Table 6.3   A modified continuum of educational approaches and cognitive responses (adapted from Davis & Harden 1998)

	Terminology	Description	Example
1. (Rul (Th))	Theoretical learning	Information provided about the theory	Traditional lecture. Standard textbook
2. (Rul (PT))	Problem-oriented learning	Practical information provided	Lecture with practical information. Protocols or guidelines
3. (Rul) → [Eg]	Problem-assisted learning	Information provided with the opportunity to apply it to practical examples	Lecture followed by practical or clinical experience. Book with problems or experiences included
4. [Eg]	Problem-solving learning	Problem-solving related to specific examples	Case discussions and some activities in practical classes
5. (Rul) → [Eg] → (Rul)	Problem-focused learning	Information is provided, followed by a problem. The principles of the subject are then learned	Introductory or foundation courses of lecture. Information in study guide
6. (Rul) → [Eg] [Eg] → (Rul)	Problem-based mixed approach	A combination of problem-based and information-based learning	Students have the option of an information-oriented or problem-based approach
7. [Eg] → (Rul)	Problem-initiated learning	The problem is used as a trigger at the beginning of learning	Patient management problems are used to interest the student in the topic
8. [Eg] → (Rul (Sp))	Problem-centred learning	A study of the problem introduces the student to the principles and rules specific to the problem	A text provides a series of problems followed by the information necessary to tackle the problems
9. [Eg] → (Rul (Sp))	Problem-centred discovery learning	Following the presentation of the problem, students have the opportunity to derive the principles and the rules	Students derive the principles from the literature or from work undertaken
10. [Eg] → (Rul (G))	Problem-based learning	The development of the principles includes the generalisation stage of learning	The investigation of patients with thyrotoxicosis is extended to a more general understanding
11. [Eg (T)] → (Rul)	Task-based learning	The problem is the real world	A set of tasks undertaken by a health care professional are the basis for the problem presented to the student

Key: Eg = example; G = generalisation; PT = practical; Rul = rule; Sp = specific; T = task-based; Th = theoretical learning

SELF–DEVELOPMENT ACTIVITIES

The Kolb learning style inventory (LSI) is located in Kolb et al (1974). Find out your learning style:

■ Does this match your observations of your own learning experiences and practice?
■ Discuss these with a trusted friend or colleague.
■ What are the implications for your education activities?

Having reviewed some of the theories of learning and looked at some of the variables in the teaching–learning process, what aspects can you apply in your own clinical education activity?

■ For example, you could focus on adapting your teaching style to cater to other learning styles.
■ You may like to focus on ways of encouraging elaboration in your students.
■ You may devise ways of bridging the gap between clinical learning and academic learning.

An excellent self-assessment tool for looking at your own habitual leadership style that in large part can be substituted for supervisory style is Hersey & Blanchard's (1982) *leadership effectiveness and adaptability description* (LEAD). We find this tool a simple way of providing ourselves with feedback about what styles we have and how effectively we use them. Please refer to Hersey & Blanchard (1982) for the actual LEAD tool.

Another way is to collect three or four samples of your pre- and post-supervisory discussion sessions with different students. Videotaping is ideal but remember to get your students' permission first. Now review the tapes and answer the following questions:

■ Who set the goals for the sessions: supervisor, student, both?
■ Who decided on the supervisory focus for the sessions: supervisor, student, both?
■ Who evaluated the session/provided feedback: supervisor, student, both?
■ Who did the majority of the talking: supervisor, student, equal?
■ Who filled out the evaluation form (if applicable): supervisor, student, both?
■ What type of questions were being asked by you: open-ended, closed?
■ What was the focus of the feedback session: client's performance, student's performance, student's deficiencies, student's strengths?
■ Who set the priorities for the next session: supervisor, student, both?

Now have a look at the pattern of your answers.

Is it always *you* (the clinical educator) who is performing the above functions? If so, it is likely you are adopting a directive/telling style in supervision. This style has its place, particularly with students at the beginning of their course and inexperienced in clinical situations, but may be very inappropriate for students who already have some competencies and a lot to contribute to the supervisory process. Check the backgrounds of the students in your tapes. Were they new to the experiences offered in your clinic, stressed, pleading for direction? If so, your supervisory style would have worked well with them. If not, you are likely to have left them feeling misunderstood and having learnt little.

Is it always the *student* who is performing the above functions? If so, it is likely you are adopting an indirect/advising style. This style works well with advanced students who are seeking confirmation that they are on the right track but may be very inappropriate for novices who require direction to get going and need confidence-building and modelling. This style can leave the novice feeling anxious and without direction. Again, check the backgrounds of the students – were they novices, advanced, outgoing or introverted in their communication?

Did you get a *mix* of student and clinical educator? You are probably evidencing a variety of supervisory styles. This is useful because at least you have these different behaviours in your current repertoire! However, you need to check that you used the most appropriate one at a particular time. Go back through your records and check the level of development of your students and then what style you were using with them.

To extend your range of supervisory styles:

- Be familiar with the different types of supervisory styles that have been described in the literature. Read one of the references included at the end of this section.
- Identify which styles you do not typically use at this point. What behaviours characterise these styles – write for your self-objective descriptors of the styles. What, if anything, might prevent you from utilising the styles you have identified? For example, fear of being too pushy or not being in full control, relinquishing power, no experience with that type of communication, thinking that you always had to get students to think for themselves.
- Can you challenge any beliefs that may prevent you from developing different styles?
- Talk to a colleague, write *for* and *against* lists for developing versus not developing different styles.
- Practise (on tape, or role-play with colleague) different styles. Ask for feedback about the different ways you handled situations. Try it out! Does it work?

REFERENCES

Best D, Edwards H 2001 Learning together: fostering professional craft development in clinical placements. In: Higgs J, Titchen A (eds) Practice knowledge and expertise in the health professions. Butterworth-Heinemann, Oxford

Biggs J 1989 Institutional learning and the integration of knowledge. In: Balla J, Gibson M, Chang A (eds) Learning in medical school: a model for the clinical professions. Hong Kong University Press, Hong Kong

Billet S 2001 Learning in the workplace: strategies for effective practice. Allen Unwin, Crows Nest

Bleakley A 2002 Pre-registration house officers and ward based learning. Medical Education 36:9–15

Boud D, Pascoe J 1988 In: Higgs J (ed) Experience based learning. ACEE, Sydney

Boud D, Keogh R, Walker D 1985 Turning experience into learning. Kogan, London

Boud D, Cohen R, Walker D 1993 Using experience for learning. SRHE, Buckingham

Carter R, Martin J, Maylin B et al 1984 Systems, management and chance. Harper & Row, London

Coleman J 1976 Differences between experiential and classroom learning. In: Keeton M et al (eds) Experiential learning: rational characteristics and assessment. Jossey-Bass, San Francisco

Coles C 1989 The role of context in elaborated learning. In: Balla J, Gibson M, Chang A (eds) Learning in medical school: a model for the clinical professions. Hong Kong University Press, Hong Kong

Coles C 1990 Elaborated learning in undergraduate medical education. Medical Education 24:14–22

Davis M, Harden R 1998 The continuum of problem-based learning. Medical Teacher 20:317–322

Dochy F, Segers M, Van den Bossche P et al 2003 Effects of problem-based learning: a meta-analysis. Learning and Instruction 13:533–568

Dunn R, Dunn K 1993 Teaching secondary students through their individual learning styles: practical approaches for grades 7–12. Allyn & Bacon, Boston

Entwistle N 1987 A model of the teaching learning process. In: Richardson J, Eyensk M, Warren Piper D (eds) Student learning. Open University Press, Milton Keynes

Entwistle N, Odor P, Anderson C 1988 Encouraging reflection on study strategies: the design of a computer-based adventure game. In: Ramsden P (ed) Improving learning: new perspectives. Kogan Page, London

Farmer S, Farmer J 1989: Supervision in communication disorders. Merrill Publishing, Ohio

Fish D, Twinn S 1997 Quality supervision in the health care professions. Butterworth-Heinemann, Oxford

Hersey P, Blanchard K 1982 Management of organisational behaviour: utilising human resources, 4th edn. Prentice-Hall, Englewood Cliffs, p 107 (Note: 3rd edn includes the LEAD questionnaire)

Higgs J 1993 Managing clinical education: the programme. Physiotherapy 79(4):239–245

Honey P, Mumford A 2003 The learning styles questionnaire – 80 item version. Peter Honey Publications, Maidenhead

Hutchinson L 2003 ABC of learning and teaching: educational environment. British Medical Journal 326:810–812

Klein P 2003 Rethinking the multiplicity of cognitive resources and curricular representations: alternatives to "learning styles" and "multiple intelligences". Journal of Curriculum Studies 35(1):45–81

Kolb D 1984 Experiential learning: experience as the source of learning and development. Prentice-Hall, Englewood Cliffs

Kolb DA, Osland JS, Rubin IM 1995 Organizational behavior: an experiential approach, 6th edn. Pearson Education, NJ

Kolb D, Rubin I, McIntyre A 1974 Organisational psychology: an experiential approach. Prentice-Hall, Englewood Cliffs

Lave J 1996 Teaching as learning in practice. Mind, Culture and Activity 3(3)

Marton F, Säljö R 1984 Approaches to learning. In: Marton F, Hounsell D, Entwistle N (eds) The experience of learning. Scottish Academic Press, Edinburgh

Maslow A 1970 Motivation and personality. Harper and Row, New York

Mawdsley B, Scudder R 1989 The integrative task-maturity model of supervision. Language, Speech and Hearing Services in Schools 20(3):305–315

Newble D, Entwistle N 1986 Learning styles and approaches: implications for medical education. Medical Education 20:162–175

Park C 2000 Learning style preference of southeast Asian students. Urban Education 35(3):245–268

Ramsden P 1984 The context of learning. In: Marton F, Hounsell D, Entwistle N (eds) The experience of learning. Scottish Academic Press, Edinburgh

Ramsden P 1988 Improving learning: new perspectives. Kogan Page, London

Regehr G, Norman 1996 Issues in cognitive psychology: implications for professional education. Academic Medicine 71(9):988–1001

Rogoff B 1990 Apprenticeship in thinking: cognitive development in social context. Oxford University Press, New York

Rogers C 1969 Freedom to learn. Charles Merrill, Ohio

Rose M, Best D 1996 Quality supervision. W B Saunders, London

Tuomi-Grohn F, Englestrom Y 2003 Between school and work: new perspectives on boundary-crossing. Elsevier Science, Oxford

Chapter 7

Reflection, practice and clinical education

Marilyn Baird and Jane Winter

The goal of practice is wise action. Wise action may involve the use of specialised knowledge, but central to it is judgment in specific situations, with conflicting values about which problems need to be solved and how to solve them. An essential genre of knowledge used in practice is practical knowledge – "knowing how" – which is embedded in practical reasoning. It involves knowing-in-action, reflection-in-action and reflection-about-action using repertoires of examples, images, and understandings learned through experience.

(Harris 1993, p. 26–27).

This chapter examines the idea of reflection as a means of enhancing the quality of clinical education and the delivery of health services to patients and clients. The chapter will introduce educators to ways of incorporating reflection into everyday work practices and supervisory practices. It will also demonstrate how reflective activities can bridge the perceived "gap" between what students learn during their on-campus studies with what they learn during clinical studies.

WHAT IS PRACTICE? TECHNICAL KNOWLEDGE VERSUS PROFESSIONAL CRAFT

Practice is the craft-like experience embodying the affective and cognitive, artistic and scientific, personal and social experiences developed over many years

(Clegg et al 2002, p. 144).

When we are in the midst of the semi-structured chaos that characterises the delivery of health services (Kowal et al 1997), it is often hard to see our practice for what it is. We simply get on with the work and assure our students when they marvel at our capacity to know instinctively what to do and how to modify the textbook to suit the patient that it will all come together with time and experience (Cross 1993). Health professionals are constantly involved in a process of working out what needs to be done in the here and now and how this can be practically achieved given the constraints of the context in which they work (Baird 1996).

Since the landmark work of Donald Schön (1983, 1987), educators are now acknowledging practice depends upon recourse to a range of "non-logical processes" such as "knowing-in-action", "reflection-in-action" and "reflection-about-action". Educators are increasingly structuring their undergraduate health science courses around the notion of reflection and reflective practice. Correspondingly, the health professions now regard the development of a reflective practitioner as a crucial ongoing professional activity (Brown et al 2003). In many ways the increasing importance accorded to reflection and reflective processes by educators and the professions marks a sea change in the way we think about professional practice. So why has this occurred and what is its relevance to supervision?

Traditionally the warrant for professional status rests upon the extent to which a practice utilises science in the delivery of its services (Johnson 1972, Freidson 1989). Thus, despite acknowledgement by professions of the co-existence of an "indeterminate" form of knowledge or professional "artistry" that defies codification (Atkinson 1981, Schön 1983, Fish & Twinn 1997), professions have maintained their faith in the traditional understanding of a practice as a service firmly grounded in pure and applied science. The work undertaken by professionals is understood to be an objective, rational and dispassionate human service that replicates scientifically based rules, techniques and procedures irrespective of the social and political context within which it is situated (Schön 1983, Fish & Twinn 1997, Romer 2003). Clinical issues and problems are therefore pre-specified in the classroom with students taught a range of solutions they are expected to apply during the practicum.

This so-called technocratic model of practice conveniently ignores the fact that it is often very difficult to define the true nature of the clinical problem accurately and that a great deal of what practitioners do is surrounded by uncertainty (Schön 1983, Bennett & Fox 1993). The model also falsely assumes practitioners can use scientifically verified knowledge off-the-shelf (Eraut 1985) in the way one can follow the instructions on a can of soup. More importantly, the traditional model disregards the fact that the quality of the service experienced by patients is defined by the values and beliefs of the practitioners themselves (Schön 1983, Baird 1998, Johns 2000).

Another reason for our increasing unease with the technocratic model is the persistent belief by its exponents that "good practice is generalisable, unproblematic and achievable by all" (Fish & Twinn 1997, p. 96). As students discover, the reality of practice often challenges the profession's view of itself and its practitioners. In the following vignette, a first-year radiography student is struggling to reconcile what she has been taught about ethics and radiation protection in the university setting with the reality of what she witnessed during her four-week placement in a busy clinical radiology department.

> *The use of radiation protection and safety for the patient can be an ethical dilemma if not adhered to. In the past few weeks on a number of occasions I observed that there was not much use of radiation protection on patients ... It could be justified that based on the standard of equipment, less protection was needed ... however the text books and profession tell us that radiographers have a duty of care to their patients and consequently have a responsibility to provide a standard level of protection to patients and themselves. What was evident was that the irregular safety procedures could be attributed to the inexperience of the radiographer or the lack of awareness of protection measures. Also, in some cases, even the lack of time became a factor – "too many patients and no time".*

(Dee, a 2003 first-year radiography student).

In the vignette, Dee is demonstrating a capacity to think about what she has seen. She is beginning to engage in a process of reflection-upon-action that her educators are hoping to develop over the time she is in the clinical setting. Dee is also beginning to understand the complexity of professional practice and the way in which organisational structures can inhibit good practice. She is appreciating that the quality of health care delivery is just as susceptible to the impact of human failing and foibles as any other aspect of life. If Dee were to be asked whether the technocratic model of practice accurately depicts practice, she would probably disagree. As indicated by Harris (1993) at the beginning of the chapter, in the real world, scientific and technological knowledge makes a relatively small contribution to the delivery of competent professional service. In arriving at justifiable practical decisions, practitioners rely heavily upon practical knowledge gained through sustained and reflective practical experience (Schön 1983, 1987, Balla 1989, Harris 1993, Johns 2000, Brown et al 2003). The technocratic model can therefore only offer a partial account of practice.

In contrast, the professional artistry, or reflective, model of practice (Fish & Twinn 1997) argues that, in the context of busy clinical departments, practitioners do not consciously and deliberately apply pure and applied research to their practice. Rather, clinical practice is characterised by a tacit and largely spontaneous "knowing-in-action" (Bines 1992). As expertise develops, practitioners increasingly rely upon their own knowledge, skills and experience to guide them in knowing what to do in the situation (Balla 1989, Benner et al 1992). From the perspective of Dreyfus & Dreyfus (1985, p. 8) human decision-making therefore represents "a mysterious blending of careful analysis, intuition and the wisdom and judgement distilled from experience".

It is the way in which expert practitioners define and solve clinical problems that distinguishes the expert from the novice practitioner. A long time ago John Dewey (1938) convincingly argued that experience of itself will not necessarily result in wise action. Rather, if experience in the practice setting is to lead to expert patient care then it must be accompanied by a special kind of thinking he named reflective thinking. Effective practice requires the appropriate use of science; at the same time it needs engagement by practitioners in a range of reflective processes. Indeed, what we now understand is that, unless practitioners engage in reflective thinking, their practical knowledge will be incomplete and, as we will see in the next section, the delivery of quality patient care will be compromised.

CHARACTERISTICS OF A REFLECTIVE PRACTITIONER

As a reflective practitioner I nurture my "knowing self", a self that is sensitive yet critical of self within the caring moment. Through reflection I learn through the experience and transcend previous ways of knowing.

(Johns 2000, p. 68).

In the following extract from another first-year radiography student critical learning experience report, we are introduced to the kind of approach to patient care that is a consequence of a habitual approach to practice that appears to lack any engagement in reflective thinking on the part of radiographer A.

... Radiographer A did not communicate with patients well. The radiographer routinely takes patients to the room and immediately directs them to assume a position. There is no attempt to build rapport through smiling or even asking how the patient is. The only communication was one-sided: the radiographer giving the patient directions. There was no general conversation with patients unless the patient spoke first. From my perspective I took the behaviour to imply the radiographer lacked a real concern for the patient, simply wishing to get the job done as quickly as possible. Radiographer B was the complete opposite. This practitioner has a genuine concern for patients and treats them as individuals, not just another "hand x-ray". I saw this radiographer build rapport from the moment of greeting the patient. This was done by forming eye contact, smiling and saying, "Hi, my name is ..." Throughout the examination I noted the radiographer being kind, polite and showing empathy. The radiographer chatted about general topics and often stood by the table and talked to the patient without setting up equipment so eye contact could be made and genuine interest shown. Whilst communication does not alter the quality of the images and it might slightly increase the examination time, when performed well, the total experience is pleasant for the patient and satisfying for the radiographer.

(2003 first-year radiography student following completion
of a four-week clinical rotation).

There is little doubt the student believed the patient was better served by practitioner B. In contrast to practitioner A, practitioner B is a thoughtful radiographer who has gone beyond a focus upon the technical aspect of his or her work. Radiographer B is demonstrating a concern with the ethical and moral dimensions of practice as well as contextual, interpersonal and integrative competence (Johnston 1995). Yet can we ascribe to the actions of this radiographer the label of reflective practitioner?

Certainly, radiographer B has taken the first step in the process envisaged by Dewey (1933), by making a conscious decision to direct his or her actions in an intelligent and creative way. This practitioner seems to have the particular attitudes of mind that Dewey (1933) believed are a precursor to reflective thinking, namely:

- open-mindedness
- whole-heartedness
- responsibility.

It is only when these attitudes are embraced that Dewey (1933) believed practitioners could engage in that form of thinking that frees them from impulsive or taken-for-granted and habitual approaches to their practice.

What kind of thinking are we talking about? Fish & Twinn (1997) argue the reflective practitioner actually moves beyond the common-sense view that practitioners should think about their actions during and after the delivery of a professional service. Reflective thinking is not idle navel-gazing and imagining how practice could be different (Bolton 2001). Reflective thinking is deliberative and orderly (Wales et al 1993). Furthermore, it is not a self-absorbed process that solely focuses upon self-reflection and self-monitoring without seeking feedback from colleagues (Bolton 2001).

Reflective thinking is a serious intellectual activity that means taking a step back before, during or after we act with a view to improvement or change. Engagement in reflective thinking means a commitment to a structured and critical review of one's practice leading to refinement and new understandings (Fish & Twinn 1997). Thus, in contrast to habitual or conformist practitioners, reflective practitioners:

- have the capacity to be open to new ideas and approaches to practice
- seek to improve the quality of their work for the benefit of the patient
- are enthusiastic and passionate about their work
- see what they do as worthwhile and meaningful
- act in an intellectually and morally responsible manner, recognising the role values and beliefs play in shaping the quality of patient care
- adopt a problem-solving and holistic approach to their practice, seeking collaborative solutions to practical workplace issues and concerns
- acknowledge their limitations and level of competence
- know how to engage in a critical conversation with their practice and their inner self and in the process gain new knowledge and insight into the meaning of their practice.

The reflective practitioner is unashamedly "enticed and engaged by thinking" (Loughran 1996, p. 5), always wanting to know why something is worth believing. Such practitioners openly question and possibly challenge the dominant institutional, political and economic imperatives that intrude upon practice and in the process seek to mitigate their impact upon the delivery of quality patient care (Smyth 1986, Bolton 2001).

Is the goal of reflective practice achievable? Have we painted a utopian ideal that lacks application to the busy and somewhat chaotic clinical world? We think not. After all, existing professional practice already depends upon knowledge that can only be gained through reflective action. However, the problem is that if these processes remain at the tacit or hidden level of understanding, genuine professional growth is stunted (Schön 1983, 1987). The idea of professionalism demands that practitioners acquire the ability to become aware of their thinking processes and at the same time "exert control over them" (Biggs 1986). What we aim to do in the next section is facilitate a more holistic and explicit understanding of the reflective process.

WAYS OF MODELLING THE REFLECTIVE PROCESS

The crucial importance of one's attitude in determining the extent to which engagement in reflection is possible cannot be overemphasised. Practitioners need to allow themselves to view their practice with an element of surprise or anticipation so that practice problems can be seen as challenges to be solved through the application of the reflective process (Schön 1983, 1987).

Dewey and the reflective process

For Dewey (1933), the reflective process comprise the five phases of:

1. suggestions
2. intellectualisation or "problem-setting"
3. hypothesis or guiding idea
4. reasoning
5. testing.

These phases constitute a structured process of problem definition, problem analysis, formulation of an action theory and subsequent testing of this theory. In the *pre-reflective stage* various ideas flood into the mind in the process of seeking resolution to a particular practice challenge. However, we must resist implementing the first idea that comes into our head and instead use the following process:

Phase 1. Ideas are converted into *suggestions* that are scrutinised to the extent they become the impetus to further inquiry.

Phase 2. The *problem-setting stage* is the process whereby the difficulty or puzzle is placed within a larger picture so its true nature can be ascertained and "courses of action may be more fully thought through and intellectualised" (Loughran 1996, p. 5).

Phase 3. Through the process of *intellectualisation*, the nature of the problem, initial insights and suggestions are restated in the form of a *working hypothesis* that allows for the measured and controlled consideration of more information or observations and testing.

Phase 4. The *reasoning* phase encourages practitioners to extend their thinking about the issue so that as many possibilities are considered as allowable in the time available.

Phase 5. The process of *testing* the proposed solution is essential if one is to know "how well one has thought through the problem situation" (Loughran 1996, p. 6). It is important to note that the possibility of failure is overtly acknowledged in the reflective process and viewed as a positive learning experience.

In summary, practitioners who really understand the process of reflective thinking:

> *delay action long enough to understand the situation as fully as possible, to consider the end that they hope to achieve, to generate and weigh up as many options as they can and to plan before they take action*

> (Wales et al 1993, p. 182).

Schön and reflection-in-action

Schön (1987) is also concerned to show us how practitioners can effectively use reflection to delineate, criticise and restructure the knowledge implicit in their actions for use in subsequent actions. His special contribution to our understanding about reflective thinking lies in his distinction between the reflective thinking that occurs during action, which he calls reflection-in-action and the reflective thinking that occurs after action. In essence, "reflection-in-action" is characterised by an interactive three-stage process:

Stage 1. Practitioners allow themselves, in the context of a situation in which they feel unsure or uncertain as to how to act, to "experience surprise, puzzlement or confusion".

Stage 2. The next stage involves bringing to the surface our implicit understandings of the situation and consciously analysing them with a view to restructuring our thinking about the situation.

Stage 3. Now the practitioner is in the position of conducting an "on-the-spot experiment" that will result in new understanding about the situation and effect a positive change to the situation in the course of the delivery of the service.

Such an inquiry in the midst of action itself may also result in unintended changes and therefore start another round of reflection-in-action.

Key points

What can we glean from the discussion so far? Firstly, some kind of stimulus needs to awaken within the practitioner the need or desire to engage in the decision-making process (Stockhausen & Kawashima 2002). Next, the nature of the problem must be identified and the desired goal or outcome articulated. Ideas are generated. A plan of action is developed and subsequently implemented and evaluated (Wales et al 1993).

The reflective process provides educators with a powerful model with which to shape student learning during the practicum. If we are to develop reflective practitioners, Wales et al (1993) strongly believe students must be allowed and encouraged to question, probe, suggest ideas, create plans and engage in intelligent action. We will now briefly examine models that educators use to guide the development of strategies for encouraging student reflection during the clinical attachment.

Reflection on practice

The steps in Figure 7.1 outline the promotion of reflection during the clinical attachment, as envisaged by Boud et al (1985). Because it is the students'

Figure 7.1 The promotion of reflection during clinical attachment (adapted from Boud 1993)

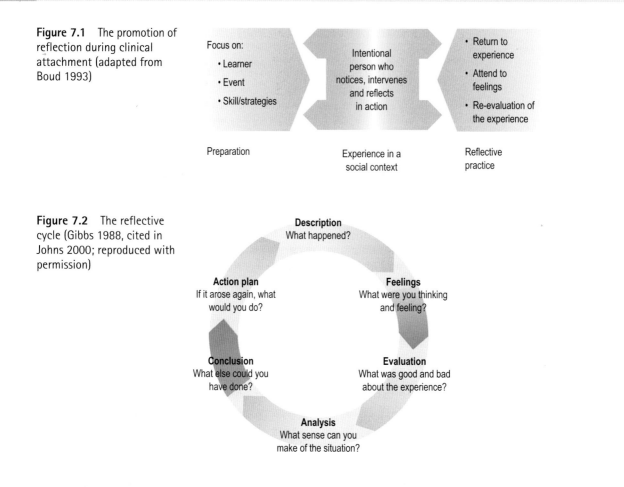

Figure 7.2 The reflective cycle (Gibbs 1988, cited in Johns 2000; reproduced with permission)

intentions and their prior experience that have the greatest impact on learning, they argue attention must be given to the pre-reflective stage. Students must be adequately prepared for the experience and equipped with the necessary learning strategies to help them to learn how to reflect on their practice.

The next stage in the cycle is direct clinical experience, during which students will engage in an active process of constructing their own understanding and knowledge of clinical practice. However, because there is not the time to step back from the action and critically evaluate practical action, time must be set aside for re-examination and reflection on practice. The third segment in Figure 7.1 represents the time for students to return to their experiences so that they can tease out, in concert with their peers, those aspects of practice which puzzled them or which possibly served to illuminate theoretical concepts.

The Gibbs model (1988, cited in Johns 2000) ensures attention is paid to feelings as well as to future actions. This model, illustrated in Figure 7.2, envisages reflection on practice as comprising six phases: a description of the learning event, an account of how the event affected the learner, an evaluation, analysis, and a conclusion, followed by the creation of an action plan to guide future interventions.

Figure 7.3 The experiential learning cycle divided into three main elements (reproduced with permission from Driscoll 2000)

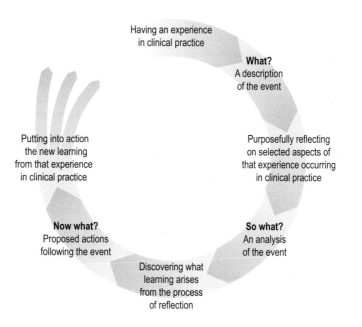

Having an experience
in clinical practice

What?
A description
of the event

Putting into action
the new learning
from that experience
in clinical practice

Purposefully reflecting
on selected aspects of
that experience occurring
in clinical practice

Now what?
Proposed actions
following the event

So what?
An analysis
of the event

Discovering what
learning arises
from the process
of reflection

A similar cyclical model (Fig. 7.3) has been proposed by Driscoll (2000), in which the experiential learning cycle is divided into three main elements:

1. *What?* A description of the event.
2. *So* what? Analysis of the event, including feelings and effects.
3. *Now* what? Proposed actions to modify or improve practice.

Although this model does not specifically focus on the preparation stage, it is particularly helpful in structuring reflective practice and converting thoughts into actions. The description of each phase of the cycle, whilst similar to the other models, is easily understood by students from an early stage in their experience and can be applied to their clinical practice. However, it is important not only to reflect on critical incidents or negative experiences but also to reflect on normal practice to ensure that we do not slip into complacency until a crisis occurs!

USING THE REFLECTIVE PROCESS TO ENHANCE SKILLS AS A CLINICAL EDUCATOR

> *Quality supervision involves a detailed understanding and appreciation of how we learn new practice and therefore how the learner can be supported in doing so.*

(Fish & Twinn 1997, p. 59).

Generally, clinical educators are considered to have a wide range of knowledge that will help students to develop their practice. However, educators should not just be content experts. They should also act as facilitators assisting students to learn for themselves by reflecting on experiences (Fish & Twinn 1997). How can educators do this?

Role modelling

One of the most crucial elements in clinical education is that of the role model. If we expect students to develop the characteristics of a reflective practitioner, they need to see those characteristics modelled. If their clinical educators demonstrate a structured approach to reflective practice in their own work, then students can start to see how it relates to them as novice practitioners. Titchen & Higgs (1999, p. 183) suggest that educators should first ensure that students have the opportunity to observe their everyday work, and then "intentionally create opportunities in which they can articulate particularly the more embedded, tacit and usually unexplicated aspects of their practice". This has also been identified in teacher education by Lazarus (2000), who suggests that teachers change their teaching strategies based on their "intuitive knowing", and unless these actions are explicitly expressed in dialogue, they will remain tacit to an observing student teacher. Mentors, supervisors and educators need to "deconstruct a fluid performance" (Lazarus 2000, p. 114) to assist students to understand reflection-in-action.

Improving practice as a clinical educator rather than as a clinician

Many experienced practitioners are presented with the task of being a clinical educator with very little preparation. Just as we need to develop our skills as dietitians or speech pathologists, we need to use reflective practice to develop these skills as an educator.

EXERCISE

Recall a session with a student where you were giving feedback or instructing on a new technique.
Use one of the models in the previous section to revisit and reflect on the experience.
Are you able to see why it did or didn't go well?
Are there things that you can work on to improve that type of student interaction in the future?
If so, how will you go about achieving those things?

Fostering students to be reflective practitioners

For an effective student–educator relationship that promotes and encourages reflective practice, Driscoll (2000) has identified that both parties need:

- a willingness to learn from what happens in practice
- to be open enough to share aspects of practice with others
- a belief that there is no end-point in learning about practice
- to be aware of the conditions necessary for reflection to occur.

However, students are not necessarily reflective by nature; rather they need to learn the skills to become reflective practitioners, and clinical educators have the opportunity to provide students with the tools to develop the characteristics described in the previous section. It also needs to be recognised that reflective practice can be an extremely difficult and foreign concept for some students (and practitioners!) and, whilst support, encouragement and tools for reflection can be provided, not all students will choose to engage in reflection. They may also be using avenues outside the clinical education setting to reflect and debrief (e.g. contact with university staff, other mentors, colleagues) and therefore focusing on evidence of reflective practice on placement may not be appropriate.

EXERCISE

Consider the last time you were supervising a student:
Did you actively encourage reflective practice by the student?
If so, how did you encourage it?
If not, can you think of ways to encourage reflection next time you are a clinical educator?

FACILITATING STUDENT REFLECTIVE PRACTICES

> *Simply being encouraged to reflect is likely to be as meaningful as a lecture on cooperative group work*

(Loughran 2002, p. 33).

Students need to understand why they are being asked to reflect on their experiences and professional practice to help them then use the various tools of reflective practice. Some of the reasons why educators encourage reflective practice have been documented by Westberg & Jason (2001). These include enabling learners to:

- identify and build on their existing knowledge
- identify deficits in their knowledge and errors in their thinking
- generalise from particular experiences and apply this new knowledge to later situations
- integrate new information
- identify unexamined assumptions and biases that can interfere with learning and patient care
- be in touch with their feelings so that they can provide compassionate, comprehensive care
- have ownership of insights that emerge from their own discoveries
- become competent and be encouraged to continue learning throughout their professional careers.

It seems also that reflecting on experiences is particularly important for the development of clinical reasoning skills. Reflection and communication of those reflections are valuable mechanisms for exploring the student's knowledge and reasoning skills (Higgs et al 1999). As we have previously seen, reflective practitioners are likely to provide a better standard of patient care and therefore it is a crucial part of the educator role to assist students to develop the skills of reflection.

A range of learning tools are used by universities to facilitate reflective thinking and practice by students during their clinical placement. These include reflective practice journals, critical incident reports, reflective portfolios or essays, assignments requiring students to interview clinicians to hear their reflections of client management and reflective summaries in written case management plans. Students therefore come to the placement with an awareness of reflective practice that should be nurtured to assist them bridge the theory–practice gap.

What are some of the ways that reflective practice can be further developed during placement experiences?

Reflective practice models: cycles of reflection

The models of reflective processes described above are a useful starting point in helping students to develop a framework for their reflections. Students need to be able to devote time to these processes, however. They need to be able to prepare for a patient interaction, as well as have time after the interaction to work through the analysis of the session and their plans for what they need to do prior to their next interaction. Students early in their experience may need more guidance in reflecting on their experiences and providing some trigger questions or prompts may assist with understanding what is required when reflecting on their actions. Westberg & Jason (2001) suggest that clinical educators can foster reflection in the following ways:

- Before the experience: discuss learning goals and plans.
- During the experience: help learners to consider alternative approaches if appropriate, and support the learner's relationship with patients.
- After the experience invite learners' reflections on:
  - their overall impressions
  - new issues or goals
  - what went well
  - key decision points
  - assumptions or biases that influenced their practice.

Verbal debriefing/feedback

A formal feedback session with the clinical educator is an important opportunity for student reflection and care should be taken to allow students to reflect on their patient assessment or management rather than just listening to the educator's observations. For further details on feedback see Chapter 4, part 3.

Reflective writing

Journal writing is one form of reflective writing which according to Boud (2001, p. 9) is a "device for working with events and experiences in order to extract meaning from them". Reflective writing can assist students to make sense of the chaotic and very unfamiliar work environment and world of patient interaction. Reflective writing is the primary way the universities get students to engage in reflective practice. It also allows students to revisit their experiences.

I found reading my previous journal entries useful and helped me to reflect on previous comments made. In many ways, I have come to realise that I have more questions for myself as each week goes by, due to being exposed to new and stimulating experiences. This has renewed my yearning to look for answers.

(Dietetic student in first clinical placement).

This student early in her placement experience already has the makings of a reflective practitioner and can use her journal to see the progress in her own professional development.

One needs to be mindful of inhibiting factors in reflective writing, and one of the most powerful is the reader. If the journal is open to others then that can shape the content of the writing and limit the scope of reflection. However, having the writing open to a tutor or mentor allows some feedback and encouragement.

I used to do it every Thursday night and I really liked it and I'd get a response back every Friday … I used to like getting home from uni and seeing what she'd said [university tutor]. We had a good thing happening and I think I'm going to miss it.

The above quote from a final-year student and the subsequent extracts from a focus group discussing the value of reflective journals by dietetic students appear to support the concept of having the reflective journal open to another person.

As a result of writing, the support [from the university supervisor] was really good so I think it was important to write what I was feeling.

I was really comfortable with relaxing and letting H know all that I was going through and I think the relationship between you and your supervisor has a huge impact.

The other major inhibitor is whether the journal is an assessable part of the placement or practicum. As assessment tends to equate to the importance of the task in students' thinking; reflective practice journals may be an assessment task at some universities in an effort to demonstrate to students that reflective practice is highly regarded. This has the benefit of encouraging students who may not otherwise engage in reflection at least to participate in some way, but again may constrain honest reflections by some students.

CRITICAL LEARNING INCIDENTS

The idea of having practitioners recall situations that provoked surprise, concern, confusion or satisfaction for reflective learning purposes has a long history (Benner 1984, Talbot 2002). Depending on its purpose in the teaching and learning programme, the incident can be a practice situation that:

- made a significant difference to the patient outcome
- exceeded expectations
- did not go well
- challenged the accepted way of doing things
- affirmed the value of academic theory to practice
- demonstrates the need for integration of theory with practice.

Once the situation has been identified as a significant incident, practitioners or students must then describe what happened, what happened to them, their thoughts about the situation and, most importantly, why the incident was critical to their learning (Benner 1984).

Griffin (2003, p. 208) strongly argues the use of a critical learning incident has the capacity to facilitate a much deeper level of reflection "because it goes beyond a detailed description of an event that attracted attention, to analysis of and reflection on the meaning of the event". She believes the use of this technique in undergraduate education has the capacity to assist students truly to engage in Dewey's reflective process.

We have already seen the power of critical learning incidents earlier in the chapter with the observations made by Dee. First-year radiography students are asked to select a communication, ethics or infection control situation and to reflect their observations against theory covered in class. The value of the exercise for students in encouraging reflection on practice is obvious from these extracts:

> This critical learning experience has really opened my eyes to the importance of infection control in the workplace.

> This incident taught me the importance of the referring doctor clearly explaining to the patient why he thought the procedure was necessary … the radiographer handled the situation very professionally and in accordance with the ethical principles of informed consent and autonomy.

REFLECTIVE PRACTICE IN SUMMARY

This chapter has aimed to provide some insights into the theory and practice of reflection. Some of the key points to take from this chapter include why reflection is important in professional practice, how we can foster reflection by students and what tools are available to assist clinical educators in this process.

Why reflect?

- potential to transform practice
- enhances the capacity to critique habitual practices whether as an educator or a practitioner
- to generate practice knowledge
- to facilitate an ability to adapt to new situations
- to resolve conflicts and contradictions in our professional practice
- to enhance self-esteem and satisfaction
- as a means of valuing, developing and professionalising practice.

How to foster reflection by students

1. Model reflective practice:
   - talk out loud about decision-making, patient management
   - share a critical incident
   - keep a reflective journal and share an excerpt with students.

2. Value students' reflections:
- practise active listening
- assist students to understand their reflections and link the theory with practice.
3. Provide an environment conducive to reflective practice:
- allow time for reflection before, during and after a learning experience
- demonstrate a collaborative work environment by reflecting with colleagues
- recognise individual student differences in ability or willingness to reflect
- encourage student reflection but respect their privacy.

CONCLUSION

A long time ago Lawrence Stenhouse (1975) argued the journey is more important than the destination. Practitioners have finished their journey; students are still making their way in unfamiliar territory. We will finish this chapter with an extract from a first-year radiography student account of the implementation of her week-two action plan:

> *I have improved on the aspects of practice that needed additional effort. I have made more of an effort of asking more clinical history of the patient. I have learned better how to adjust exposure factors.*

Her supervising practitioner wrote in response:

> *After a slow start Mel has progressed well. Like all students she seems to be very hesitant when addressing the patients. Her communication skills and personal interaction with the patients is now first rate.*

Thus students will achieve their goals provided practitioners embrace their learning needs and support them.

REFERENCES

Atkinson P 1981 The clinical experience: the construction and reconstruction of medical reality. Gower Publishing, Westmead

Baird M A 1996 The idea of a reflective practicum: overcoming the dichotomy between academia and the practice setting. Radiography 2:119–138

Baird M A 1998 The preparation for practice as a diagnostic radiographer: the relationship between the practicum and the profession. Unpublished PhD, La Trobe University

Balla J I 1989 Changing concepts in clinical education: the case for a theory. In: Balla J I, Gibson M, Chang A M (eds) Learning in medical school. Hong Kong University Press, Hong Kong

Benner P 1984 From novice to expert: excellence and power in clinical nursing. Addison-Wesley, CA

Benner P, Tanner C, Chesla C 1992 From beginner to expert: gaining a differentiated clinical world in critical area nursing. Advances in Nursing Science 14(3):13–28

Bennett N L, Fox R D 1993 Challenges for continuing professional education. In: Curry L, Wergin J F et al (eds) Educating professionals: responding to new expectations for competence and accountability. Jossey-Bass, San Francisco

Biggs J B 1986 Enhancing learning skills: the role of metacognition. In: Bowden H A (ed) Student learning: research into practice. University of Melbourne, Melbourne

Bines H 1992 Issues in course design. In: Bines H, Watson D (eds) Developing professional education. SRHE & Open University Press, Buckingham

Bolton G 2001 Reflective practice: writing and professional development. Chapman, London

Boud D 1993 Experience as the base for learning. Higher Education Research and Development 12(1):33–44

Boud D 2001 Using journal writing to enhance reflective practice. In: English L M, Gillen M (eds) Promoting journal writing in adult education. New directions in adult and continuing education, no. 90. Jossey-Bass, San Francisco, p 9–18

Boud D, Keogh R, Walker D 1985 What is reflection in learning? In: Boud D, Keogh R, Walker D (eds) Reflection: turning experience into learning. Kogan Page, London

Brown G, Esdaile S A, Ryan S E 2003 Becoming an advanced healthcare practitioner. Butterworth-Heinemann, Edinburgh

Clegg S, Tan J, Saeidi S 2002 Reflecting or acting? Reflective practice and continuing professional development in higher education. Reflective Practice 3(1):31–146

Cross V 1993 Introducing physiotherapy students to the idea of 'reflective practice'. Medical Teacher 15(4):293–307

Dewey J 1933 How we think: a restatement of the relation of reflective thinking to the educative process. D C Heath, Massachusetts

Dewey J 1938 Experience and education. Collier Books, New York

Dreyfus H L, Dreyfus S E 1985 Mind over machine – the power of human intuition and expertise in the era of the computer. Free Press, New York

Driscoll J 2000 Practising clinical supervision. A reflective approach. Edinburgh, Baillière Tindall

Eraut M 1985 Knowledge creation and knowledge use in professional contexts. Studies in Higher Education 10(2):117–133

Fish D, Twinn S 1997 Quality clinical supervision in the health care professions. Butterworth-Heinemann, Oxford

Freidson E 1989 The theory of professions: state of the art. In: Windt P Y et al (eds) Ethical issues in the professions. Prentice Hall, Englewood Cliffs

Gibbs G 1988 Learning by doing: a guide to teaching and learning methods. Oxford Brookes University, Oxford

Griffin M L 2003 Using critical incidents to promote and assess reflective thinking in pre-service teachers. Reflective Practice 4(2):208–220

Harris I B 1993 New expectations for professional competence. In: Curry L, Wergin J F et al (eds) Educating professionals: responding to new expectations for competence and accountability. Jossey-Bass, San Francisco

Higgs J, Jones M, Refshauge K 1999 Helping students learn clinical reasoning skills. In: Higgs J, Edwards H (eds) Educating beginning practitioners. Challenges for health professional education. Butterworth-Heinemann, Oxford

Johns C 2000 Becoming a reflective practitioner. Blackwell Science, Oxford

Johnson T J 1972 Professions and power. Macmillan, London

Johnston R 1995 Two cheers for the reflective practitioner. Journal of Further and Higher Education 19(3):74–83

Kowal E, Secomb E, Chew J 1997 Students, examine thyselves. Arena Magazine 29(June–July):9–10

Lazarus E 2000 The role of intuition in mentoring and supporting beginning teachers. In: Atkinson T, Claxton G (eds) The intuitive practitioner. On the value of not always knowing what one is doing. Open University Press, Buckingham, p 107–121

Loughran J 1996 Developing reflective practice: learning about teaching and learning through modeling. Falmer Press, London

Loughran J 2002 Effective reflective practice. In search of meaning in learning and teaching. Journal of Teacher Education 53(1):33–43

Romer T A 2003 Learning process and professional content in the theory of Donald Schön. Reflective Practice 4(1):85–93

Schön D 1983 The reflective practitioner: how professionals think in action. Basic Books, New York

Schön D A 1987 Educating the reflective practitioner. Jossey-Bass, CA

Smyth J 1986 The reflective practitioner in nurse education. Keynote address to Second National Nursing Education Seminar. South Australian College of Advanced Education, Adelaide

Stenhouse L 1975 An introduction to curriculum research and development. Heinemann, London

Stockhausen L, Kawashima A 2002 The introduction of reflective practice to Japanese nurses. Reflective Practice 3(1):118–129

Talbot M 2002 Reflective practice: new insights or more-of-the-same? Thoughts on an auto-biographical critical incident analysis. Reflective Practice 3(2):226–229

Titchen A, Higgs J 1999 Facilitating the development of knowledge. In: Higgs J, Edwards H (eds) Educating beginning practitioners. Challenges for health professional education. Butterworth-Heinemann, Oxford

Wales C, Nardi A H, Stager R A 1993 Emphasising critical thinking and problem solving. In: Curry L, Wergin J F et al (eds) Educating professionals: responding to new expectations for competence and accountability. Jossey-Bass, San Francisco

Westberg J, Jason H 2001 Fostering reflection and providing feedback. Helping others learn from experience. Springer, New York

SECTION 3

Challenges in clinical education

SECTION CONTENTS

Chapter 8

The challenging learning situation

Susan Ryan

This chapter presents several different scenarios of learning challenges that can happen on placement. These have been taken from real-life experiences and the excerpts from students' narratives illustrate the dilemmas. I have been involved in many of these stories and they are supported by evidence from the professional education literature, adult learning theories, clinical reasoning studies and psychological tests, as well as from research studies. These exemplars could raise awareness of the individuality of problems and the complexity of causes. Ways of handling these challenges are presented. The outline of the chapter is as follows:

- Catching difficulties before they become problems
- Working and learning together
- Following good practice – pre-empting difficulties
- Capturing emerging problems
- Analysing and interpreting the problem
- Working through the problem.

CATCHING DIFFICULTIES BEFORE THEY BECOME PROBLEMS

A difficulty has turned into a problem. It happened during a practice placement between a therapist and a student. The delay, caused by the late realisation from the parties concerned that things were not going well, turned a normally difficult situation into a challenging problem. But, whose problem is it? How far into the placement has this situation happened before it was detected or acknowledged? Is it rectifiable? When the dynamics of a learning situation are going wrong one of the greatest challenges for all the parties concerned (therapist/clinical educator, student/learner, university staff/mediator) is to pinpoint the difficulties and to ascertain when one or both parties realised that degeneration of learning was occurring. It is not an easy situation to deal with. It helps to seek out feedback early on in the placement and to recognise the symptoms sooner rather than later so that they can be dealt with proactively and positively.

WORKING AND LEARNING TOGETHER

Contemporary literature in professional education and in adult learning theories that focus on learning in the practice setting place great emphasis on the two parties learning together (Best & Edwards 2001, Knowles et al 1998, McAllister 2003). Both people are considered to be in a learning partnership and on a similar plane where two-way enquiry is promoted (Ryan 1996). However, in reality, many people attribute the problem to the student as it is assumed that the therapist/clinical educator is knowledgeable and "right". In fact, by viewing the situation at the start from a stance of equality, a broader perspective emerges. Also, at this point in time, when it is realised that there is a challenge to constructive learning, feelings from both parties are usually running at a high level of frustration, anxiety and anger and this reactive situation needs to be acknowledged and diffused. Both parties are usually trying hard to resolve any conflict but the situation is not improving and some kind of intervention appears to be necessary. In this state of tension it is not easy for either party to be objective and diagnostic.

If the situation is recognised sooner rather than later, or if the clinical educator has sought out feedback from the student earlier, then it is possible that the two individuals can deal with the challenge themselves. If the difficulties have been allowed to run their course and they are only acknowledged at a later critical stage then a mediator may be required. In either of the events above third parties can be useful as they do bring a balanced, less reactive view to bear on both sides of the situation. It is useful for individuals to share their story or version of events with someone of their choosing. The following section will describe two ways to "catch" the problem early and to do something about it by analysing the facts from both sides.

FOLLOWING GOOD PRACTICE – PRE-EMPTING DIFFICULTIES

Quality assurance procedures in universities in the UK (Quality Assurance Agency 1998) have cued educators into making *early evaluations* of learning situations. The same procedures could usefully be employed in the practice setting. The therapist/clinical educator concerned, being the one who works in this setting, should initiate this procedure. Ideally, he/she should ask a third party to meet the student and to talk to him/her. It can be anyone who is working in the setting. Approximately one-third of the way through a placement the student(s) could be interviewed to see how the learning experience is going. Questions should be open-ended to allow the learner to elaborate. Possible questions are given in Box 8.1.

Box 8.1   Questions to ask the learner

- Tell me about this placement (This question allows the learner to give an overview of the experience to date – follow-up questions can deal with positive then negative aspects from this account)
- Did you feel your induction was well planned?
- Was your learning contract discussed and agreed mutually?
- Do you feel supported in your learning?
- Are there other things that could be done to help your learning?
- Have you sufficient access to learning materials (files, journals, internet)?
- Are you meeting regularly with your supervisor?
- Have you both worked out ways of communicating that suit both of you?
- What else could *you* do to improve your learning opportunities?

All being well, this meeting need not take more than 15 minutes of someone's time. Students can be invited to write their thoughts down, to answer a series of questions or, simply, to tell their story. But, whichever way is used, notes should be made. This timely intervention will catch difficulties early so they may be acted upon before they become problems. Oftentimes, this feedback is simple and difficulties can be easily rectified in the last two-thirds of the remaining time on placement. This work could form the basis for an evaluative research report. Evaluating a learning experience after the event can only improve the learning situation for the next student(s) if not for this one. It is also too far removed from the experience for the people involved to gain much learning from it.

Sometimes challenges are relatively simple. The student might not know what to do and difficulties are just happening in certain stages of the intervention process. Things like reading cues correctly or executing strategies effectively or establishing patient–client rapport might be the focus of what is going wrong. Maybe the students did not like to ask or maybe they do not realise they are not working well enough or safely enough. These difficulties can be resolved with more coaching, demonstrating, discussing and reflecting. It is when things have been left to become more serious that real problems emerge.

CAPTURING EMERGING PROBLEMS

When problems rather than difficulties arise then catching them and re-mediating them needs to happen quickly. Writing things down, as suggested above, clearly brings some measure of early diagnostic evidence to the situation. Writing immediate responses diffuses some of the negative feelings of frustration and can be cathartic. Writing is better than talking in this more serious situation as it has some degree of coherence. The writing does not have to be formal; it can flow freely or be put into note form. It does not have to be presented perfectly as the idea is to get the problem down on paper and out in the open. In my experience, the best way to do this is to write things down without considering grammar or spelling or any other aspect of formal writing that inhibits free expression.

But, when either side recognises that strong emotional feelings are involved, it helps to share your written response with others, discussing it with them, and considering the situation collectively. Only after a period of time (one day at least) should a response be made and then shared with each other. With this time lapse the whole situation can be viewed reflectively so that feelings as well as facts are recognised (Boud & Walker 1991). It is at this point in time that realisations as to the possible cause or causes can be pinpointed – but this will not occur unless there is some insight into the problems. The following sections illustrate, through practice examples and from the literature, some possible reasons for problems on placement. Less complicated examples will be presented first. Reading through these sections may bring new understandings to the challenge and so make it easier to go forward.

Having communication difficulties – is this the problem?

Although this heading sounds simple, problems with *the quality* of communication or with *the timing* of communication periods can be crucial factors. Communicating effectively in an educational way is an art (Alsop & Ryan 1996, Brown & Ryan 2003, Henry 1985). Whatever the adult learning literature says about being equal learning partners, with assessment looming at the end of the placement and with a judgement being made on the student's performance actual equality remains difficult to achieve. Furthermore, the student is only a part of the therapist/clinical educator's work. Creating a learning environment that is conducive to learning from each other needs considerable thought, planning and educational knowledge that is often greater than that which is received in short preparatory courses for placement educators.

Working on a learning contract together from the start can encourage both parties to formulate ground rules about how and when to ask questions. Some students are hesitant to ask directly or to ask in the midst of actual practice (Schön 1987). Ways of signalling help or of exiting the situation to think about what is occurring need to be discussed. Situated feedback directly *after* an occurrence enhances immediate learning, and, if this is coupled with giving considered feedback during supervision or when viewing a debriefing videotape, then deeper levels of understanding are reinforced (Fish & Twinn, 1997).

From the student's perspective, knowing the criteria by which you are being judged helps in negotiating learning situations so that a measure of self-assessment of performance starts occurring early in the placement. The criteria and outcomes should be worked out and agreed together and they can also be re-adjusted as the placement progresses.

Having different learning styles or levels – is this the problem?

Many recent studies have highlighted the differences between education and training (Higgs & Edwards 1999, Higgs & Titchen 2001, Ryan 2001, 2003, Taylor 1999). It is known that present ways of educating students are very different from those used in the past and this is so in some schools and disciplines more than others. If the therapist/clinical educator came from an era where training was the norm, and if that person has not experienced other ways of learning since then, it is likely that there could be dissonance between each other's styles of learning. The concept of facilitation as opposed to that of imparting information or "telling" will be at odds. A student, Anna, described how she felt when she was constantly "told" things by her educator:

> *She was an absolute font of knowledge, she knew everything about – about everything. Never mind OT but sort of general knowledge as well. But it got to the point that it detracted from my sort of feelings about myself because you never, I never felt that anything I said was original because she had already thought of it or she already knew ten articles about it in journals. She knew exactly where to look so you just thought – what's the point of, why am I thinking this.*

(Ryan 2003).

However, in a contradiction to the scenario above, uncertain students may feel that they need to be "told" what to do, especially in critical and difficult situations. Both these possibilities could cause problems if the factors are not appreciated and understood as each person will have different needs and expectations of the other.

Another difference in learning styles is, perhaps, more simple to deal with. The four styles proposed by Honey & Mumford (2003) – the activist, the theorist, the reflector and the pragmatist – reveal ways of thinking and working that could be construed as incompatible if they are not understood or recognised. Either party may have "black and white" thinking while the other needs to ponder, reflect and conceptualise information in an elongated process-led fashion. While I believe that learning styles do not need to be matched, they do need to be respected. Adjustments to these ways of information-processing will need to be made. During induction it could be useful to talk about each other's preferred ways of learning. Some people are more visual, some like asking people questions, while others prefer to study first and ask questions later.

Having different starting points – is this the problem?

One of the most frequent yet misunderstood problems on placement arises from a mismatch between the learner's and the clinical educator's levels of "knowing". Each is operating on a different plane and consequently has different expectations of the other and, therefore, different starting points. Perhaps the clinical educator expects students to know much more than they actually do. This situation often arises when the levels of learning and expectations of knowing are at odds with each other. From clinical reasoning studies of the last decade it is now well known that experienced therapists have different knowledge schemas from novice learners (Benner 1984, Boshuizen & Schmidt 2000). Mattingly & Fleming (1994) explain that experienced therapists have assimilated their knowledge in what the literature terms a *tacit way.* This knowledge is chunked or clustered together and so experts are able to see seemingly obvious problems in clinical situations. Slater (1991) explains the differences between the two parties:

> *Experienced therapists appear to have an ability to tease out relevant infor-*
> *mation from an abundance of complex data and make sense from it, while*
> *novice therapists have tremendous difficulties knowing where to start, what*
> *to do, and how to put it all together.*

Given the above situation the educator does need to understand how clinical reasoning is built up in a novice therapist. Knowing about this, the clinical educator will allow more *time* for the learner to work out what to do; he/she will help to *make links with prior experiences or theoretical knowledge* in order to enhance comparative practice (Ryan 2000). Talking about levels of knowledge and each other's expectations while getting to know each other and during the formulation of the learning contract will help this. Mary's story, below, illustrates the difficulties she was experiencing on her neurological placement:

> *Mary was not clear if there was any dementia as she had previously had*
> *experience in her other placements working with this condition. She decided*
> *that it was the cognitive effect of the stroke that had affected her insight,*
> *problem solving and concentration, a combination of all the little things.*
> *She came to the conclusion that any assessment should be functional. And,*
> *when her lady started to do things she would talk to herself in order to con-*
> *centrate and Mary could hear her voice coming along the corridor. Other*
> *patients would put headphones on or turn away because she made such a*
> *noise. So she was quite isolated socially. Mary thought all this was so com-*
> *plicated; every time she dug down she discovered more. She felt that she*
> *could not apply the anatomy or physiology that she had learnt. She even*
> *started saying to herself, "I'm a good therapist, I'm going to get through*
> *this or at least half-way in the right direction." But what she was seeing she*
> *did not know how to recognise as anything meaningful. She was not sure*
> *if it was because her lady could not physically do it or if it was a mental*
> *problem. She said, "it completely threw me and I felt I was thrown in at the*
> *deep end".*

(Ryan 2003).

In this story Mary's clinical educator had assumed a level of knowledge and pathways of connected knowing that were simply not there. Furthermore, this educator had given Mary a "difficult" stroke patient in order to "stretch her" although Mary had not had a neurological placement before. It would have been preferable to start with someone with a relatively simple stroke and once the basics were understood only then to progress to working with people with complex manifestations of a cerebral vascular accident. The clinical educator had not supported Mary nor had she taken the time to work with Mary. She only gave ideas later in post-session discussions and Mary still did not understand or see the connections as this feedback was not in situ. This placement was a disaster, resulting in Mary wishing to leave the profession.

Recent research in physiotherapy (Potter 2001) has presented an alternative idea about the levels of knowledge of the two parties. Contrary to popular opinion Potter (2001) has shown that if clinical educators are recently qualified, within the last 18 months or two years, then their knowledge schemas are more similar to that of the student. They are only beginning to mass their knowledge into chunks and it has not become tacit yet. Then, if they work out interventions together with the student so that they make their reasoning transparent, this is often more beneficial for the student's learning. Alternatively for the student, having a peer on the placement at the same time gives other possibilities for working together and supporting each other's learning. Both these possibilities happen because each is at a similar level of understanding and their knowledge schemas are better matched (Molineux 1999).

Working with different knowledges – is this the problem?

During the past few years, work emanating from Australia and the UK in nursing, occupational therapy and physiotherapy, has laid emphasis on using different forms of knowledge (McKay & Ryan 1995, Higgs & Titchen 2001). Previously, health disciplines talked about and used only book knowledge or propositional knowledge. Now, it is recognised that a wealth of life experience and personal and intuitive knowledge could usefully be used and recognised in practice, providing that it is orchestrated well by the facilitator and that it is relevant. This new paradigm of professional learning sits outwith the prior positivistic, scientific knowledge and is situated in the post-modern era where there is a greater understanding of the vagaries and frailties of human responses to therapeutic interventions. Clearly, this mismatch of professional understanding is complicated and can only be relieved by further study of a deeper nature than a short course. Postgraduate education programmes are addressing these issues but many therapist/clinical educators are not operating at this level. Recently qualified clinical educators are more likely to have encountered this phenomenon in their undergraduate courses as the use of narratives and other qualitative work is now used more frequently in some disciplines.

Using different frameworks or schemas – is this the problem?

Another aspect of learning that differentiates present-day students from those qualified one or two decades ago and who have not updated their knowledge is the use of theoretical frameworks or conceptual models of practice. When health science colleges moved into the university sector their aim was to educate a more scholarly student. Furthermore, this move happened in different decades in different countries. Nowadays, there is a greater emphasis on journal reading and abstracting knowledge at, according to some therapists, the expense of skill-based abilities (Creek & Feaver 1993). Previously, a biomedical framework was taught whereas now a variety of more holistic frameworks are presented. The art of client-centred practice is to decide what framework(s) is best to use in the current situation (Hagedorn 1995, Sumsion 1999). The story below illustrates this problem and the resulting confusion:

> *Hazel thought about her practice in a biomedical way. It was the way she had been taught and was the only way that she worked. In the past year while she was working with people with profound learning disabilities she*

had designed a programme that used behavioural modification feedback to assist the person to reach forward to grasp a hairbrush. This was painstaking work and the results were slow and minimal. Peter came on this placement just before he was due to qualify. He had been educated to look at practice holistically. He disagreed with the entire programme as he thought the therapist's time could be more productive if she worked with the carers to improve the clients' daily routines and living schedules. Peter was using a completely different and incompatible framework to that of his supervisor. This problem had to be mediated by the university staff as it was apparently irreconcilable to either person. One could not see into or understand the other's world. Both were 'stuck' in their frameworks.

(Personal communication 1996).

However, there is another side to this problem of theoretical understanding. In my research (Ryan 2003) I found that some students who studied in a problem-based learning curriculum had sought out information that they believed was relevant. But, they had omitted to learn the solid scientific foundation of knowledge to help them to make connections between what they were seeing in actuality and what was happening physiologically and neurologically. Examining the knowledge bases used in a particular practice context in great detail is a very useful exercise that a service could prepare before a student arrives on placement (Alsop & Ryan 1996). I have found that this exercise is perceived as long and laborious and I suggest different members of staff prepare each section. This will reduce the tedium, make explicit the knowledge bases and theories that are being used in that setting and promote a focus for collaborative discussions as gaps in knowledge may also surface during the exercise. The framework is presented in Table 8.1.

All the above scenarios and Table 8.1 illustrate the importance of both facilitator (clinical educator) and student discussing, working and learning together from a point in time that starts even before the beginning of the placement. Looking from the stance of equality, it is clear that current students could bring much knowledge to the practice situation, providing they are allowed and given the opportunity to do so.

Behaving differently – is this the problem?

Literature from psychology and pedagogical education informed work on supervision conducted by Frum & Opacich (1987). These authors found that there were stages in behavioural development of a learner that could often be the cause of problems. These stages are stability, confusion and integration. These three areas are not unlike parts of the learning cycle, where disorientation and confusion result from learning and seeing new things in different and "other" ways. Table 8.2 highlights the various attributes for each stage.

Reading through this work and understanding where the two players are in the problem can be very beneficial. It may not be the student who is "stuck" in his/her thinking. This work illustrates how a learning contract may not be working or it shows how the relationship may be seen from either party. This work is extremely useful. The authors then formed a matrix with other qualities of a learner's needs, such as competence, emotional

Table 8.1   Examining contextual knowledge

Definitions used in this setting	Client information	Family and social structures	Work environment	Professional and personal characteristics
List abbreviations used in notes	Medical knowledge base	Family options	Physical environment	Synthesising research findings and new information
	Specific knowledge base	Learning styles suitable for family	Social environment	Ability to observe
	Influencing factors	Client–family interactions	Other persons working in this environment	Ability to bring about change
	Knowledge of unique factors	Transitions from practice to home	Organisational culture	Understanding interpersonal skills
	Knowledge of approaches and theories	Specific skills related to family (culture/attitudes/ interests/strengths/ priorities/preferred communication styles/skills family need to develop)	Specific skills in adapting the environment	Academic interest and commitment
	Specific skills	Interactions and interpretations		Provisions from educational programmes
	Inter/multidiscipline plans and discharge	Adaptations to the intervention process		Insight into pro-fessional limitations
				Ability to value and collaborate with others
				Ability to articulate one's values, attitudes and reasoning

awareness, autonomy, identity, respect for individual differences, purpose and direction, personal motivation and professional ethics. Making a profile of the learner by using this matrix can be another way of examining a challenging problem. This can be done together or as a form of self-assessment.

ANALYSING AND INTERPRETING THE PROBLEM

The sections above have given examples and illustrations of some of the likely causes of problems on placement. There are many others but the ones outlined above could be those that are more profound and fundamental to the learning situation. The challenge is to analyse, interpret and diagnose the situation. This is a starting point.

Analysing

As notes have been written down it becomes easier to do an analysis. Read through both the sets of individual notes that were written about the problem. Then read through the sections above, highlighting any words, phrases or instances that appear to match. These can be colour-coded to match sections.

Table 8.2 Stages of development (adapted from the text of Frum & Opacich 1987)

Stability	Confusion	Integration
• Initial learning stage • Learners are unaware of what they don't know (naïve, innocent) • Learners may be "stuck" in their knowledge • A false sense of security develops • Thinking can be rigid, simplistic, black and white • Problems are seen through a narrow tunnel • Learners may devalue what they know • Learning needs should come from another (dependency) • Educator may be idealised or be seen as irrelevant • This is a time of rest, latency and potentiality • Mutual goal-setting can be difficult	• This stage is characterised by instability, disorganisation, conflict and disruption – a stage of unfreezing • Thinking in a black and white mode is no longer sufficient – awareness that something is not right happens • Fluctuation between being positive and feeling negative • Opposing attitudes to the supervisor prevail – either as all-knowing or inadequate (learner can respond with anger or disappointment) • Learner may be in an emotional turmoil, and so may the educator if he/she gets caught up with feelings	• "Calm after the storm" • Reorganisation, integration and flexibility from the new knowledge perspectives • Greater cognitive understanding • Clarity and wholeness prevail • Creative flexible views are seen as possibilities • Educator is seen as being more realistic with weaknesses as well as strengths • Educator is seen as a peer and colleague who can help develop him/her • Learner takes an active role in the learning process. Expectations of others are more reasonable • There is a fluidity of thought and work is seen as a process, not a product • A commitment to professional development happens • This process does not end with formal education

Interpreting

Interpretation is subjective and it does need to be treated with caution. Having done an analysis and being aware of personal biases, as well as having other parties involved in the discussions and readings, should bring insight into the challenging situation. It is at this stage that it may be possible to make a diagnosis.

WORKING THROUGH THE PROBLEM

This section will present different ways that an awkward challenge can be handled once an idea of the diagnosis has been formed. Likely ways could be:

1. *Working it out together*. This could be in the form of writing down each other's present perspectives; discussing and reading each other's work; changing seats by trying to understand the other's point of view; making a new learning contract together and re-deciding on short- and long-term goals and mutually agreed criteria for making decisions about each aspect of the contract; deciding when to review this new scenario.
2. *Bringing in another party*. This person could be from the same setting or from the university – this will help to ensure equal rights and representation for both sides. This person should be appraised of both sides of the situation either by looking at the prior work or by talking to both parties alone and together. Reflective frames of reference could be useful tools to assist in this process.

3. *Stopping the placement*. This solution is more extreme but sometimes it takes great courage from all the parties concerned to acknowledge that it is the best course of action. Transferring to another venue immediately or re-doing the placement at another site on another occasion are the options available to the learner. If this happens then the third party involved should make sure that the feelings and situation from both sides have been resolved to a satisfactory level so that there is less likelihood of the challenge happening again.

4. *Disclosing information at the following site*. The situation of whether to keep confidence at the new site or whether to disclose the previous situation at the new place brings in the question of ethics as well as the question of safety. This is a delicate decision. It is preferable to be guided by professional bodies, the literature and by having a process in place in the university regulations. Much depends of the cause of the problem.

5. *Bringing in a mentor to work with both parties*. This may happen after the challenging situation so that perceptions and experiences can be worked through by someone not connected or involved in the previous encounter. Rather than analysing the past challenge it is advisable to move on and to learn ways of understanding the encounter. Again, reflective frameworks help this to happen.

6. *Writing up the account*. For all the people involved in this drama, writing about the encounter can be a cathartic exercise but it can also become a case study where people beyond the situation can learn from and develop. This could form a book chapter (Brown & Ryan 2003, Molineux 1999) or a journal article (McKay & Ryan 1995) or a topic for research (Ryan 2003).

CONCLUSION

This chapter has highlighted some of the root causes for difficulties and problems on clinical placements and it is obvious that these are complex. Oftentimes the various players are not aware of these subtleties, hence the need to elaborate on them and to publish them so that they may be discussed in open forums when clinical educators are learning how to facilitate students' knowledge development. Also, from the opposite side, this chapter has been written to enable students to tease out any difficult situation they find themselves in.

REFERENCES

Alsop A, Ryan S (eds) 1996 Making the most of fieldwork education: a practical approach. Chapman and Hall, Cheltenham

Benner P 1984 From novice to expert: excellence and power in clinical nursing practice. Addison-Wesley, Menlo Park, California

Best D, Edwards H 2001 Learning together: fostering professional craft knowledge development in clinical placements. In: Higgs J, Titchen A (eds) Practice knowledge and expertise in the health professions. Butterworth-Heinemann, Oxford

Boshuizen H, Schmidt H 2000 The development of clinical reasoning expertise. In: Higgs J, Jones M (eds) Clinical reasoning in the health professions, 2nd edn. Butterworth-Heinemann, Oxford

Boud D, Walker D 1991 In the midst of experience: developing a model to aid learners and facilitators. Paper presented at the National Conference on Experiential Learning: Explorations of Good Practice. University of Surrey, 16–18 July 1991

Brown G, Ryan S 2003 Enhancing reflective abilities: interweaving reflection into practice. In: Brown G, Esdaile S, Ryan S (eds) Becoming an advanced healthcare practitioner. Butterworth-Heinemann, Oxford

Creek J, Feaver S 1993 Models for practice in occupational therapy: part 1, defining terms. British Journal of Occupational Therapy 56(1):4–27

Fish D, Twinn S 1997 Quality clinical supervision in the health care professions: principled approaches to practice. Butterworth-Heinemann, Oxford

Frum D, Opacich K 1987 Supervision: the development of therapeutic competence. American Occupational Therapy Association, Rockville, MD

Hagedorn R 1995 Occupational therapy: perspectives and processes. Churchill Livingstone, Edinburgh

Henry J 1985 Using feedback and evaluation effectively in clinical supervision model for interaction characteristics and strategies. Physical Therapy 65(3):354–357

Higgs J, Edwards H (eds) 1999 Educating beginning practitioners: challenges for health professional education. Butterworth-Heinemann, Oxford

Higgs J, Titchen A (eds) 2001 Professional practice in health, education and the creative arts. Blackwell Science, Oxford

Honey P, Mumford A 2003 The learning styles questionnaire – 80 item version. Peter Honey Publications, Maidenhead

Knowles M, Holton III E, Swanson, R (eds) 1998 The adult learner. Gulf Publishing, Houston

McAllister L 2003 Using adult learning theories: facilitating others' learning in professional practice settings. In: Brown G, Esdaile S, Ryan S (eds) Becoming an advanced healthcare practitioner. Butterworth-Heinemann, Oxford

McKay E, Ryan S 1995 Clinical reasoning through story telling: examining a student's case story on a fieldwork placement. British Journal of Occupational Therapy 58:234–238

Mattingly C, Fleming M H 1994 Clinical reasoning: forms of inquiry in a therapeutic practice. F A Davis, Philadelphia

Molineux M 1999 Making changes: a clinical reasoning journey. In: Ryan S E, McKay E A (eds) Thinking and reasoning in therapy: narratives from practice. Stanley Thornes, Cheltenham

Potter J 2001 Visualisation in research and data analysis. In: Dadds M, Hart S (eds) Doing practitioner research differently. Routledge, London

Quality Assurance Agency 1998 Higher quality, nos. 3 & 4. Quality Assurance Agency, Gloucester

Ryan S 1996 The process of supervision. In: Alsop A, Ryan S (eds) Making the most of fieldwork education: a practical approach. Chapman and Hall, Cheltenham

Ryan S 2000 Teaching clinical reasoning during fieldwork education to occupational therapists. In: Higgs J, Jones M (eds) Clinical reasoning in the health professions, 2nd edn. Butterworth-Heinemann, Oxford

Ryan S 2001 Perspective on widening university access: critical voices of newly qualified occupational therapists. British Journal of Occupational Therapy 64(11):534–540

Ryan S 2003 Voices of newly graduated occupational therapists: their practice and educational stories. Unpublished doctoral thesis, University of East London

Schön D 1987 Educating the reflective practitioner. Jossey-Bass, San Francisco

Slater D 1991 Staff development through analysis of practice. American Journal of Occupational Therapy 45(11):1038–1044

Sumsion T 1999 Client-centred practice in occupational therapy: a guide to implementation. Churchill Livingstone, Edinburgh

Taylor C 1999 Occupational therapy: empowers or oppressors? A study of students' attitudes towards disabled people. Unpublished PhD thesis, Department of Sociology, University of Warwick

Chapter **9**

Clinical education and evidence-based practice

Megan Davidson

INTRODUCTION

Evidence-based practice (EBP) "is the acknowledgment of uncertainty followed by the seeking, appraising and implementation of new knowledge. It enables clinicians to openly accept that there may be different, and possibly more effective, methods of care than those they are currently employing" (Dawes et al 1999, preface).

The central aim of EBP is to optimise outcomes for patients by selecting interventions that have the greatest chance of success, and avoiding those that have little, if any, chance of success. EBP requires clinicians to reflect critically on current practice and to change practice as advances in knowledge indicate that some treatment choices, on average, are more likely to benefit patients than others. It also maintains the centrality of the patient's values and preferences in the clinical encounter. Sackett et al (2002, p. 1) define evidence-based medicine as "the integration of best research evidence with clinical expertise and patient values". Patients bring their own values and preferences to the clinical encounter while health professionals bring their clinical expertise. The research evidence is increasingly available via the internet, to both patients and professionals, as summaries packaged in the form of systematic reviews and evidence-based clinical practice guidelines. EBP can be seen as a "paradigm shift" from expert or opinion-based practice, and has the potential to increase patients' involvement in clinical decision-making and to improve health outcomes.

The "research evidence" component of EBP has attracted by far the greatest amount of attention, so much so that the other aspects – clinician's expertise and patient's preferences – tend to be overshadowed. The term "research-enhanced health care" has been proposed to move the focus from the research evidence to the patient (Haynes et al 2002).

ATTITUDES ARE POSITIVE BUT KNOWLEDGE AND SKILLS ARE UNDERDEVELOPED

The literature consistently reports that the majority of allied health professionals hold positive attitudes about EBP. A survey by Metcalfe et al (2001) of four allied health professions (dieticians, occupational therapists, physiotherapists, speech and language therapists) in England reported that almost all respondents (97%) agreed with the statement "research is important for professional practice" and only 5% said that "finding and reading research is of no interest". A similar finding by Upton (1999) was that more than 80% of respondents representing four allied health professions (podiatrists, occupational therapists, physiotherapists, speech and language therapists) in Wales agreed that "EBP is fundamental to professional practice".

Positive attitudes toward EBP have also been reported amongst general practitioners (McColl et al 1998), medical specialists (Olatunbosun et al 1998, Veness et al 2003), nurses (Retsas 2000) and physiotherapists (Jette et al 2003). While the majority of respondents in these surveys reported positive attitudes, some respondents also reported negative attitudes. Upton (1999) reported around 10% of respondents thought EBP was a "fad". Jette et al (2003) found that younger therapists had somewhat more positive attitudes to EBP than older therapists. Strauss & McAlister (2000) classified the common criticisms of EBP as limitations or misperceptions. Limitations are the lack of good or consistent evidence in many areas of practice, the challenges of applying evidence to individual patients, the need for clinicians to develop new skills and the limitations imposed by time and resource availability. Common misperceptions included that EBP is a "recipe" approach to health care, that EBP ignores the individual patient's preferences, that the true motive of EBP is to reduce health care costs, and that only systematic reviews and clinical trials are considered "evidence".

In contrast to generally positive attitudes, health professionals' self-ratings indicate that knowledge and skills in database searching and critical appraisal of research are limited. In one survey (Metcalfe et al 2001), 66% of therapists surveyed thought they were not capable of evaluating research. In another survey (Upton 1999) between 40% and 60% of podiatrists, speech and language therapists, occupational therapists and physiotherapists rated their overall knowledge of EBP as low. Therapists rated themselves relatively low on technical skills such as the ability to perform electronic literature searches, their research skills, the ability to convert information needs into a research question and to analyse critically the evidence against set standards.

Pollock et al (2000) surveyed nurses and therapists in stroke rehabilitation settings in Scotland and reported that confidence in ability to understand literature ranged from 42% (for occupational therapists) to 70% (for physiotherapists). Between 63% and 77% of respondents in each professional group agreed they needed further training in critical appraisal. Another study

(Closs & Lewin 1998) reported 61% of therapists surveyed rated the therapist's inability to evaluate the quality of the research as a substantial barrier to EBP. The inability of therapists to understand statistical analysis appears to be a substantial barrier to interpreting the clinical relevance of research (Pollock et al 2000, Metcalfe et al 2001). Jette et al (2003) reported that level of training in EBP, use of databases and confidence in searching for and evaluating research was associated with younger physical therapists with fewer years since graduation.

The relatively recent development of critical appraisal of research against set standards and the easy availability of evidence delivered online mean that students may be more "expert" than many clinical educators in the domains of searching for and evaluating the evidence. However, the clinical educator is likely to possess a more highly developed level of clinical expertise and skills in eliciting patient preferences. This provides the potential for the student–educator relationship to be highly complementary.

THE EBP PROCESS

Sackett et al (2000) proposed that EBP could be broken down into five steps:

1. Identify a knowledge need and formulate an answerable clinical question.
2. Locate the best available evidence.
3. Critically evaluate the evidence.
4. Integrate the evidence with patient's unique biology, preferences and values.
5. Evaluate steps 1–5.

Step 1: Identify a knowledge need and formulate an answerable clinical question

Step 1 requires both the recognition of a gap in knowledge and the formulation of a clinical question. Sackett et al suggest that an answerable clinical question is one that specifies the *patient* or *problem*, the *intervention* and perhaps a *comparison* intervention, and the *outcome* of interest (remembered by the mnemonic PICO). The formulation of the question in this format facilitates the second step, locating the evidence, by providing a narrow, focused set of search terms. Poorly formulated, vague questions may result in an unsuccessful step 2 in that a large volume of literature is located and time-consuming "browsing" for relevant studies fails to locate relevant material, or yields an unusable volume of material.

Because there are an infinite number of questions that could be generated, a judgement must be made as to whether the question is sufficiently important to warrant the effort of continuing to the next step. High-priority questions generally involve high-volume, high-cost conditions and treatments.

Step 2: Locate the best available evidence

The time and effort expended on step 2 depend on the speed with which an answer is required, and the information resources available. The search for the best available evidence might range from a search for "pre-appraised" evidence only, such as systematic reviews and evidence-based clinical practice guidelines, or may extend to a search for individual research reports. In some organisations, clinicians may be able to outsource steps 2 and 3, receiving a comprehensive report from the reviewing service.

Step 3: Critically appraise the evidence

Critical appraisal of the evidence seeks to answer three questions (Sackett et al 2000):

1. Is the evidence valid?
2. Is the valid evidence important?
3. Can I apply the valid, important evidence to my client?

The first of the critical appraisal questions requires a critical evaluation of the study's methodology, its internal validity, to determine whether the conclusions are believable. Critical appraisal checklists for evaluating studies of treatment, prevention, prognosis, diagnosis or screening, and economic evaluations can be found online. Such checklists allow the reader to evaluate a study against widely accepted quality criteria. Pre-appraised sources (systematic reviews and evidence-based clinical practice guidelines) can save the considerable effort of doing one's own appraisal of the original studies. Quality checklists are also available for evaluating the validity of systematic reviews and clinical practice guidelines.

A researcher seeking to answer a particular question must select an appropriate research design. The research design considered best suited to questions about therapy, prevention, aetiology or harm is a high-quality randomised controlled trial. For questions about diagnosis or prognosis cohort studies are suitable. For questions about the meaning and experience of illness qualitative designs are required. Evidence hierarchies or levels of evidence have been developed that place systematic reviews as the highest level of evidence, with individual study designs ranked in order of the confidence with which they are able to contribute to the answer. Expert opinion, if included at all, is ranked lowest, but in the absence of higher levels of evidence (which may often be the case for allied health therapies) consensus of expert opinion may be all that is available.

Quality appraisal checklists have been developed for qualitative research designs, but no evidence hierarchy has yet been proposed for qualitative designs. A systematic review remains the logical "top level" of evidence. The many qualitative theoretical frameworks and research designs that seek to describe, explain, interpret and understand the meaning of social phenomena as experienced by individuals in their contexts may not lend themselves to a hierarchy in which one design is considered to yield more confident conclusions than others. The recent development of integrated systematic reviews of controlled trials and qualitative evidence (Thomas et al 2004) may be the way forward in providing useful and clinically informative evidence summaries.

The second critical appraisal question, "is the valid evidence important?", assumes that evidence that is judged to be invalid (to have fatal methodological flaws) should not be used to inform clinical decision-making. The judgement of whether the evidence is important requires skills in interpreting research results and clinical understanding of the outcomes likely to be valued by patients (Herbert 2000a, 2000b).

The third question, "can I apply the valid, important evidence to my client?" refers to the external validity of the study. Put more simply, this question asks: "is my client like the participants in this study?" If the client is not represented in the sample (for example, people like this have been explicitly excluded from the study sample) then the evidence cannot be applied to them.

Step 4: Integrate the evidence with patient's unique biology, preferences and values

Clinical expertise and experience are essential to this step. Research evidence provides an indication of the "average" response to treatment, but therapists are working with individuals who may respond better or worse than the average. A patient's unique biology, comorbidity and socioeconomic status must be taken into account when considering the likely outcomes for the individual. The patient's expectations, beliefs, values, fears and preferences are given a high priority. A treatment plan is developed in consultation with the patient who is sufficiently informed of the potential benefits and harms of any particular treatment option to make an informed choice. A patient-centred approach requires the therapist to begin by eliciting the patient's preferences, by asking patients what they want and expect from treatment, before presenting treatment options and strategies (Bridson et al 2003).

Step 5: Evaluate steps 1–5

This step asks the clinician to reflect on the processes, abilities and outcomes for patients of steps 1 through 4. Reflection may identify professional development needs (such as computer skills or database search skills) or insights gained from the process. A logical extension of this step is to share the information, skills and insights gained from the process with colleagues.

CHALLENGES FACING EBP

EBP has revolutionised the way in which research is evaluated. Before the development of standardised methods of locating and appraising the quality of evidence, clinicians were restricted to reading individual research reports or narrative (non-systematic) reviews of the literature. The systematic review seeks to minimise or eliminate biases (such as self-confirming bias) that are inevitable in the narrative review.

Most of the work to date has focused on systematically reviewing the research evidence on treatment efficacy. The Cochrane Library contains only systematic reviews of the research evidence on the efficacy of treatment and prevention interventions. The Cochrane Collaboration has announced that systematic reviews of diagnostic tests will be included in future (Deeks et al 2003).

The model established by systematic reviews – the systematic approach of locating and critically evaluating the evidence – can equally be applied to research designs that answer clinical questions other than those relating to treatment efficacy. A benefit of the systematic evaluation of research has led to internationally agreed reporting standards for some research designs – the CONSORT statement for randomised controlled trials (Moher et al 2001), the STARD statement for studies of diagnostic tests (Bossuyt et al 2003). The AGREE standards have also been widely adopted as a framework for evaluating clinical practice guidelines (AGREE Collaboration Writing Group 2003). It is likely that standards for other quantitative and qualitative research designs will follow.

A central assumption of EBP is that it results in better patient outcomes, but there is currently little evidence to support this assumption (Norman 1999). The main challenges to be faced if EBP is to deliver on the promise of better patient outcomes are that:

- there is a lack of good-quality evidence in many areas of practice
- changing practice, or getting evidence into practice, is difficult.

EVIDENCE-BASED EDUCATION AND SUPERVISION

The systematic review has also been applied to questions not directly related to patient care. For example, the effectiveness of different interventions for changing health professionals' behaviour or improving professional practice (Bero et al 1998, NHS Centre for Reviews and Dissemination 1999) and the effectiveness of teaching critical appraisal skills (Hyde et al 2000). One systematic review has appeared on supervisory practice (Ellis et al 1996). It is systematic in that it describes explicit methods of locating all relevant studies and has explicit inclusion and exclusion criteria and multiple independent raters. The findings of this systematic review and two more recent narrative reviews (Goodyear & Bernard 1998, Kilminster & Jolly 2000) are shown in Table 9.1.

All three reviews agree that the methodological quality of published research on supervision efficacy is generally poor. Fong & Malone (1994) also noted the poor quality of counselling research in their analysis of the research papers published in one journal in 1992. Poor methodology results

Table 9.1 Reviews of research evidence of supervisory practices

Author and year	Title	Discipline	Type of review	Studies included	Conclusion
Ellis et al 1996	Clinical supervision research from 1981 to 1993: a methodological critique	Counselling	Systematic	2,017 potential articles located; 144 studies were included	Methodological quality of research is very poor
Goodyear & Bernard 1998	Clinical supervision: lessons from the literature	Counselling	Narrative	Not stated	No evidence from comparative studies of supervisory models
Kilminster & Jolly 2000	Effective supervision in clinical practice settings: a literature review	Medicine, nursing, social work, teaching, psychology and counselling	Narrative	300 papers and books	Little theoretical or empirical basis for current supervisory practices

in studies of very low internal validity and therefore the conclusions of such studies are not credible.

Goodyear & Bernard (1998) suggested there were three major barriers to determining the effectiveness of supervisory models:

1. confusion in the definitions of "supervision" and "training"
2. an absence of comparative studies (due to lack of theories, supervision protocols and the need to protect clients)
3. reliance on trainee satisfaction as the outcome of interest.

Ellis et al (1996) identified the most common research errors as:

- low statistical power (small sample size)
- failure to adjust for multiple tests
- use of unreliable measures
- sampling errors.

It seems that at present the research evidence does not allow us to draw conclusions about the comparative efficacy of supervisory models.

Kilminster & Jolly (2000, p. 827) suggested that "the supervision relationship is probably the single most important factor for the effectiveness of supervision, more important than the supervisory methods used". Supervision is an "interpersonal exchange" and as such it is a complex phenomenon for which "adequate research methodologies have yet to be established" (Kilminster & Jolly 2000, p. 828).

DEVELOPING AN EBP CULTURE

Clinical educators are important role models for students. Clinical educators' attitudes, beliefs and behaviours are observed by students and influence their professional development. Behaviours that students acquire at university but that are not valued and reinforced in the clinical setting are unlikely to be continued. For students to value EBP and the skills learned in their university studies, they need to see the relevance of these skills to patient care. A key starting point of EBP is to recognise a knowledge gap and to seek to fill that gap. An EBP culture is one where even very experienced clinicians recognise gaps in their knowledge and examine their clinical practice in the light of emerging research evidence.

The size and type of the workplace, the mix and experience of staff and access to resources impose constraints on suitable strategies for developing an EBP culture. The following lists provide a starting place for reflection on how clinical educators and workplaces can actively engage in a process of developing an EBP culture.

The following attributes have been identified as contributing to the development of an EBP culture in individuals and organisations:

- patient-centred practice
- ability to recognise gaps in knowledge
- willingness to examine current practice
- willingness to change practice
- valuing of evidence over opinion.

> **Box 9.1   Learning resources**
>
> **Centre for Evidence-Based Medicine**
> http://www.cebm.net/ (online learning resources covering the five steps of EBP)
>
> **Critical Appraisal Skills Programme Learning Resources**
> http://www.phru.nhs.uk/casp/resourcescasp.htm (offers a range of EBP learning resources)
>
> **Dawes et al 1999**
> *Evidence-Based Practice: A primer for health care professionals*, Churchill Livingstone, Edinburgh (one of many basic texts available)
>
> **Greenhalgh T 1997**
> *How to Read a Paper: The basics of evidence-based medicine.* BMJ, London (the book of the series of "How to read a paper" articles that appeared in BMJ in 1997)
>
> **Netting the evidence**
> http://www.shef.ac.uk/~scharr/ir/netting/ (provides comprehensive links to EBP-related sites)
>
> **Physiotherapy Evidence Database (PEDro)**
> http://www.pedro.fhs.usyd.edu.au/index.html (an online tutorial on evaluating the validity and importance of clinical research)

Some suggested strategies for developing an EBP culture are to:

- allocate time for updating knowledge
- provide adequate computer and internet access
- provide access to key databases and journals
- provide access to EBP self-learning resources (Box 9.1)
- identify and apply high-quality evidence-based clinical practice guidelines
- train staff in searching and critical appraisal skills
- set up an EBP journal club (a forum for identifying important clinical questions, sharing the results of searching and the critical appraisal of evidence; a detailed description of an EBP journal club can be found in Sackett et al 2000, p. 198)
- develop a collection of critically appraised topics (CATs – a CAT is a summary of the evidence and an answer to the question)
- develop a research culture by:
    - inviting researchers to present seminars
    - developing relationships with researchers/universities
    - collecting data for multi-site research projects
    - benchmarking outcomes for clinical groups against results in clinical trials
    - supporting staff to undertake research-based higher degrees.

Strategies that have been suggested for teaching EBP in clinical settings include:

- plan and structure EBP activities
- help students to formulate answerable clinical questions

- ask students to search for and evaluate evidence and report their findings
- be a co-learner with the student
- help the student accept that there are big gaps in the currently available evidence
- tolerate ambiguity (answers are rarely clear-cut)
- do not interpret lack of evidence as negative evidence
- discuss research and its relevance to practice
- assist students to integrate evidence with patient preferences and unique circumstances.

Although the amount of research evidence may vary considerably between professions, the development of an EBP culture allows practitioners to appreciate explicitly the extent to which current practice is based on evidence. In many cases a traditional or widespread clinical practice will be found not to be based on evidence, that is, there is either no evidence or the evidence is of such poor quality that no conclusions can be drawn from it. Such absence of evidence provides no reason to abandon the practice, but only indicates where research efforts need to be directed. In the absence of research evidence on which to base a decision to continue or abandon current practice, evidence of clinical effectiveness, provided by monitoring patient health outcomes with standardised assessment tools, provides some confidence that the intervention is justified.

REFERENCES

AGREE Collaboration Writing Group 2003 Development and validation of an international appraisal instrument for assessing the quality of clinical practice guidelines: the AGREE project. Quality and Safety in Health Care 12(1):18–23

Bero L A, Grilli R, Grimshaw J M et al on behalf of the Cochrane Effective Practice and Organisation of Care Review Group 1998 Getting the research findings into practice. Closing the gap between research and practice: an overview of systematic reviews of interventions to promote the implementation of research findings. British Medical Journal 317:465–468

Bossuyt P M, Reitsma JB, Bruns D E et al for the STARD steering group 2003 Towards complete and accurate reporting of studies of diagnostic accuracy: the STARD initiative. British Medical Journal 326: 41–44

Bridson J, Hammond C, Leach A, Chester M R 2003 Making consent patient centred. British Medical Journal 327:1159–1161

Closs S J, Lewin B J P 1998 Perceived barriers to research utilization: a survey of four therapies. British Journal of Therapy and Rehabilitation 5:151–155

Dawes M, Davies P, Gray A, Mant J, Seers K, Snowball R 1999 Evidence-based practice: a primer for health care professionals. Churchill Livingstone, Edinburgh

Deeks J, Gatsonis C, Clarke M, Neilson J 2003 Cochrane systematic reviews of diagnostic test accuracy. Cochrane Collaboration Methods Groups Newsletter 7:8–9. Online. Available: http://www.cochrane.de/newslett/MGNews_2003.pdf 5 Dec 2003

Ellis M V, Ladany N, Krengel M, Schult D 1996 Clinical supervision research from 1980 to 1993: a methodological critique. Journal of Counseling Psychology 43(1):35–50

Fong M L, Malone C M 1994 Defeating ourselves: common errors in counseling research. Counselor Education and Supervision 33:356–363

Goodyear R K, Bernard J M 1998 Clinical supervision: lessons from the literature. Counselor Education and Supervision 38:6–22

Haynes R B, Devereaux P J, Guyatt G H 2002 Physicians' and patients' choices in evidence based practice: evidence does not make decisions, people do. British Medical Journal 324:1350

Herbert R D 2000a How to estimate treatment effects from reports of clinical trials. I: Continuous outcomes. Australian Journal of Physiotherapy 46:229–235

Herbert R D 2000b How to estimate treatment effects from reports of clinical trials. II: Dichotomous outcomes. Australian Journal of Physiotherapy 46:309–313

Hyde C, Parkes J, Deeks J, Milne R 2000 Systematic review of effectiveness of teaching critical appraisal. UK national R&D programme: evaluating methods to promote the implementation of R&D. Project Reference 12-8

Jette D U, Bacon K, Batty C et al 2003 Evidence-based practice: beliefs, attitudes, knowledge, and behaviours of physical therapists. Physical Therapy 83:786–805

Kilminster S M, Jolly B C 2000 Effective supervision in clinical practice settings: a literature review. Medical Education 34(10):827–840

McColl A, Smith H, White P, Field J 1998 General practitioners' perceptions of the route to evidence based medicine: a questionnaire survey. British Medical Journal 316:361–365

Metcalfe C, Lewin R, Wisher S, Perry S, Bannigan K, Moffett J K 2001 Barriers to implementing the evidence base in four NHS therapies: dietitians, occupational therapists, physiotherapists, speech and language therapists. Physiotherapy 87:433–441

Moher D, Schulz K F, Altman D G for the CONSORT Group 2001 The CONSORT statement: revised recommendations for improving the quality of reports of parallel-group randomised trials. Lancet 357:1191–1194

NHS Centre for Reviews and Dissemination 1999 Getting evidence into practice. Effective Health Care Bulletin 5(1)

Norman G R 1999 Examining the assumptions of evidence-based medicine. Journal of Evaluation in Clinical Practice 5(2):139–147

Olatunbosun O A, Edouard L, Pierson R A 1998 Physicians' attitudes toward evidence based obstetric practice: a questionnaires survey. British Medical Journal 316:365–366

Pollock A S, Legg L, Langhorne P, Sellars C 2000 Barriers to achieving evidence-based stroke rehabilitation. Clinical Rehabilitation 14(6):611–617

Retsas A 2000 Barriers to using research evidence in nursing practice. Journal of Advanced Nursing 31:599–606

Sackett D L, Straus S E, Richardson W S, Rosenberg W, Haynes R B 2002 Evidence-based medicine. How to practise and teach EBM. Churchill Livingstone, Edinburgh

Strauss S E, McAlister F A 2000 Evidence-based medicine: a commentary on common criticisms. Canadian Medical Association Journal 163(7):837–841

Thomas J, Harden A, Oakley A et al 2004 Integrating qualitative research with trials in systematic reviews. British Medical Journal 328:1010–1012

Upton D 1999 Clinical effectiveness and EBP 2: attitudes of health-care professionals. British Journal of Therapy and Rehabilitation 6(1):26–90

Veness M, Rikard-Bell G, Ward J 2003 Views of Australian and New Zealand radiation oncologists and registrars about evidence-based medicine and their access to internet based sources of evidence. Australasian Radiology 47(4):409–415

Chapter 10

Ethics in clinical education

Louise Brown

INTRODUCTION

This chapter will explore how students and clinicians develop ethical competence. The role of the clinical educator in nurturing and assisting this development and the ethical issues related to the student/learner role within the clinical environment will be discussed. Ethical practice is a core consideration throughout clinical work and therefore is also central in clinical education. Some of the values and development of professional attitudes and socialisation within the workplace have already been considered (Chapters 5 and 6). In subsequent chapters issues relating to power in the supervision relationship and issues of confidentiality when collaborating in student supervision will be discussed. In fact, ethical considerations are relevant in all areas of clinical education.

When I work as a clinician and a clinical educator, there are numerous values and ethical issues that impact on my work. To be an effective guide of clinical development in others, I need to be aware of how my values and ethical interpretations of the clinical situation impact on my clinical reasoning and therapeutic presence. I need to reflect on these components of my practice in order to be able to model them and discuss them with my colleagues and students.

As you start to read this chapter, take a moment to reflect on five questions:

1. What is your role in the development of the student's ethical competence?

2. What are the *values and ethical standards or behaviours* that are expected or demonstrated in your workplace?
3. What are the *ethical issues and problems* that the student may encounter during a placement?
4. What ethical issues have you encountered or might you anticipate occurring during a student's clinical placement?
5. What have you done, or would you do, with a concern arising about an ethical matter during a student's placement?

DEFINITIONS

To commence this discussion, it is useful to ensure a shared understanding of some of the many terms that are used in discussing ethical practice in allied health.

Values and morals are culturally and individually developed broad notions of "right and proper" behaviours and beliefs. These are the beliefs that influence our decision-making and judgement in all areas of our lives. Our values might relate to justice in our dealings with others or to our sense of caring for people. Other values include respect for client rights and individual dignity, non-discrimination and objectivity (Speech Pathology Australia 2000). A source of potential difference in value judgements relates to the relative strength of people's views on two key ethical approaches (Beauchamp & Childress 1994). "Utilitarianism" is a term derived from the writings of Bentham, 1748–1832, and Mill, 1806–1873, and relates to doing good for the greatest number. "Deontological" or "obligation-based" practice is based on the writings of Kant, 1724–1804, and supports the notion of carrying out an action because it is intrinsically right. Thus, a clinician who believes it is best to maximise the general welfare of the majority may allocate budget to screening programmes, whereas a clinician with a stronger sense of moral duty towards each client may argue for an expensive procedure that will impact on only a small number of people.

Ethics is the study of the social behaviours, morals and values discussed above. This area of study is replete with complex terminology such as beneficence (do good), non-maleficence (do not do harm), veracity (tell the truth), fairness (justice), autonomy (self-determination) and professional integrity (fidelity). The application of these concepts in areas related to health care is the focus of biomedical ethics (Beauchamp & Childress 1994).

Professional etiquette is described as expected behaviours or conventions, for example, the professional role delineations in your agency (Johnson 1990, 1999). These expectations are determined by cultural, situational and professional factors. Professional etiquette may be thought of as the source of some of the Standards of Practice set out in mandatory Codes of Ethics (for example, rules of professional advertising and requirements for referrals).

Codes of professional ethics are "rules of practice [which] typically describe duties professionals must perform, conduct they must forgo and situations they must avoid" (Fulwinder 1996). They represent the combination of aspiration and prescription for "the cultivation of moral character" (Lichtenberg 1996), expectation for professional etiquette and sanctions for transgression (Fulwinder 1996, Speech Pathology Australia 2002).

Ethical behaviour or situations need to be differentiated from *ethical dilemmas*. The former refers to those occasions in which moral/ethical behaviour is normally demonstrated in the working day. Examples include respect for patient confidentiality and acceptance of culturally diverse values. Ethical dilemmas are situations in which moral, ethical or legal positions are unclear or in conflict. Examples include situations where the patient's wishes are at odds with evidence-based practice or where management of waiting lists (resource allocation) is difficult or controversial.

WHAT DO WE KNOW ABOUT MORAL AND ETHICAL DEVELOPMENT?

Some of the most interesting literature about moral development was written in the 1980s when a controversy emerged between Kohlberg and his colleague Gilligan. Kohlberg (1981) studied the moral development of a group of children for 15 years and identified an invariant and hierarchical sequence of six stages of moral development. His work has also resulted in the view that a sense of justice is a relatively universal moral principle (Johnson 1999).

Gilligan (1982) published a paper recognising that Kohlberg's results should not be generalised to females because his empirical study was conducted only with males. She challenged his notion of an invariant sequence and proposed that women undergo moral development in which similar morals are seen, but not in the invariant sequence described for males (Johnson 1999). Gilligan (1982) proposed that there are two major components of moral growth:

1. morality of rights and formal reasoning – the justice perspective as described by Kohlberg
2. morality of care and responsibility – the care perspective (Beauchamp & Childress 1994, Johnson 1999).

Recent studies have confirmed the importance of including both the care perspective and issues relating to justice in ethics education with speech pathology students (Kenny et al 2004, Smith 2004).

YOUR ROLE IN THE DEVELOPMENT OF THE STUDENT'S ETHICAL COMPETENCE

Students will arrive at your clinic keen to do the right thing, but perhaps not well equipped to meet the ethical demands of our increasingly complex clinical working lives. They will probably have been to classes in which codes of ethics and some standards of ethical behaviour have been discussed. They may have participated in discussions about the place of ethics in clinical reasoning (Chapparo & Ranker 2000, Ersser & Atkins 2000, Jones et al 2000, Ranker & Chapparo 2000, White 2001). To assist you in helping students to develop ethical clinical practice three approaches to this facilitation are outlined below.

The use of modelling

It has been claimed that, for many students, the greatest part of their learning and application of ethical practice has occurred in the clinical setting

(Davis & McKain 1975). Modelling is one key to how this learning is optimised: "Daily interaction with our students does more to develop their appropriate attitudes than any other form of teaching" (Davis & McKain 1975). Modelling with reflective discussion is particularly suited to the development of the morality of care and understanding discussed above.

Clinicians' ethical views and values are demonstrated for students in our interactions with staff, clients and the students themselves. A certain amount of learning therefore will occur by "osmosis" as students absorb the qualities of the interactions and exchanges which occur around them and consolidate areas they have learnt about before coming to the clinic. For example, when a clinician collaborates with the client in setting goals for therapy, principles of patient autonomy and respect are being modelled. These confirm what students have learnt in class.

Passive "osmosis", however, is insufficient and may lead to the student failing to develop the required ethical competencies. For example, if students in the situation above have not learnt about the notion of patient autonomy and how this philosophy differs from a paternalistic style, they may fail to learn anything about ethical practice from the clinician–patient discussion.

It has been claimed that practices failing to demonstrate ethical behaviour can lead to "ethical erosion" in students (Feudtner et al 1994). This erosion of the ethical beliefs students bring to the clinic may result from the students observing apparently unethical behaviour which is not discussed, and which appears to be accepted practice. For example:

1. In many settings, the (un)professional "shorthand" used is demeaning to the patient:
   - "Is the new patient a feed?"
   - "I've just seen the fracture in bed 21"
   - "He's nursing home."
2. Students may not be present to see the clinician asking the patient if they consent to being observed or treated by a student.

In some cases the behaviour observed may be flagrantly inappropriate. Brennan (2000) cites the larger than life (but unfortunately sometimes still true to life) Sir Lancelot Spratt, fictional consultant surgeon in the film "Doctor in the House" who, during a ward round, drew a large incision line on the belly of a terrified patient, saying: "Don't worry my good man; this is absolutely nothing to do with you."

These examples highlight the fact that the learning of ethics is too important to be thought of as an incidental outcome of participation in clinical experience. It is important for clinicians to reflect on the ethics and values that are entrenched in their own practice and then to discuss these reflections and observations with students. It is especially helpful when clinicians are prepared to discuss the positive examples of ethical practice and the occasions when ethical practice could be improved.

Using an ethical model or decision-making protocol

Lovett & Seedhouse (1990) captured the complexity of ethical health practice in a multifaceted and multicoloured grid. The major components of their

Table 10.1   Considerations within ethical practice (based on Lovett & Seedhouse 1990)

Level of practicality	Are resources available? Estimate the likely effectiveness and efficiency of action	What is the risk? Which codes of practice relate?	What is the degree of certainty of the evidence on which the action is taken (evidence-based practice) Are there disputed facts?	Is there a relevant law or legal precedent? Have you considered the wishes of others?
Level of consequences	Most beneficial outcome for the client	Most beneficial outcomes for one's self	Most beneficial outcome for a particular group	Most beneficial outcome for society
Level of duties	Keep promises (fidelity)	Tell the truth (veracity)	Minimise harm (non-maleficence)	Do most positive good (beneficence)
Basis of care	Respect persons equally (fairness)	Respect autonomy	Serve needs first (justice)	Create autonomy

Table 10.2   Considerations for ethical clinical practice for students

Level of clinical readiness	Has the student studied and had practical experience with this situation?	Does the student feel confident and prepared?	What is the likelihood the student may cause harm for the patient? and the client?	Is it likely that this will be a positive experience for the student?

grid are included in Table 10.1. You can use this sort of model working with students for identifying and analysing the contributing components in ethical situations and dilemmas and to help students structure their understanding of these situations and thus enhance their learning.

It is reasonable in the clinical education context to consider an additional layer in this model. This new layer relates to the level of reasonable expectation for the outcome for the client of working with a student. This additional layer may be constructed as shown in Table 10.2.

It may also be useful to employ an ethical decision-making model to assist learners to work within an ethical framework. These models are of most use when ethical principles are apparently in conflict, or where an ethical position is not consistent with a legal or organisational standard. There are numerous examples of the application of these decision-making models, for example:

- the use of the CELIBATE model is described in a rehabilitation setting (Kornblau & Starling 2000)
- Kerridge et al (1998) applied their ethical decision-making model to a question of provision of nutrition and hydration for a patient after a severe stroke.

In the Speech Pathology Australia (2002) *Ethics Education Package*, the following decision-making model (prepared by Brown & Lamont) is applied to several clinical dilemmas (Box 10.1). One scenario explores the situation of a speech pathology student who is asked to provide therapy for children while working as an assistant in a child care setting.

> **Box 10.1 Decision–making protocol (reproduced with permission from Speech Pathology Australia (SPA) 2002)**
>
> 1. The facts
>   - What are the facts and how did you learn about them?
>   - Who is involved?
>   - What are the client-related factors?
>   - What are the external considerations?
>   - Do you need any other facts or information?
> 2. Is there a problem that requires action?
>   - List possible actions which are you are considering at this early stage of your ethical reasoning
>   - What are the practical alternative actions and likely outcomes?
> 3. The problem
>   - Which ethical principles apply?
>   - beneficence (benefit others) and non-maleficence (prevent harm)
>   - truth
>   - fairness (justice)
>   - autonomy
>   - professional integrity (fidelity)
>   - Which duties, obligations or rules are not being met?
>   - standards of practice set out in the SPA code of ethics, competency-based standards
>   - laws, employer's policies
>   - other
>   - What is the conflict?
>   - where and what is the conflict (e.g. between ethical principles, between duty versus outcome, between ethics and external factors)?
> 4. Proposed decision and action plan
>   - make a decision and indicate your action plan
> 5. Evaluation plan
>   - consider how you will evaluate and reflect on this process and its outcome

Identifying and using learning opportunities

At the commencement of the placement, you will need to decide what predictable opportunities exist in your agency for learning about ethics. There will be certain mandatory ethical behaviours students need to understand and adhere to from the commencement of the placement. These may include issues of confidentiality and security of client files. Later, when the student observes a team meeting, respect and patient autonomy may be discussed. There will be many opportunities throughout the placement for discussion of mandatory ethical behaviours as well as for modelling of some of the aspirational components, such as facilitating client autonomy, treating colleagues and clients with dignity and making fair and just decisions.

As placements progress, "teachable moments" may arise in which modelling or use of a decision-making model with reflection and discussion may be possible. These teachable moments are those occasions "in a learning experience when the learner is more receptive to accepting and using new information, accepting new attitudes, or learning new skills" (Lassman 2001, Leist & Kritofolo 1990). Teachable moments may occur when the student has observed or participated in actions that were not consistent with ethical expectations. For example, the student may observe treatment of a patient that appeared insensitive to the patient's dignity or privacy. An unfortunately frequent example is the shouted question: "Have you had your bowels open today dear?" The student may have observed this treatment and thought it was accepted or even expected in this setting, or appropriate to the client's needs, and therefore have treated the patient in a similar manner. This situation provides an ideal teachable moment to discuss patient dignity and how important it is to respect this dignity and privacy.

Other teachable moments may relate to the dramatic dilemmas or exceptional controversies that may occur. Ethical dilemmas are useful because they create an awareness that a value-based or ethical judgement must be made in order to act (or to explain distress or contention about an action). They usually occur when two or more ethical obligations appear to conflict with each other. These will be particular to each work and team setting, and may be best addressed by using a decision-making tool. If this approach is taken with a patient-based dilemma, it is important to include a discussion with the student about the implications of the various options for the quality of care the patient receives. This will ensure there is a focus on justice and reasoned decision-making but that it is done within a framework of care-based practice (Gilligan 1982, Kenny et al 2004, Smith 2004).

PRACTICAL APPLICATIONS

The aim of the following sections is to revisit the questions asked at the start of this chapter to support your review of the ethical teaching opportunities that exist in your agency and to consider the application of some of the suggestions.

Expected values and standards

- What do you consider to be the values and ethical behaviours or standards that are expected or demonstrated in your workplace?
- Which of these do you expect the students to understand from the commencement of their placement? How can you demonstrate or teach those that are important for the placement?

In preparation for placements it will be helpful for the clinical educators to establish what level of ethical competence is required for this placement. It will also be useful for those involved in the clinical experience to examine the (often covert) ethical and moral milieu of your department and agency. Your awareness and description of the ethical and moral basis of your practice in the workplace are one of the most useful ways to assist students' development of ethical awareness.

The ethical competencies that students require for acceptable practice in your agency may be derived from multiple sources, including:

- Professional codes of ethics
- Vision and values articulated for your agency or service area

- Professional etiquette, as practised in your agency
- Workplace morals and values, such as attitudes to ethical issues which arise as a predictable part of patient care
- Personal morals and values. It can be useful for staff or students to reflect about their own values and morals by using questions such as: who/what have been the three most important influences on your understanding of right and wrong? Name three things that you value the most and why? (adapted from Purtilo 1993).

At the commencement of the placement, it is advisable for the clinical educator to confirm shared understanding with the student about competencies that will be required during the placement. You need to clarify:

- Which competencies need to be demonstrated from the commencement of the placement (e.g. confidentiality of patient information)
- Which competencies can be learned during the placement (e.g. how to obtain consent for relevant procedures).

Ethical issues and problems anticipated

- What are the ethical issues and problems that you or the student may encounter during this placement? For example, are there issues relating to:
  - dual role and conflict between your role in educating the student clinician and your role in caring for your client?
  - resource allocation, such as waiting lists, equipment needs and budgeting?
  - end-of-life issues such as palliative care, not-for-resuscitation orders, advanced directives?
  - client and family disagreeing with the recommendations of treating team, or not following team members' recommendations?
  - complex patient consent issues?
  - differences in values amongst workers in your agency?
- How can you help students learn from these issues and problems? For each issue, consider how and when you will address these situations with students. For example, will you:
  - discuss a situation and the underlying principles before it occurs?
  - use a decision-making model to clarify the issues and outcomes?
  - use "teachable moments" to model, then discuss the situation and outcomes?
  - use other forms of debriefing, reflection and discussion, particularly when considering issues of care and personal reactions?

Issues and problems experienced

- What ethical issues have you encountered or might you anticipate occurring during a student's clinical placement?
- What have you done, or would you do, with a concern arising about an ethical matter during a student's placement?

Some time ago, in an unpublished study, speech pathology, nursing, occupational therapy and physiotherapy students on placement in a rehabilitation setting were asked the following question: "In your opinion, what is the most unethical thing you could do, as a student, or your clinical educator could do?" Their responses are grouped in themes in Box 10.2.

The information in Box 10.2 may help you to identify topics of concern to students, and thus issues you may wish to target in discussions with students. You could also use this list to focus staff discussions about how they would plan to manage these issues, should they occur.

Box 10.2   Ethical issues – student perspectives

Personal and professional limitations
- continuing to treat a patient when unsure without asking for advice
- undertaking a procedure you don't know and not seeking guidance
- not performing the job you are supposed to do
- ignoring the clinical educator; making own decisions

Doing good, not harm (beneficence, non-maleficence)
- ignoring or neglecting a client; harming patient; jeopardising patient safety
- not letting patients fulfil their potential
- compromising patient's health
- "leaving the patient for dead" (i.e. harming)

Ethical attitudes and values
Respect; confidentiality; fidelity, veracity (truth), autonomy:
- totally ignoring patient and not aware of doing so
- teasing patients about their condition
- violating patient's rights
- lying or falsifying information

Professional integrity, respect
- speaking badly about peers, workmates and patients
- breaking confidentiality; talking about patients with other patients around
- going out with client; coming on to patients or other staff
- not documenting in the medical record

Power
- (clinical educator) abusing position of power
- using position of authority in an influential way

Ethical dilemmas (or lack of them)
- euthanasia
- refusing to treat
- drug-induced restraints
- "I couldn't see anything drastic a physio could do"

Additional
Topics raised by clinical educator, but not students, and may be worth discussing:
- resource allocation, limitations imposed by service requirements
- role clarity, professional integrity in team work
- a wider range of ethical dilemmas

CONCLUSION

"The clinical instructor is placed in a powerful position by the student. With that power come some rather obvious responsibilities" (Davis & McKain 1975). The premise of this chapter is that awareness and preparation for the ethical component of a clinical placement need to be as carefully planned and implemented as other areas of professional development. This process requires reflection and discussion by members of the department prior to clinical placements commencing and evaluation following completion of the placement.

Acknowledgements

Much of this chapter reflects collaborative research, discussion and workshop presentations with Sue Lamont, Manager of Rehabilitation in the Home, Peninsula Health, Victoria, Australia.

REFERENCES

Beauchamp T L, Childress J F 1994 Principles of biomedical ethics, 4th edn. Oxford University Press, New York

Brennan S 2000 Ethics and attitudes In: Dent J, Harden R (eds) A practical guide for medical teachers. Churchill Livingstone, New York

Chapparo C, Ranker J 2000 Clinical reasoning in occupational therapy. In: Higgs J, Jones M (eds) Clinical reasoning in the health professions, 2nd edn. Butterworth-Heinemann, Oxford

Davis C, McKain A 1975 Clinical education: awareness of our "not OK" behaviour. Physical Therapy 55:505–506

Ersser S, Atkins S 2000 Clinical reasoning and patient centred care. In: Higgs J, Jones M (eds) Clinical reasoning in the health professions, 2nd edn. Butterworth-Heinemann, Oxford

Feudtner C, Christakis D, Christakis N 1994 Do clinical clerks suffer ethical erosion? Students' perceptions of their ethical environment and personal development. Academic Medicine 69(8):670–679

Fulwinder R 1996 Professional codes and moral understanding. In: Coady M, Bloch S (eds) Codes of ethics and the professions. Melbourne University Press, Melbourne

Gilligan C 1982 In a different voice: psychological theory and women's development. Harvard University Press, Cambridge, MA

Johnson A G 1990 Pathways in medical ethics. Edward Arnold, London

Johnson A G 1999 Bioethics – a nursing perspective, 3rd edn. Edward Arnold, London

Jones M, Jensen G, Edwards I 2000 Clinical reasoning in physiotherapy. In: Higgs J, Jones M (eds) Clinical reasoning in the health professions, 2nd edn. Butterworth-Heinemann, Oxford

Kenny B, Lincoln M, Reed V 2004 Building students' ethical reasoning skills: does a model of ethical decision making help? In: Murdoch B, Vidler K (eds) 26th World Congress of the International Association of Logopedics & Phoniatrics. Speech Pathology Australia, Brisbane

Kerridge I, Lowe M, McPhee J 1998 Ethics and the law for health professionals. Social Science Press, Katoomba, NSW

Kohlberg L 1981 The philosophy of moral development: moral stages and the idea of justice. Harper and Row, San Francisco

Kornblau B, Starling S 2000 Ethics in rehabilitation. Slack, Thorofare, NJ

Lassman J 2001 Teachable moments – a paradigm shift. Journal of Emergency Nursing 27:171–175

Leist J, Kritofolo R 1990 The changing paradigm for continuing medical education: impact of information on the teachable moment. Bulletin of the Medical Library Association 78:173–179

Lichtenberg J 1996 What are codes of ethics for? In: Coady M, Bloch S (eds) Codes of ethics and the professions. Melbourne University Press, Melbourne

Lovett L, Seedhouse D 1990 An innovation in teaching ethics to medical students. Medical Education 24:37–41

Purtilo R 1993 Ethical dimensions in the health professions, 2nd edn. W B Saunders, Philadelphia

Ranker J, Chapparo C 2000 Teaching clinical reasoning to occupational therapists. In: Higgs J, Jones M (eds) Clinical reasoning in the health professions, 2nd edn. Butterworth-Heinemann, Oxford

Smith H 2004 Teaching professional ethical practice. What do students learn? In: Murdoch B, Vidler K (eds) 26th World Congress of the International Association of Logopedics & Phoniatrics. Speech Pathology Australia, Brisbane

Speech Pathology Australia 2000 Code of ethics. Speech Pathology Australia, Melbourne

Speech Pathology Australia 2002 Ethics education package. Speech Pathology Australia, Melbourne

White K 2001 Professional craft knowledge and ethical decision making. In: Higgs J, Titchen A (eds) Practice knowledge and expertise in the health professions. Butterworth-Heinemann, Oxford

Chapter 11

Power issues in clinical education

Dawn Best

INTRODUCTION

Clinical educators new to the role may see this chapter on power as somewhat unrelated to their tasks. Its relevance may be clouded by the challenge to include the additional responsibility of clinical education to an already full workload. However, more experienced clinical educators will recognise that many of the fundamental issues in clinical education relate to power. My own personal experience over the last 25 years as a health care practitioner, a physiotherapy academic and a medical educator within an acute health care setting has highlighted its importance. Certainly power is the one topic that has presented me with the greatest challenges and pain in all workplaces as both an educator and learner. On the other hand it has also provided me with the most valuable opportunities for learning and personal growth. Indeed, the challenge to manage the power issues inherent in organisations today has the potential to be truly transforming.

The chapter aims to:

- recognise the underlying power issues which impact on clinical education
- raise awareness of personal attitudes which impact on learning effectiveness
- apply principles of group dynamics to facilitate effective learning
- relate principles of conflict resolution to potential power issues which arise in clinical education

- empower and increase confidence of individuals for more effective outcomes
- encourage communication which is honest, sensitive and assertive of individual needs
- recognise the legal rights of individuals
- provide some guidelines for dealing with personal situations.

Power issues

Power issues relate to a number of different topics critical to clinical education. Many of these are based on personal assumptions that individuals may never have clarified before. When the power challenge arises it may come as such a surprise that it is difficult to understand and respond appropriately, let alone discuss calmly and openly. Power issues have emerged in many other chapters of this text and may relate to:

- the tension between individual professional autonomy and the university agenda (see Chapter 1)
- economic factors related to changes in funding to health care and education (see Chapter 1)
- the partnership between health and education (Ferguson & Edwards 1999, see Chapter 1)
- different ways of knowing – the very different assumptions and values associated with propositional knowledge and practice knowledge (see Chapter 5, as well as multiple chapters of Higgs & Titchen 2001)
- the dichotomy of the qualitative and quantitative research paradigms (eloquent arguments which support each paradigm are presented in Chapters 9 and 20).

In addition, clinical educators are challenged to resolve:

- the conflict between patient-centred health care delivery and student-centred learning
- misconceptions or different perceptions of the balance between the enabling function focused on individual learning and development, and the ensuring function associated with credentialing competence and staff appraisal
- the tension between individualisation and different organisation practices and values.

Each workplace has its own aims, values, structures and assumptions. Engestrom (1998) explains that cognitive scientists focus on expertise in a given field as individual mastery of the discrete tasks and skills, with the potential for gradual achievement with the assistance of a more experienced practitioner or worker. This focus on the individual fails to acknowledge the social and cultural structures which impact on all environments. Engestrom identifies that professionalism, bureaucracy and corporatisation are powerful influences on expertise and "leave little room for construction from below" (1998, p. 199). In other words, the work environment places powerful barriers to individualisation.

Plant (1984) attributes any change in power to a balance between specific forces within the individual and forces within the organisation. We expect a lot of our students when we schedule them from university to clinical facility and from one placement to another with little preparation for the very different politics and functioning of the different work environments they will enter. Integration into a new working environment to a level that enables a deep understanding of meaning takes considerable time (see Chapter 6). Learning the specific interpretation of "professionalism, bureaucracy and corporatisation" in any organisation is not a quick lesson, as anyone who has moved from one workplace to another will have discovered.

UNDERSTANDING THE CONCEPT OF POWER

When we think about power we may identify feelings associated with getting or not getting something we want. Whether we are students or clinical educators, we may have felt totally overwhelmed by the futility of a situation that renders us helpless and immobile or we may have felt the heady enthusiasm and excitement of achievement and success when things have met our expectations. Within the organisation behaviour literature, power is understood as the ability to get someone to do something you want or the ability to make things happen in a way you want. It relates to control over the behaviour of others (Bailey et al 1991).

Street (2001) rejects this view of power as an object that is held or not held by someone. She promotes a more liberating view of power as a dynamic force where power can be used but not held. Such power relates to social and personal circumstances and is available to any of us, although she does concede that some people have greater opportunities than others. Brislin (1991) interviewed successful power holders and identified that these people used resources, skills, strategies and tactics in order to get things done and achieve goals. They also recognised the effect of power, used their networks very effectively, shared resources with others, developed sophisticated tactics which managed emotional responses and saw power as only one of the very important aspects of life.

TYPES OF POWER

Aguinis et al (1996) studied power relationships between academic staff and students engaged in postgraduate supervision and the relationship between student perceptions related to the trustworthiness with and credibility of their supervisor. Trustworthiness was established if supervisors:

- gave credit for student contributions on the research project
- did not take the students' ideas as their own
- did not prescribe unrelated tasks
- did not manipulate students to their own end.

Credibility was achieved when supervisors:

- demonstrated that they kept their word
- did what they say they would

- made accurate and honest statements of fact to students
- told the truth.

These perceptions were related to the following five different types of power.

1. *Expert power* related to technical knowledge and advice that resulted in student perceptions of trustworthiness and credibility.
2. *Reward power* was recognised by students as the special benefits and rewards a supervisor may be able to grant.
3. *Legitimate power* related to the supervisor's ability to encourage the student to accept personal responsibility for tasks and commitment.
4. *Referent power* related to the supervisor's ability to foster feelings of acceptance and value.
5. *Coercive power* related to any punishment from the supervisor, even when it was justified.

The different types of power identified in the Aguinis et al (1996) study related to either the position of authority held by the supervisor or to personal attributes of the individual person.

Power is inherent in the role of clinical educator. Students perceive that getting on with the clinical educator is the single most important factor related to success in clinics. If one of the tasks of the clinical educator is also the role of assessor then this will increase the student's perception of power due to the greater opportunity for reward or punishment. On the other hand, the clinical educator's ability to create a supporting learning environment and establish a trusting relationship, along with highly developed clinical skills, expert knowledge and professional reputation, balances and further increases the power of the clinical educator (see Chapter 5, part three).

In summary, position power is related to the formal authority of roles, especially to the ability to reward or coerce. Personal power is related to the specific knowledge, skills and abilities of the individual supervisor. However, it is important to acknowledge that expertise in one area may have a halo effect in other areas. Gale & Grant (1998) note that experts are given greater credibility in all matters, even those well outside their expertise. Although both position power and personal power contribute to an overall perception of one's power base by others, it is interesting that in communication with a higher authority, personal power has the greater influence whereas position power as well as personal power is more effective in communication with subordinates (Bailey et al 1991). This may explain the challenge voiced by some clinical educators to establish a trusting relationship with students who have poor self-esteem and limited self-confidence. No matter what personal skills we may bring to the role, we need to remember that our students still see the inherent power advantage of the educator role.

POWER GAMES AND THE CLINICAL EDUCATION RELATIONSHIP

Game-playing is inherently related to power but may be either conscious or unconscious. The psychoanalyst Eric Berne (1964, p. 44) defined a game as "an ongoing series of complementary ulterior transactions progressing to a well defined, predictable outcome". Hagler & Casey (1990) define game-playing as inappropriate behaviours that have a pernicious influence on the

Table 11.1   Games in supervision

Impetus for game	Game	Implication
Reduce responsibilities	"You are doing just fine"	Time and effort are not needed to observe and question
Maintain an image	"It's a good idea – if I have it first"	Hides any educator knowledge deficit
Meet unfulfilled needs	"I can do anything better than you" (clinical educator interrupts student–client interaction)	Meets the educator's need for self-esteem

task in hand and are thus symptoms of an unhealthy relationship. Games arise from fear about losing face and fear of failure or criticism and serve to avoid a situation rather than deal with it openly. Kadushin (1968) elaborated on the potential for game-playing within supervision in social work and identified the potential for four different categories of games that sought to manipulate demands, redefine relationships, reduce power disparities and control the supervisory conference.

It is not surprising that students may seek to minimise threats and penalties and maximise rewards and resort to game-playing. It is just as understandable that supervisors would seek to do the same. Both may be tempted to play a game of seduction by flattery for ulterior motive, such as a version of: "be nice to me and I'll be nice to you" (Kadushin 1968, p. 25). It is understandable that the potential for game-playing would increase with responsibilities associated with assessment or appraisal.

A small study by Hagler & Casey (1990) asked speech pathology and audiology students to identify games their supervisors initiated. Games were identified which served to reduce supervisors' responsibilities, maintain an image or to meet unfulfilled personal needs (Table 11.1).

Over many years in university clinical briefing sessions with physiotherapy undergraduate students it was interesting to observe that fourth-year students, without any knowledge of the literature on games, were able to identify game-playing behaviour in their clinical placements. When invited to brief third-year students about to embark on placements it was not unusual for fourth-year students to advise them to:

- "find out what the game is so that you'll get good marks"
- "watch out for clinicians who use questioning to play the game of 'guess what's in my head/match my list'."

Although these examples focus on educator games, any experience in clinical education will quickly enable the identification of common games initiated by students.

Minimising game-playing

In playing games the supervisee (or player) loses – by winning.

(Kadushin 1968, p. 32).

Game-playing serves to avoid an issue rather than confront it or solve it (Hagler & Casey 1990). Hence it is essential that clinical educators are aware of the potential for game-playing and accept their own responsibilities to minimise such ineffective behaviours. In refusing to play games they are able to model honest direct communication which addresses the underlying issue.

It is important that all clinical educators accept that gender and cultural differences provide the potential for serious abuse of power and very dangerous game-playing. Skaine (1996, p. 11) defines sexual harassment as:

> *unwelcome sexual advances, requests for sexual favours and other verbal or physical abuse of a sexual nature when submission or rejection of this conduct explicitly or implicitly affects an individual's employment or work performance or creates an intimidating, hostile, offensive work environment.*

Students need to be aware of the appropriate processes available to them within the placement or university should they encounter any unwanted touching or verbal harassment. It is essential to recognise that there are always choices to be made and using personal networks and accepting help from others provide valuable support.

Although the following strategies were devised for victims of sexual harassment (Skaine 1996, p. 364), they provide wise direction for others in need of empowerment:

Informal approaches

- recognise the behaviour
- don't blame yourself
- keep a diary of what happened
- consider confrontation to empower yourself.

Formal approaches

- know the policies, procedures and the law
- be aware of time limits
- file a grievance
- seek legal advice and be prepared to file a legal suit.

GROUP DYNAMICS AND LEADERSHIP

Heron (1989) defines group dynamics as the combined configuration of mental, emotional and physical energies in a group at any one time. These factors include:

- the qualities of the members – their abilities, experiences, personalities and motivations
- the quality of the task – the clarity of the task or goal, the difficulty of the task, deadlines, criteria for success, resources
- the qualities of the group – previous experience within the group, cohesiveness, size and values
- the quality of the relationship with other groups – contact with other groups, outside sources of expertise, conflicting loyalties
- the group structure – power relationship, roles, group norms and climate (Best & Rose 1996, Jaques 1984; see also Chapter 14).

Although the leadership and authority held by the clinical educator are only one of the influences on overall group functioning, nevertheless it is a strong predictor of learning outcomes:

When power is applied as force and consented to out of fear the group dynamics will focus on submission.

(Stacey 1992, p. 192).

Without consent it will result in rebellion. However, if group members accept the authority of the organisation then dependence and conformity are the likely outcomes. Stacey (1992) advises that none of these outcomes is likely to provide the complex learning required for transformation. The dynamics for such a group require the flexible facilitation of argument and conflict with consensus, and chaos with clarity. In such a group there is no place for dependence or authority:

The true skill of the enabling leader lies in the ability to design the best use of power in each situation, based on experience, reflection and judgement.

(Stacey 1992, p. 193).

CONFLICT RESOLUTION

Conflict arises within every workplace and in any relationship and, as already acknowledged, it provides the opportunity for creative solutions and stimulating discussion. However, conflict situations may arise from the misuse of power. Students may become defensive because of authoritarian tactics, condescension, loaded words and flaunting power (Kreidel, cited in Downs 1992).

The following suggestions for dealing with hostile and oppositional students over a decade ago were devised for academic teachers in the USA; however they have universal application for us as clinical educators. With few exceptions, which relate to the educator role, they also provide strategies for use in situations of disempowerment. Steps towards harmony:

1. Ask yourself if you have done anything to contribute to the conflict.
2. Confer with the student/other person on your own in a neutral setting.
3. Look for a common ground.
4. Try a series of cooperative learning exercises and discuss social skills.
5. Try not to become defensive or to make personal attacks.
6. Talk with colleagues about their similar experiences and their strategies for management.
7. Integrate problem-solving and social skills within your education sessions.
8. Use direct confrontation as a last resort (Downs 1992, p. 107–108).

In addition, clinical educators are advised to:

- learn to recognise burnout and look after themselves (see Chapter 19)
- know the ethical implications (see Chapter 10)
- look up the relevant state and federal legislation related to sexual harassment, discrimination and equal opportunity
- remember that power is only one of many other very important aspects of life!

In determining ways to achieve transformation from conflicts, Cloke & Goldsmith (2000, p. xiii) offer the following advice:

Follow your intuition, be guided by your heart, expand your empathy and be willing to risk deep and compassionate honesty about whatever you see.

EXERCISE

Learning activities

1. *Understanding your power as a clinical educator*

   The following self-assessment exercise is adapted from Lambert (1996, p. 120–122). It aims to clarify your perceptions of your own power bases as a clinical educator. Think about which of the following statements is true for you. Mark those that are true with a tick and those that are false with a cross.

   1. Resource power: Students may do as I want because I control resources that they value
   2. Position power: I have power over students because of the position I hold within the organisation
   3. Proxy power: Students may do as I want because I have friends (or relatives) in high places
   4. Reward power: Students may do as I want because I can reward those who comply
   5. Sanctions (coercive) power: Students may do as I want because I can punish those who don't
   6. Expert power: Students may do as I want because they respect my professional knowledge and clinical expertise
   7. Personal power: Students may do as I want because they like me and want to model their behaviour on mine
   8. Status power: Students may do as I want because I have status within the group – I may be the oldest, the longest-serving, the only one with a postgraduate degree, research grant, etc.
   9. Charisma power: Students may do as I want because they are influenced by my vision, enthusiasm, charm or personality
   10. Favour power: Students may do as I want because I build a bank of favours and call on them when I need compliance

   Reflect on:
   Which of these power sources do you use most frequently?
   Which are you least comfortable with?
   If asked, do you think a work colleague would agree with your analysis?
   If asked, do you think a family member would agree with your analysis?
   What are your surprises about this knowledge?
   Next time I have a new student in the clinic I will....

2. *Games in clinical education*
   What student games can you identify in your workplace?
   What is the motivation for this game?
   What clinical educator games can you identify?
   What is the motivation for each?
   Can you recognise any personal favourites?

REFERENCES

Aguinis H, Nesler M S, Quigley B M, Lee S, Tedeschi J T 1996 Power bases of faculty supervisors and educational outcomes for graduate students. Journal of Higher Education 67:267–297

Bailey J, Schermerhorn J, Hunt J et al 1991 Managing organisational behaviour. John Wiley, Brisbane

Berne E 1964 Games people play. Penguin, Middlesex

Best D, Rose M 1996 Quality supervision: theory and practice for field university clinical educators. W B Saunders, London

Brislin R 1991 The art of getting things done: a practical guide to the use of power. Praeger, New York

Cloke K, Goldsmith J 2000 Resolving conflicts at work: a complete guide for everyone on the job. Jossey-Bass, San Francisco

Downs J 1992 Dealing with hostile and oppositional students. College Teaching 40(3):106–108

Engestrom Y 1998 The tensions of judging: handling cases of driving under the influence of alcohol in Finland and California. In: Engestrom Y, Middleton D (eds) Cognition and communication at work. Cambridge University Press, Cambridge

Ferguson K, Edwards H 1999 In: Higgs J, Edwards H (eds) Educating beginning practitioners. Butterworth-Heinemann, Oxford

Gale R , Grant J 1998 Managing change. In: Jolly B, Rees L (eds) Medical education in the millennium. Oxford University Press, Oxford

Hagler P, Casey P 1990 Games supervisors play in clinical supervision. ASHA 32:53–56

Heron J 1989 The facilitator's handbook. Kogan Page, London

Higgs J, Titchen A 2001 Practice knowledge and expertise in the health professions. Butterworth-Heinemann, Oxford

Jaques D 1984 Learning in groups. Croom Helm, London

Kadushin A 1968 Games people play in supervision. Social Work 13:23–32

Lambert T 1996 The power of influence: intensive skills at work. Nicholas Brealey, London, p 120–122

Plant R 1984 Managing change and making it stick. Fontana Collins, London

Skaine R 1996 Power and gender: issues in sexual dominance and harassment. McFarland, Jefferson

Stacey R 1992 Managing the unknowable. Strategic boundaries between order and chaos in organization. Jossey-Bass, San Francisco

Street A 2001 Professional craft knowledge and power relationships. In: Higgs J, Titchen A (eds) Practice knowledge and expertise. Butterworth-Heinemann, Oxford

Chapter 12

Clinical educators as cultural guides

Louisa Remedios and Gillian Webb

This chapter is about assisting your students to become acculturated to the clinical culture of the health professional and the clinical environment they are learning in. We believe that the ability to learn the culture of health practice is an important fundamental early step for all students, and that access to this cultural knowledge may be more challenging for overseas-educated (OSE) students. We refer to international students or those who have studied predominantly in another culture as OSE students, recognising that it is cultural difference that is often at issue when learning in a new cultural environment.

Without knowledge of the dominant culture that is operating in the clinical environment, miscommunication becomes commonplace and learning possibilities are reduced. This chapter is therefore about increasing awareness of the role that culture plays in clinical education and suggests strategies for dealing with some of the more commonly encountered problems. It is based on our experience over the last 14 years in developing and implementing a voluntary extracurricular preclinical preparation programme for physiotherapy students in a four-year undergraduate programme within a medical school. All students were invited to attend. Some local students chose to join OSE students in the programme and many of the suggested activities are equally appropriate for local students.

UNDERSTANDING CULTURE

One of the earliest and most commonly referred to definitions of culture comes from Gerte Hofstede, who referred to it as the:

> *mental software learned throughout a lifetime and dependent on the group of people and the shared values surrounding the person. It is the collective programming of the mind which distinguishes the members of one group or category of people from another.*

(Hofstede 1994, p. 5).

The essence of culture is that it is a learned-value system that is deeply embedded into the thinking and behaviours of a "large" social group. Typically broad definitions of cultural groupings have included a range of variables such as ethnicity, nationality, religion, language, age, gender and education, as well as both formal affiliations to family or organisations and informal affiliations to ideas and a lifestyle.

Minas & Klimidis (1994) drew attention to culture as guidelines for behaviour and understanding in social contexts. They cite Goodenough's conceptualisation of culture as:

> *whatever it is one has to know in order to operate successfully and in a manner acceptable to its members [of a given society]. It is the form of things that people have in mind, their models for perceiving, relating, and interpreting. Culture consists of standards for deciding what is … for deciding what one feels about it … for deciding what to do about it.*

(Goodenough, cited in Minas & Klimidis 1994, p. 139).

Minas & Klimidis (1994) go on to describe culture as shared ideas, rules and meaning, which function as a code, mainly submerged beneath consciousness, which enables individuals within a community to communicate, live, work and anticipate and interpret behaviour. Culture then is the lens through which people see and judge the world around them. In shaping their fundamental beliefs and values, it guides their expectations, attitudes, behaviours and practices (Minas & Klimidis 1994).

The key points here are the pervasiveness of culture as providing guidelines for all aspects of what we think and do as well as what we feel. It also shapes what we anticipate and interpret as appropriate in social interactions and sometimes becomes established as stereotypes. Culture pervades all social context, including the clinical environment. The culture of clinics is the context in which students build their understanding of the cognitive, behavioural, affective and communication demands that are placed on them. Aspects particularly pertinent are the patterns of thinking, feeling and acting, which are essentially learned behaviours.

This concept of guidelines, codes, fundamental beliefs and values is often portrayed as an inflexible system which is so powerful, deep-seated, collective and binding as to limit individuals' freedom to act outside the bounds of their culture (Gudykunst et al 1988, Hofstede 1994). It is not uncommon to hear of "culture" being discussed as a great divide between people, and as limiting individuals' ability to cope outside their own cultural boundaries. In some instances, when behaviours are labelled as cultural, the implication is that individuals are unable to recognise when a meaning is not shared or are unable to learn and change their behaviours to comply with the "demands" of a new culture.

We are more sympathetic with an alternative construction of culture presented by Keesing (1974). This position proposes that, within any culture, individuals internalise its rules and nuances to a different extent, and act out varying attachment to cultural values. Further, these values are constantly being reorganised in response to the context and to the degree to which the meanings in the context are explicit. So, while we all carry well-embedded cultural beliefs and values, we are capable of learning how to modify these as we are exposed to different social contexts. It is important not to view culture as a narrow domain or of cultural beliefs as a rigid and inflexible system that cannot be modified. Culture is dynamic, and we are all exposed to multiple cultures. We can view ourselves as multicultural with a greater or lesser attachment to different aspects of our culture. We can successfully negotiate different cultures as long as the important rules are made explicit (Schirato & Yell 2000).

THE CLINICAL CULTURE

It is currently well accepted that all individuals operate within a number of cultures and subcultures (Eisenhart 2001, Spack 1997). In our own situation as clinical educators we are operating within the broader culture of our country, our ethnic group, as well as our professional environment. The clinical environment has its own culture, as do the professions that function within the clinical cultures. As we develop our clinical identity we tend to internalise the culture of the professional group, sometimes forgetful that its rules are not clear to outsiders.

It is also accepted that most established social contexts have developed a culture. For example, the concept of classroom cultures (CC) has been described in the literature. If we substitute clinics for classrooms and clinical educators for teachers, the following description of CC helps our understanding of clinical culture. Marilyn Nickson (1992) describes CC as "the invisible and apparently shared meaning that teachers and pupils bring to the ... classroom and that governs their interaction in it". It includes the "knowledge, beliefs and values that are held by the actors in the setting ... unseen beliefs and values, of both student and teacher" (p. 102).

The idealised theoretical model, envisaged in the mind of clinical educators, with all its learning objectives and intentions clearly visible, is not necessarily innately understood by the student. Students develop their theories of the codes of the clinics, some of which are visible and explicitly established by their clinical educators and some of which are invisible. These theories are used to shape their own choices of how they should behave in the clinics. Cultural literacy is about the need to understand the "rules" and beliefs operating within the dominant culture, in this case the clinical environment students are learning in.

CULTURAL LITERACY

The concept of cultural literacy has been defined as a knowledge and understanding of meaning systems and a way to negotiate these meaning systems appropriately in different cultural contexts (Schirato & Yell 2000). This concept can be framed in terms of reading what is important in different situations, in being able to sum up the priorities of the time and then acting in a way that best suits the situation as well as having the choice to act in a way that allows you to achieve what you would like. It involves understanding the rules of the culture, both explicit and implicit.

Cultural literacy is also about knowing what is appropriate in different but similar circumstances. It is not always easy, and subtleties are often hidden in social contexts. It should be recognised that, to a local student who has a high level of cultural literacy, what may appear to be straightforward and obvious could be riddled with complexity and be a minefield of potential misunderstandings for a newcomer to the culture. Lack of experience or knowledge of a culture may result in an inability to read the meaning of the social context and individuals may respond in a way that is viewed as inappropriate to locals who have previously learnt the rules of the context.

For example, apparently similar but different situations can lead to problems. Think about the similarities and differences between greeting a patient, a doctor, a fellow student or the head of the department. The formality, the demonstration of respect and the time taken for the greeting typically vary. We need to know who initiates the greeting, the length of time involved in the exchange and how to conclude the conversation appropriately. Misunderstanding any of these often hidden rules can make for an uncomfortable situation, which some students manage by avoiding greetings altogether.

When thinking about cultural literacy we need to consider both the literacy of the clinical educator and the students. Clearly the educator has a more sophisticated literacy about the culture of the clinical environment and the profession that the student is entering. One of the major objectives of clinical education should be to develop the cultural literacy skills of students and to acculturate them to their professional culture.

THE CULTURAL CONTINUUM

It is important to remember that all students, local and OSE, need to become culturally literate in the clinical culture. All students experience similar difficulties and anxieties in their encounters with patients and with learning the rules of professional functioning in a clinical environment. However, difficulties may be more apparent for those students who come from different cultural backgrounds to those operating in the clinical environment. Further, for a number of OSE students, language difficulties may exacerbate the cultural difficulties they experience.

One aim in clinical education is to make the major operating values fundamental to practice more explicit to the student. Educators need to be aware of their own deeply held cultural assumptions and be open to appreciating that these are learnt and not simply acquired as a part of common sense.

In shifting from the preclinical learning environment to the clinical one, students are also exposed to a new culture. In the preclinical learning environment, students are typically exposed to expectations and routines that are similar to those they experienced in previous classroom learning environments and the role of student is a familiar one. In contrast, the shift to a more professional identity in a health system with its own expectations and codes of practice may be challenging for students. Some of the cultural values that operate within the clinical environment may be so embedded that they are never made explicit to students. If you think a student is behaving "inappropriately" it may be because he or she does not understand the cultural rules that you value highly.

UNDERSTANDING POTENTIAL DIFFICULTIES CONFRONTING THE OSE STUDENT

From our experience in developing strategies for supporting OSE students who are having difficulty in the clinical environment we have found it useful to refer to a flow chart (Fig. 12.1) that categorises some of the more common themes. The two major categories are those of predominantly language and cultural issues. These are further subdivided into subsections that require different approaches. It should be noted that language difficulties can dominate experiences and may often camouflage more complex cultural issues.

Language issues

It can be anticipated that some students learning in a second language may have serious difficulties with communicating effectively and confidently with the language of the profession in a clinical environment. It is helpful to view language difficulties as follows:

- expressive communication, both verbal and non-verbal, that is, the ability to communicate a message clearly
- written communication, both reading and writing
- receptive communication, that is, the ability to understand the verbal and non-verbal information that is being communicated by another.

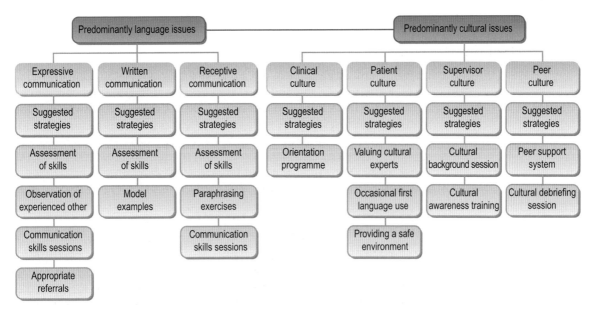

Figure 12.1 Understanding difficulties confronting the overseas-educated student

It should be noted that language issues often interlink with cultural elements and it is sometimes difficult to isolate a language problem from a cultural issue. For example, a student who does not appear to understand what is being said, that is, the receptive element, may in fact be having difficulty listening to a young female clinical educator, since in some cultures females and young people are considered to have a lower status in social hierarchies. They may not be giving the information the attention that is required or responding as expected. The language might be understood but the underlying cultural knowledge may not be available to these students.

Expressive communication: verbal

In Australia, students are expected to have a high level of sophistication in languages when communicating in the clinical environment. They are typically required to be fluent in English as used for daily interactions, including colloquialisms, the professional language used for reporting and communicating with other health professionals, as well as the ability to switch from formal to informal language as the context demands. The students may have inadequate language skills in terms of vocabulary, pronunciation, ability to recognise the demands of the context or of the individual with whom they are communicating. The difficulty of communicating with English-speaking patients may be further exacerbated when communicating with patients who also do not have English as a first language.

Expressive communication: non-verbal

Expressive communication is both verbal and non-verbal (Box 12.1). Non-verbal cues such as body language and elements such as tone and volume of voice as well as speed of delivery add considerable meaning to verbal expression. These non-verbal behaviours are often not taught explicitly or given only limited attention when students are studying a second language and these skills may be slow to develop even when the vocabulary itself is quite advanced. Different cultures use different non-verbal cues to communicate and students will fall back on these, especially during stressful times. For example, the nodding head or the smiling face when receiving negative feedback may indicate the student's defence mechanism rather than disrespect.

Box 12.1   Suggested strategies for developing expressive communication skills

Assessment of skills
We suggest that students at the beginning of their clinic be asked to rate their confidence in their English-language skills for tasks, such as the ability to write a report, interview a patient and report their findings. These self-assessment ratings need to be verified by the clinical educator early in the clinic. It may be useful to ask the student to give verbal summaries of patient histories and to practise interview skills with a fellow student or an empathetic patient in the first instance.

continued over

This allows the student and the clinical educator to have confidence in more difficult situations should they arise

Observation of experienced other
The student who is having difficulty with asking appropriate questions may benefit from observing a competent junior member of staff. This will clarify expectations as well as provide the opportunity to see the task is achievable. Following this the student may be asked to summarise the key factors that contributed to the effective interaction, before having an opportunity to interview another patient

Communication skills sessions
We have found informal communication skills sessions, for both local and international students, to be invaluable. These may take place prior to clinics and also during clinics and allow students to practise verbal and listening skills in a safe environment. It encourages the use of language of the clinical environment in a non-threatening atmosphere. Videos and role-plays are also used to familiarise the students with the different clinical environments and tasks expected of them

Appropriate referrals
We have found that, if any difficulties around pronunciation are identified prior to students attending clinics, they can be managed early. This may require a referral to an English as a second language (ESL) teacher or a speech pathologist. This is an important early step to be taken that will build student confidence in their verbal skills

Written communication (Box 12.2)

Students may experience difficulties with both the reading and writing required of them. For example, recording patient histories, letters of referral and other forms of professional documentation may be especially problematic as students struggle to find the appropriate language and grammar to maintain their professional credibility.

Box 12.2 Suggested strategies for developing written communication skills

Assessment of skills
As for expressive skills, we suggest that students be asked at the beginning of their clinic to comment on their confidence in their ability to read and write the various forms of documentation required for the clinics. It may be useful to ask students to write short summaries of parts of a patient's history and referral letters to develop these skills as early as possible. This will also help them in writing in a timely manner

Model examples
For a student who is having trouble with writing an effective summary, several model examples could be provided

Receptive communication: verbal and non-verbal (Box 12.3)

Receptive skills include listening, interpreting and understanding both the verbal and non-verbal messages being communicated. In our experience this is one of the key difficulties experienced by OSE students who have difficulty with local accents, shortened, fast speech and the use of colloquialisms. This is often the cause of misunderstandings between clinical educators, patients and students. The students may appear to be engaged in the interaction or even signal an understanding but have in fact misinterpreted, failed to understand or only partially understood the conversation. It may be culturally difficult for the student to acknowledge any "failure" to understand, and raise concerns about the implied criticism of the speaker as well as a reluctance to question an individual in authority. Silence or nodding in following a conversation therefore does not always indicate full comprehension.

Box 12.3   Suggested strategies for developing receptive communication skills

Assessment of skills
It is an advantage if the ability to understand verbal communication fully is established as early as possible. Students can be asked to quantify with the use of percentages how much of a conversation they have understood. Clinical educators can ask questions to confirm students' understanding of all issues under discussion. Educators should also make an effort to curb any tendency to use colloquialisms, or if they use them, to do so with an explanation. When the supervisor is unsure of a student's understanding the student may be asked to paraphrase appropriate explanations and instructions

Paraphrasing exercises
Also following conversations between students and supervisors, such as feedback sessions, *all* key messages may be confirmed by explicit questioning. That is, the clinical educator could ask the student to repeat what has been heard, what is understood and what needs clarification. Misinterpretations are often the basis of clinicians feeling that the student is not listening to feedback

Communication skills sessions
Specific sessions where students have the opportunity to paraphrase their understanding of fellow students and to clarify their understanding in role-plays provide very useful learning opportunities

Increased interaction time
It would be helpful if students are given more opportunities to practise their communication skills in a non-pressured environment. Perhaps they could be given extra time to observe, listen and rehearse and/or opportunities for self-study, using both videotapes and transcripts

---

Cultural issues

As outlined previously, culture can play a powerful role in all clinical interactions and affect the students' learning. It is again helpful to break down cultural issues into a number of categories, so that targeted strategies are implemented to resolve difficulties.

Culture of clinical environments (Box 12.4)

Most students who have not been previously exposed to the western health care system will have less knowledge of the structures and values operating within the system. This may again affect their interpretations of how to behave in different environments. Although it is rare for the values and health beliefs of institutions to be made explicit to students, they are expected to have the cultural literacy to deal with these appropriately. For example, in paediatric health care the family is considered to be central in the decision-making processes surrounding care for their child. This may appear to the student as if the therapist is no longer taking the responsibility for the decision-making and may be very different to existing concepts of the role of the health professional.

Patient autonomy may be a culturally difficult concept for some students. The framework of health beliefs in other countries may be in marked contrast to this. Alternatively the student may accept statements from people that they consider to be in authority without questioning.

Box 12.4   Suggested strategies for learning about the culture of clinical environments

Orientation programme

In any orientation programme the clinician must ensure that all students have a clear understanding of the expectations of that particular environment. This is particularly important for overseas-educated (OSE) students, as they are unlikely to have knowledge of the local context. This may include professional behaviours, social interactions and ways of addressing their clinical educator. If there is a hierarchy operating that the students need to attend to, this must be made explicit. For example, will the student report to the doctor, the nurse in charge and/or to their clinical educators?

The clinical educator needs to make all these issues especially clear to the OSE students, as they may not have the underlying cultural knowledge to interpret the situation. This may mean that at times you need to be prepared to answer questions that appear to be naïve and obvious. The orientation sessions may need to be spread across the first week to allow for the students to assimilate the information and to feel that it is appropriate for them to continue to ask questions. In the following weeks brief discussions may need to be held to ensure that the knowledge of the rules and expectations of the clinic have been fully understood and that the acculturation of the students is progressing effectively.

Culture of patients (Box 12.5)

Once again, the communication between people with different attitudes and cultural beliefs may affect all aspects of clinical interactions. For example, students dealing with an older person of their own cultural background may experience difficulties due to the fact that the patient is not willing to be treated by such a junior person, which the patient may see as a sign of disrespect. Sharing information with a young person is not culturally appropriate in some countries.

It should also be remembered that local students might not be sensitive to issues of different health beliefs and customs. Lack of understanding and appreciation of different religious beliefs may lead to conflict in patient interactions: for example, issues of gender, where it is unacceptable for a male health professional to examine a female patient without a member of the family present. Students should also be aware of and respect prayer times and religious festivals and how they may impact on treatment choices.

Some students may also experience racism from patients and other health professionals. This is often in the form of stereotyping people from particular cultures. It may be overt or subtle, such as refusing to be treated by a student because he or she comes from another country or not respecting advice given by a student on health care management. This issue needs to be dealt with as soon as it is apparent.

Box 12.5 Suggested strategies for learning about the culture of patients

Valuing cultural experts
Overseas-educated (OSE) students may be able to act as cultural experts to inform the local students on cultural beliefs and practices of patients from similar cultural backgrounds to their own. This will give credit to the knowledge of the OSE student and build confidence as well as increasing the clinical knowledge base of local students

Occasional first-language use
An excellent strategy to give students confidence in their interpersonal skills and their view of their own professional identity is to allow them to speak to patients of their own cultural background in their own language. Although we may not be able to confirm what is being said, it gives the students a chance to feel at ease with their language and their professional role and may also put the patient at ease

Providing a "safe" environment
Clinical educators need to be vigilant in watching for any evidence of racism, gender bias or cultural inappropriateness that may be affecting an interaction and be willing to withdraw the student immediately. Students need to feel confident that their concerns regarding any of these issues are listened to seriously

---

Culture of the clinical educator (Box 12.6)

In some cases the culture of the clinical educator may negatively influence the learning experience of the student. At a personal level conflict may arise when the clinical educator is not flexible in world-view and values and does not readily accept alternative cultural beliefs and understandings. At a professional level, it is common for the clinical educator to expect the student to have a framework of learning that is similar to his or her own. Clinical educators may expect the students to think as they do, to be independent in their learning and to be able to speak about their own learning. Clinical educators may expect students to value themselves as, for example, critical thinkers and autonomous learners. This may well be in contrast to what has been expected of the student previously, where content knowledge may have been valued more than the skills of problem-solving and clinical reasoning.

Box 12.6   Suggested strategies for understanding the culture of the clinical educator

Cultural background session
At the commencement of a clinic it is important for the clinical educator to take time to understand the cultural background of the students and how this may affect their practice. Students from diverse backgrounds can contribute to the clinical educators' understanding of other cultures as these students often have knowledge of the health professions in their own countries

Cultural awareness training
We would recommend that cultural awareness training be part of the requirements for clinical educator training. This will allow the individuals to understand their own cultural beliefs and how these may impact on their students. Most university departments and health facilities run cultural awareness programmes that can be readily accessed

---

The culture of fellow students (Box 12.7)

In most clinical environments, fellow students assist in the acculturation of their peers into the clinic culture as well as the learning of professional skills. Students from different cultures may feel socially isolated and lack this form of support. The literature suggests that cultural comfort or cultural congruence is helpful in developing friendships (Campbell 1996, Volet & Ang 1998). Cultural dissonance between students may have major consequences for the OSE student's ability to learn successfully.

Box 12.7   Suggested strategies for learning from the culture of fellow students

Peer support system
A peer support system such as "buddying" students in clinical environments is an effective strategy (Ladyshewsky 2000). Students work in groups of two or three and share and support each other through their clinical learning. When this strategy is employed it is important that the clinical educator is aware of cultural congruence between students so that the students are able mutually to support each other

---

continued over

> **Cultural briefing session**
> We recommend an introductory session where students, both local and overseas-educated, talk about themselves, their cultural backgrounds and the health beliefs in their countries. It would be of value for clinical educators to participate and share knowledge of their own cultural backgrounds. This acknowledges and values the role of culture in health care, the richness and diversity of culture, as well as the need for students to learn about the dominant culture they are currently learning within

CONCLUDING COMMENTS

It is our assumption that all clinical educators reading this chapter will have had some experience working with students from different cultural backgrounds and that at times they may have encountered difficulties. Finally, it must be remembered that all students (local and OSE) may benefit from the suggested strategies. Our position is that:

- all students and clinical educators bring to their clinical encounter both cultural similarities and cultural differences
- cultural differences may interfere with clear communication and effective supervision
- a culturally sensitive approach will facilitate all encounters and will enhance the learning experience of all students.

REFERENCES

Campbell A 1996 Frogs and snails and puppy dog tales: creating cultural comfort zones. Keynote address at the 7th National ISANA Conference: Waves of Change

Eisenhart M 2001 Changing conceptions of culture and ethnographic methodology: recent thematic shifts and their implications for research and teaching. In: Richardson V (ed) Handbook of teaching, 4th edn. AERA, Washington, DC, p 209–225

Gudykunst W B, Ting-Toomey S, Chua E 1988 Culture and interpersonal communication, vol. 8. Sage series in interpersonal relationships. Sage Publications, Newbury Park

Hofstede G 1994 Culture and organizations: software of the mind. McGraw-Hill, London

Keesing R 1974 Theories of culture. Annual Review of Anthropology 3:73–77

Ladyshewsky R 2000 A quasi-experimental study of the effects of a reciprocal peer coaching strategy on physiotherapy students' clinical problem-solving skills. PhD thesis, Curtin University of Technology

Minas H, Klimidis M 1994 Cultural issues in post-traumatic stress disorders. In: Watts R, Horne D (eds) Coping with trauma: the victim and the helper. Australian Academic Press, Brisbane

Nickson M 1992 The culture of mathematics classrooms: an unknown quantity? In: Douglas A, Grows D (ed) Handbook of research on mathematics teaching and learning. Macmillan, New York, p 101–114

Schirato A, Yell S 2000 Communication and cultural literacy: an introduction. Allen and Unwin, St Leonards

Spack R 1997 The rhetorical construction of multilingual students. TESOL Quarterly 31:367–774

Volet S E, Ang G 1998 Culturally mixed groups on international campuses: an opportunity for intercultural learning. Higher Education, Research and Development 17:5–22

Chapter 13

From a distance: the challenges of clinical education

Maggie Roe-Shaw

DEFINING DISTANCE CLINICAL EDUCATION

This chapter explores distance education in the context of health science clinical education. The concept of distance learning is an interesting and complex one in the context of clinical education experiences. How different is the experience of being in a clinical placement that is distant? The word distant comes from the Latin *distantia* (di-stare, *stand apart*). How does one define distance? The Oxford English Dictionary defines distance as "not closely related to, the state of being separated in space or time, remote". Implicitly, by definition this indicates that the clinical experience is away from something or somewhere else. The concept is relative. In most western heath science programmes (including speech language pathology, occupational therapy, nursing and physiotherapy), the undergraduate clinical education programme includes some clinical placements that are distant. The notion of distance in this context is from the university, the academic staff and university clinical educator staff employed to visit the students in clinical placements.

The main players in the clinical education model are the triad of the university clinical educator, the field university clinical educator and the student. Distance learning and distance supervision create challenges and provide innovative opportunities for university clinical educators, field university clinical educators and students (Pickering & McAllister 1997). The challenge is to develop context-specific tools to develop these opportunities fully.

However, the theoretical literature that informs the theory of distance education tends to focus on the effectiveness of different distance delivery methods that include two-way audio conferencing (Reed 1997) and the changes in information technology (Woodward 1995).

PREPARING STUDENTS FOR DISTANCE CLINICAL EDUCATION

From the student's perspective, going away from the main centre of clinical education for a six-week block of clinical experience can produce high levels of anxiety (Mitchell & Kampfe 1990). This anxiety can be detrimental to the student's ability to make most effective use of the experience of being at a distant clinical placement, so a small study was undertaken in 2000 (Roe-Shaw 2004) with three cohorts of undergraduate physiotherapy students. These students were being sent to musculoskeletal, cardiopulmonary and neurorehabilitation placements in hospitals, community settings and schools, which required distance supervision by a university clinical educator. The purpose of the study was to describe and understand their concerns, and to determine the most effective strategies to deal with these concerns. These concerns, identified prior to beginning the placement, were:

- what would be expected of them?
- how would they get on with their field clinical educator? (a field clinical educator is a registered physiotherapist who is employed by a health care facility but also oversees the clinical experiences of a student)
- what would they do if they had difficulties?
- would their missing out on contact supervision from a university clinical educator affect their grades? (a university clinical educator is a registered therapist – occupational therapy, speech language pathology, physiotherapy – employed by a university to coordinate placements, organise clinical exams, and troubleshoot problems within the placement with either the field clinical educator or the student)
- would the placement provide adequate learning opportunities?
- would the placement provide a wide variety of patients?
- would they be able to pass the clinical practical exam?

Following this survey, a rural and remote package was developed for those students who would be receiving distance clinical education, so they would know what was expected of them. The package gave them strategies to help them maximise their clinical education experience. This package is explained later in this chapter.

PREPARING THE FIELD UNIVERSITY CLINICAL EDUCATOR FOR DISTANCE CLINICAL EDUCATION

The preparation for distance clinical education begins with the university clinical educator preparing the field clinical educator who is responsible for the clinical education of the student in the distant placement. There are a number of ways that the university clinical educator can engage with the field clinical educator to ensure the clinical placement has support from the university, albeit from a distance. Some of the topics that have been used with physiotherapy students include:

- orientation to the placement outcomes, including the content and process of the clinical practical exam
- outline of the expectation of their role
- outline of the role of the university clinical educator
- outline of the process of distance clinical education and these experiences
- outline of the structures and supports in place for the field clinical educator
- communication strategies
- how to provide effective written and verbal feedback.

COMMUNICATION

Communication lines for management of the distance placement between the university clinical educators and the field clinical educators are important to establish prior to commencement of the placement. There are several strategies to assist with communication. These include:

- The development and use of a communication sheet (Table 13.1). The communication sheet can go directly from the student to the field clinical educator, or directly to the university clinical educator.
- Regular exchange of the communication sheet between field clinical educator, student and university clinical educator through fax or e-mail.
- Weekly telephone contact with the student to discuss a clinical scenario (Table 13.2).
- Peer placement review document (Table 13.3).

Another strategy to support the student is to have a telephone link with the university clinical educator at the university to discuss a clinical scenario. Prior to the telephone conversation, the student can fax through notes from the clinical encounter.

Another useful tool is for the student who has been in a distance placement to have a formal written debrief with the student following him/her into the rotation. This has benefits for the clinical placement (who can see how the students perceive their workplace), the educators (who can identify potential risks and problems) and the students (who feel more knowledgeable and prepared about the clinical placement).

INNOVATIVE STRATEGIES IN DISTANCE CLINICAL EDUCATION

The number of undergraduate health science students who require distance clinical education depends on the programme and the context. Within occupational therapy in Canada, for example, there are undergraduate and postgraduate programmes conducted within a distance supervision framework (Mitcham 2003). Within speech language pathology in Australia, Pickering & McAllister (1997) focus on the needs that are specific to the vast rural areas that include technologies such as telephones, fibreoptic networks, microrelays, satellite downlinks or compressed videos.

Table 13.1 Sample communication sheet
Student name: John New Zealand Placement: Hospital X, musculoskeletal physiotherapy

Date	Student comment	Field clinical educator comment	University clinical educator comment
18/7/05		I know this is only week one of the placement but I am finding it impossible to leave John alone with a new patient. He is having difficulty knowing how to use his subjective history to begin the objective assessment. Any ideas how to deal with this?	Have you talked to John about what he thinks is happening? Let's see what he perceives the problem with his time management to be
		Faxed to university clinical educator at the university	*Faxed back to the field clinical educator and John*
19/7/05	I feel under pressure to try to hurry through my subjective because the next new patient is due in 40 minutes. I just get confused about how to make a quick differential diagnosis. When I do get it right, I am not sure why		Let's try the following strategies for a week: John to keep reflective log to document *where* he is learning and *how* he is learning in the clinical setting. Field university clinical educator to keep the patient numbers and visits to hourly for the next week
	Faxed back to university clinical educator at the university		John to break the assessment into quarters and time-manage each quarter. John to report briefly to the field university clinical educator with his suggestions and ideas between the subjective and the objective assessment
			Faxed back to student and supervisor

Table 13.2 Telephone clinical scenario sheet

Student name _____ Placement _____ Date _____ Patient details _____

Describe your subjective history	What were the things you did really well, and what could you improve on? Describe how you would make these changes and why
Describe your objective examination	What were the things you did really well, and what could you improve on? Describe how you would make these changes and why
Describe your communication strengths today	What would you change about your communication today?
Describe your findings and differential diagnosis	Discuss your clinical reasoning
Describe your treatment plan today	Discuss progressions of this treatment plan
Overall comment on your assessment and treatment today	

Table 13.3   Peer placement review document (sample). (All students' names are fictitious, as is the scenario in the text)

Rotation 1	Rotation 2	Rotation 3	Rotation 4
John	Anne	Margo	Shania
Paul	Annette	Richard	Sheila
Ringo	Lynnette	Kay	Jill
George	Margaret	Pat	Heather
Karen	John	Jan	Gavin
Ethan	Jim	Jack	Raymond
Tony	Janet	David	Juliet

1. *Describe the placement to the person on the next rotation to you. Include physical confines, staff support and types of patients you mostly saw*
   I had my own desk and shared a room with two other physios and the physio assistant. Everyone hangs out for lunch together and we share the tearoom with the occupational therapy department. The staff are positive. I saw mostly outpatients but I went up to the wards to orthopaedics for 2 hours a day and did many hip [sic]. There was a hydrotherapy pool at the back so did quite a lot of exercises in there with patients. Most of the patients were older but there were some rugby injuries

2. *Describe your learning experiences: clinical cases, teamwork, resources*
   I went to theatre and saw a total hip patient and followed her through, which was good. I did all the post-op inpatients so learned a lot about the different surgeons' protocols and types of prosthesis. In outpatients, they have all types of machines and equipment so make sure you use them. They have all the recent journals, including *Australian Journal of Physiotherapy* and *Physiotherapy*, to read. You get to go to team meetings and do some community follow-ups as well

3. *Describe the benefits of your clinical learning from being in this placement*
   There was a wide range of disorders and patients in inpatients and outpatients.
   You get to work mostly on your own but there are very different physios to ask for help and they are friendly

4. *Describe the things you found difficult, and make suggestions for improvement as well as the strategies you found most useful to deal with these difficulties*
   The relative isolation so I had to think and function independently from my peers was hard.
   Initially the field university clinical educator was quite stand-off and I needed to ask for appraisal/criticism.
   I found the communication sheet worked well because Maggie talked to the supervisor about my time management problems in the first week.
   Just don't be scared to ask questions because everybody is really helpful

Within physiotherapy in New Zealand I have developed rural and remote guides to learning that are physiotherapy-specific, but consultation with my colleagues within the health science divisions of podiatry, occupational therapy and speech therapy confirms that these learning guidelines are suitable for adaptation to their specific programmes. To address the physiotherapy undergraduate student's needs, three innovative strategies were introduced to make the process of distance clinical education more transparent to the clinical education programme.

Rural and remote guide to learning physiotherapy clinical practice

A ten-page booklet for those students who were going out to a clinical placement that would require distance supervision was developed in 2001 (Rural & Remote Guide to Learning Physiotherapy Practice, developed by and © Maggie Roe-Shaw 2001). The aim of this rural and remote guide was to provide the students with written material that they could draw on to assist them to develop strategies to make this a positive clinical education experience. The guide was split into sections that addressed the following:

Context of distance supervision

In the context of distance supervision, the student was given:

- Placement guidelines, which included physical maps of the facility, contact details of the supervisor, accommodation facilities and transport maps.
- Placement facilities, that included the number of physiotherapy staff employed, the range of experiences of staff and the types of facilities, such as hydrotherapy pools, canteen facilities, staff-room facilities and the type of library in situ.
- A formal facilitated debrief with the student who was in the placement the previous trimester. This peer placement review document was shown above in Table 13.3.

Framing clinical learning

The students were given a section to read which focused on:

- student-centred learning (Boud & Edwards 1999)
- the use of reflective practice to facilitate clinical learning outcomes (see Chapter 7)
- the anatomy of patient-centred performance.

This framework of clinical learning was documented in a series of learning outcomes sheets, which students kept in their portfolio. The questions on this sheet changed from week one to week six, as students made gains with their clinical competence and confidence. The clinical education learning outcomes sheet illustrated in Table 13.4 is week five out of six.

Strategies for students to maximise a distance clinical placement

The students were given a section that focused on:

- strategies to deal with stress (Fontana 1994a, 1994b)
- use of critical reflection to promote adaptation (Schön 1987)
- staff support: whom to contact at the placement if you need a mentor (an experienced local physiotherapist) or a peer (new graduate) to talk to about personal or professional issues
- each student filled in a SWOT plan (Table 13.5) prior to the distance clinical placement

Table 13.4   Clinical education learning outcomes: week 5
(This is an actual week-5 clinical supervision sheet, included with permission of the student)

What were the most important things that you have used over the past week?	Never to forget to pull the curtains around patients or wear gloves in the medical and surgical wards. That the patient's condition can vary dramatically day to day so communication is essential every time. That you are not allowed to mobilise a patient who has just had a pulmonary embolism. How to develop my order of doing the assessment and reasoning for my treatment
What was the best thing that happened to you during this week in your clinical placement?	I had a good conversation with an 81-year-old Greek man I was treating who didn't speak very good English. Before this conversation, he was reluctant to answer too many questions. After this conversation, he was much more happy and compliant with the treatment. I learnt that it is helpful to establish a relationship with patients to obtain the maximum information and to be more effective with my treatment
What were you thinking about when you completed your evaluation of the patient today?	Who is this man? What is his normal functional ability? When did his symptoms start? What are his problems now? *Evidence*: medical notes to cue what I wanted to find out information-wise about the patient. I focused on information about his previous functional ability (he was quite active) and his main problems at present
What was the most difficult thing about this patient? How did you identify this problem. What evidence did you use? How did you learn to do this?	He was very tired. *Observation*: he was reclined on the bed and looked tired. He said he was tired and didn't want to speak for too long
Tell me how you went about making clinical decisions with this patient. What was your approach?	I only took the subjective history but I would have looked at his ventilation pattern and respiratory rate to determine his shortness of breath and work of breathing before doing the treatment. I would have done breathing control and rest positions. His cough was productive of frothy pale sputum (small amounts) so I don't want to emphasise the cough so I would not have done forced expiratory techniques for treatment but reinforced the importance of mobilising
How would you rank yourself in the clinical setting at this point?	6/10
How do you know you have been effective in your evaluation and treatment of this patient today?	I am imagining since I didn't actually treat him. But the education about breathing control, resting positions and mobilising was found useful by the patient. The patient felt good after moving around as he feels after previously being so active he has "lost his muscle tone"

- the SWOT was discussed with the university clinical educator in terms of the action plan; a standard SWOT is shown in Table 13.5
- the SWOT personal action plan was developed with the university clinical educator, as shown in Figure 13.1.

Video self-evaluation forms

The students going to a distant placement were given a video self-evaluation form, which they could enclose with a video of a clinical case scenario to the

Table 13.5 A SWOT plan

Strengths	Weakness
Opportunities	Threats

Figure 13.1 SWOT action plan (developed by and © Maggie Roe-Shaw 2002)

How can I use my SWOT analysis in this next placement?

1. What do I want to focus on developing during this placement?
   Please circle one

   strengths   weaknesses   opportunities   threats

2. Why I want to focus on this _____

   _____

   _____

3. Critically examine your other three descriptors and list three characteristics you can use to help develop your focus.

   1. _____

   2. _____

   3. _____

4. How will I evaluate my action plan?
   Please circle one

   self-evaluate   ask field university clinical educator   peer view

5. How will I know when I have further developed my strengths/opportunities or strengthened my weaknesses and perception of threats? _____

   _____

   _____

   _____

   _____

university clinical educator at the university for feedback. This evaluation form was modelled on the peer-review document used by students who were in university clinical educator based settings and had the opportunity to work with fellow students. The video self-evaluation is shown in Figure 13.2.

SUMMARY

Distance supervision is a unique and exciting way of maximising clinical education opportunities for health science students. Although the examples

When you plan to use self-evaluation by video there are several things to remember:
  1. You must get **informed consent** from your patient using the video consent form
  2. You are responsible for organising this session, **not** your field university clinical educator
  3. You must go through the self-evaluation then post back to your university clinical educator
	Checklist
	
	☐ Patient informed consent
	☐ Ward/supervisor informed of session
	☐ Video camera charged
	☐ Tripod organised
	☐ Video cassette

Describe your introduction to the patient	☐ Introduced myself – comment ☐ Clarity of structure of the session – comment ☐ Patient comfort – comment
Discuss your observation of your subjective assessment today	☐ I know who this person is – comment ☐ I understand what they do, and what their functional limitations are – comment ☐ I gained all the information I needed today – comment
List the key things you gained from the subjective assessment. Which will facilitate your objective assessment?	☐ ☐ ☐ ☐
Discuss your observation of your objective assessment today	☐ The patient understood what I was doing and why – comment ☐ All my tests were appropriate and effective – comment ☐ The patient was well positioned and comfortable – comment ☐ I got informed consent – comment ☐ I summarised my findings to the patient – comment
Discuss your communication today	
Discuss your treatment plan today	☐ Why I chose this treatment – comment ☐ What alternative treatment could I have chosen? – comment ☐ Efficacy of my choice – comment ☐ Treatment outcomes – comment ☐ What was the best thing about my treatment today? – comment
Overview of today's treatment session. Write a summary	☐ Patient satisfaction – comment ☐ Time management – comment ☐ Things that went really well – comment ☐ Things I would do differently next time – comment ☐ Treatment outcomes – comment ☐ My grading of myself: 5 6 7 8 9 10 (circle)

Figure 13.2   Video self-evaluation form (developed by and © Maggie Roe-Shaw 1998)

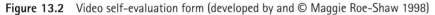

I have used in this chapter have been designed specifically for physiotherapy students in the clinical setting, consultation has determined these can easily be modified and adapted for other disciplines such as podiatry, occupational therapy and speech language pathology.

To gaze into the future, the path of sophisticated information technology will be an integral part of the distance supervision model. As costs to access technology decrease, and availability increases, the use of *Blackboard* and video-conferencing may well give students the necessary support through a visual medium to engage on a meaningful level with their educator, and to enhance their self-efficacy in the clinical setting. It may well be possible for clinical triad scenarios to be monitored through small portable projectors beamed to the university to encourage instant feedback in clinical scenarios.

REFERENCES

Boud D, Edwards H 1999 Learning for practice: promoting learning in clinical and community settings. Educating beginning practitioners. In: Higgs J, Edwards H (eds) Butterworth-Heinemann, Oxford

Fontana D 1994a Managing stress. British Psychological Society & Routledge, London, p 1–15

Fontana D 1994b Managing stress. British Psychological Society & Routledge, London, p 62–82

Mitcham M 2003 Integrating theory and practice: using theory creatively to enhance professional practice. In: Brown G, Esdaile S, Ryan S (eds) Becoming an advanced healthcare practitioner. Butterworth-Heinemann, Oxford, p 83–85

Mitchell M, Kampfe C 1990 Coping strategies used by occupational therapy students during field work. American Journal of Occupational Therapy 44:543–550

Pickering M, McAllister L 1997 Clinical education and the future: an emerging mosaic of change, challenge and creativity. In: McAllister L, McLeod S, Maloney D (eds) Facilitating learning in clinical settings. Stanley Thornes, Cheltenham, p 265

Reed K 1997 Theory and frame of reference. In: Neistadt M, Crepeau E (eds) Willard & Spackman's occupational therapy, 9th edn. Lippincott, Philadelphia

Roe-Shaw M 2001 A rural and remote guide to learning physiotherapy practice. Unpublished workbook

Roe-Shaw M The loneliness of the long distance student (in preparation)

Schön D A 1987 Educating the reflective practitioner. Jossey-Bass, San Francisco

Woodward C 1995 Internet international. The Chronicle of Higher Education June:A21

Chapter **14**

Collaboration in clinical education

Magdalen Rozsa and Michelle Lincoln

BACKGROUND

Collaboration refers to two or more people working together for a common purpose or to achieve common goals, where each person has recognised skills or qualities and where there is a respect for each person's contribution. Collaborative learning refers to pairs or small groups engaging in reciprocal learning experiences whereby knowledge and ideas are exchanged.

Collaboration in clinical education can refer to a range of situations and approaches, and in this chapter we will discuss the following: collaboration between pairs or groups of students (peers); collaboration between two or more clinical educators from the same health profession; collaboration between clinical educators or students from different professional fields; and multiple layers of collaboration between all stakeholders involved in the clinical education process, i.e. students, clients, clinical educators and university staff. For each type of collaborative learning presented the educational background of each approach will be discussed, examples of successful models given, a table summarising the advantages and disadvantages of each approach provided and the challenges inherent in each approach highlighted.

The importance of collaborative skills in the current health professional workplace

Health professionals' workplaces change rapidly in response to different demands on services, different client needs and different approaches to clinical and professional practice. For example, the change in approach in health care from "illness" care to "wellness" care has resulted in a greater emphasis being placed on clinicians' interpersonal skills and team-functioning abilities (Hunt et al 1999). Clinicians in the workplace need to be able to develop skills, incorporate new theoretical knowledge and adapt and change to ensure that their profession remains relevant in the changing health care context.

A major task of clinical educators of students from the health professions is to facilitate the development of skills, attitudes and knowledge that allow graduates to function successfully in such contexts. For beginning health science graduates there is an expectation that they will be able to interact effectively with people in a variety of contexts (Higgs & Edwards 1999), and demonstrate high-level communication and negotiation skills when dealing with clients, families, colleagues, workplace teams and organisational staff. Graduates are also expected to embrace a commitment to ongoing or life-long learning throughout their professional careers. Effective collaborative learning skills such as reflective practice, peer learning and giving and receiving feedback can all contribute to this.

The nature of successful collaboration

There are many components of successful collaboration. Collaborators need to be skilled communicators, and able to take an equal share in communication (that is, to listen actively and impart their own opinions, feelings and ideas as well as give others the chance to do the same). Respect for others is vital – for the role of others in the partnership or group, for their opinions and approaches, and their overall contribution. It is not necessary to have to agree with others within collaborative situations, but it is important to be able to demonstrate openness, acceptance of diversity and attempt to negotiate when disagreements occur. In this way, an atmosphere of trust can be fostered, where individuals are able to share their own opinions and feelings in a safe and accepting context. We would also argue that attitudes are central to successful collaboration; participants need to show a willingness to engage in the collaborative process and a commitment to the overall purposes or goals of the collaborative situation.

Learning collaboratively as a formal part of a course is more than students linking up informally to work on assignments or course projects. Establishing collaborative learning opportunities as part of the clinical education process requires careful planning and ongoing support to explicate expectations and foster relationships that will enable the benefits to be realised (Cohen & Sampson 1999).

Collaboration in clinical education and promoting collaborative professional practice

In our experience fostering collaboration within clinical education can have many benefits in terms of the quality and depth of students' learning experiences, as well as advantages for clinical educators, clients, professional colleagues and university staff. Students working and learning collaboratively can experience benefits academically, professionally, emotionally and socially and these form the basis of later professional socialisation and life-long learning (Cohen & Sampson 1999). Clinical educators can benefit from assistance with their workload and consolidate their own learning, the quality of professional care for the client may be enhanced, there may be a growth in successful teamwork experiences or communication in the workplace, as well as successful completion and achievement of the objectives of clinical placements.

In clinical education collaboration revolves around students' and clinical educators' learning relationships, and is successful when the relationship is based on mutuality, reciprocity and respect for individual difference. It is a learning journey for students and clinical educators, which occurs in the context of shared experiences and human relationships. The success of the relationship is affected by the qualities of the clinical educators (their assumptions, values and beliefs) and how these relate to the individual responsiveness and characteristics of the learners (Goodfellow et al 2001).

There has been a recent shift in the educational literature and subsequent approaches towards student-centred teaching and learning. This reflects a move away from didactic teacher–student models to models where students are active in the learning process and educators are more facilitators than teachers (Baxter & Gray 2001). Such a shift has been embraced specifically through changes in approaches to clinical education in some university departments where there is a greater emphasis on the development of students' autonomy and increased use of collaborative learning strategies in order to enhance the development of thinking and questioning practitioners (Bruce et al 2001).

There are specific differences between traditional (or "product-oriented") and collaborative ("process-oriented") approaches to clinical education, which are summarised in Table 14.1.

Table 14.1   Comparison of traditional and collaborative approaches to clinical education

	Traditional	Collaborative
Students		
	Competitive	Cooperative
	Passive learners	Active learners
	Work on own	Interaction encouraged
Clinical educator		
	Expert	Co-learner
	Control of time/response	Group control time/response
	Control content/knowledge	Group control content/knowledge
	Responsible for structure	Group responsible for structure
	Autonomous	Group interdependent
Objectives/assignments		
	Preset learning objectives	Objectives set by group
	Traditional assignments	Multidimensional activities

Adapted with the permission of Nelson Thornes Ltd from *Facilitating Learning in Clinical Settings* (McLeod et al 1997) ISBN 07487 3316 7 first published in 1997.

In their conceptual approach to collaborative learning, Johnson et al (1992) describe five key elements that are needed: positive interdependence, face-to-face interaction to promote each other's learning and success, individual accountability, cooperative skills and participation in group processes. These are consistent with the generic attributes of health care professionals that have been recently described that include interdependence, i.e. the ability to collaborate with other professionals in learning and service delivery (McAllister 1997). Hence a collaborative educational approach is consistent with contemporary goals of clinical education.

Peer learning as the foundation for collaboration

Peer learning is one type of collaborative learning where participants share both "teacher" and "learner" roles. There has been much in the literature regarding the benefits of peer learning (Lincoln & McAllister 1993, Lincoln et al 1997a). These include the development of a non-threatening learning community, decreased work-related anxiety, increased self-discovery, insight and personal growth, recognition for and promotion of professional expertise, improved staff morale and improved quality of care. Peer consultation provides an opportunity for professionals to share their expertise in clinical reasoning (Hart & Ryan 2000).

Working in groups or teams can also incorporate peer learning; however, as the number of participants increases, so does the complexity of the task as the skills, knowledge and needs of each participant have to be accounted for in the group process. Groups are often formed for particular purposes and for specifically defined time periods, and tend to move through general sequences of well-documented stages (Tuckman & Jensen 1977).

When groups are functioning well, collaboration within them can lead to very successful outcomes, in terms of the overall purpose of the group and the learning and development of individual group members. As with peer learning, the group context allows knowledge to be pooled and the educator is a facilitator or co-learner rather than instructor or supervisor.

CLINICAL EDUCATION FOR GROUPS OF STUDENTS – COLLABORATIVE STUDENT LEARNING

Description

A common approach to current clinical education practice is assigning two or more students simultaneously to one clinical placement site. Usually, the students are from the same training institution and are at the same stage of their course; however, this is not always the case.

There are a number of reasons for taking more than one student on clinical placement. Universities are increasingly finding it difficult to secure sufficient numbers of off-campus clinical placements for their students. Thus it may solve a logistical problem to send two or more students to one placement. Many clinical educators prefer having two or more students concurrently because of the advantages in terms of planning placement experiences, caseload management, timetabling and workload issues. Overwhelmingly, the practice of providing clinical education experiences for two or a group of students is consistent with the shift in educational literature that recognises the benefits of peer learning and reflects the changing roles of students as learners and clinical educators as teachers or supervisors.

Group supervision refers to the situation where a clinical educator is responsible for a student's professional development within a group of peers. It has been recognised for some time that group situations have a positive effect on learning; one of the early researchers to propose this was Vygotsky who, in 1922, proposed that cognitive skills were more effectively acquired through social interaction (cited in Hillerbrand 1989). In terms of development of cognitive skills, group supervision has been shown to be effective largely due to students being able to practise skills within a context where feedback about performance is provided, where cognitive rehearsal can occur and discussion of various perspectives may facilitate attitude change (Hillerbrand 1989).

In terms of the differences between experts and novices, groups may also be more effective learning situations than the one-to-one expert and novice teaching context. It has been found that often experts are not able to verbalise clearly their cognitive processes in a way that can be understood by novices as their clinical decisions may be more automatic or integrated. In group supervision there is interaction of several novices with an expert, and skills are enhanced by verbalisation of one novice in the presence of others, where cognitive processes are made explicit, and in a language that may be easily understood by other novices (Hillerbrand 1989).

Procedures that allow peer learning to occur include peer teaching, peer tutoring, peer evaluation (Lincoln & McAllister 1993) or group supervision. There are also different approaches to peer learning, including those that are structured (e.g. teaching clinic, peer tutoring, supervisory conferences, structured observation, supervision in absentia), and those that are unstructured (e.g. multiple student placements, observation facilities, clinical educator modeling, peer facilitation or role playing) (Lincoln et al 1997a).

Examples of successful student collaboration models

There are a number of examples from the literature where peer-learning models are described in a variety of clinical education contexts:

1. University programmes may pair a novice student with a more advanced student for the management of one or more designated clients. This arrangement facilitates the creation of a safe and less threatening learning environment for the novice student and allows the advanced student to begin developing skills in clinical education through a peer-learning process (Lincoln et al 1997a).
2. Murphy & Watson (2002) described an integrated approach to supervision developed and modified particularly to enhance clinical preparation of students in the treatment of fluency disorders which they termed blended individual–group supervision (BIGS). This approach was based on the continuum of supervision model (Anderson 1988) and the teaching clinic model (Dowling 1979).

   In the BIGS approach, group supervision is the primary context for clinical education, with individual one-to-one conferences conducted at mid-term, end of term and as needed. Preliminary activities were introduced to encourage collaborative and consultative communication with other students and the clinical educator and included a teaching clinic, client orientation, group supervision orientation, self-exploration and a goal-setting session.

   Subjective outcomes and feedback from students for the BIGS approach were reported as very positive in a number of areas (for example, administration, flexibility, communication, interpersonal skills and professionalism), with 89% preferring group supervision over one-to-one supervision, providing that access to individual supervisory meetings was available. From the perspective of clinical educators, the approach was found to be effective in terms of enhancing student learning; however, the approach was found to be less suitable for some students (for example, non-communicative students, weak students, students less willing to participate in group problem-solving or self-disclosure). These students needed a one-to-one approach to explore jointly the nature of the difficulties and course of action needed (Murphy & Watson 2002).

3. Bruce et al (2001) described a programme used with Masters students in their final year in a university clinic where students were placed in pairs or groups. In this programme the roles of clinicians and students were modified, i.e. the clinical educator's role was to guide the learning of students, and each student had two main roles – learner/practitioner and facilitator. Observations of clinical sessions and feedback on performance are the responsibility of students under the guidance of clinicians. The programme proceeds in stages, with the clinical educator providing more support and direct input for students in both learner/practitioner and facilitator roles during the beginning stages.

    Outcomes for the students were generally positive. Students reported that they found the amount of clinical responsibility difficult but that reflective practice provided them with effective coping strategies. Some students perceived that clinical educators provided less than optimal support, and some felt the process was too time-consuming. From the clinical educators' points of view, students varied in terms of their involvement in the supervisory process and their openness and commitment to the process. They felt that more flexibility in the programme was needed to account for individual student differences and needs (Bruce et al 2001).

4. Parker & Emanuel (2001) reported on a collaborative project between clinical educators and university staff that resulted in the provision of group student placements in a therapy service with high demands and long waiting lists. This programme involved groups of six students who worked either in rotating pairs, or groups of threes when an observer was required. The role of the clinical educator was that of supervisor of delegated work rather than therapist working alongside the students; thus a high level of preparation and induction of students was needed, as well as carefully planned support. The programme was modified over three years to account for feedback and suggestions from service users, students, clinical educators and university staff.

    A range of outcomes was reported for this programme. There were service provision advantages that were demonstrable to the therapy service; groups of students enabled completion of more work than possible by a single therapist. The feedback from service users was positive, as was feedback from students, clinical educators and university staff. Identified areas of improvement included the need for increased support for students' report-writing skills, and additional time for individual student feedback (Parker & Emanuel 2001).

Advantages and disadvantages of working with groups of students

Table 14.2 lists the advantages and disadvantages of working with groups of students in the clinical education context, for students, clinical educators and universities.

Table 14.2   Advantages and disadvantages of working with groups of students

Advantages	Disadvantages
Students	
• Extended learning opportunities • Emotional support and reassurance (Parker & Emanuel 2001) • Anxiety is often reduced (Baxter & Gray 2001) and students may more readily communicate their doubts and insecurities to a peer than a clinical educator (Bruce et al 2001) • Do not see themselves as alone in a new and potentially challenging situation (Borders 1991) • Successful experiences of peer supervision may lead to continuing peer collaboration in later work settings (Borders 1991) • Engaging in and sharing self-reflection may lead to deeper insights • By reflecting on their own and others' experience, vicarious learning can occur from taking on the role of observer and provider of feedback • Practise skills relevant to the profession and practise technical language • Analyse their own and others' ways of learning, develop responsibility for own and each other's learning and work • Discuss and critique literature, identify and try to apply relevant evidence and understand the relationship between theory and practice (Cohen & Sampson 1999) • Appreciate different viewpoints, and become life-long learners (by engaging in self-directed and peer-assisted learning)	• Mismatch between level of competency of students, leading to comparison and competition (Murphy & Watson 2002) • Differences in personality, confidence or cultural dimensions • Some students may be unwilling to establish interpersonal relationships within their learning context • Some students may perceive difficulties with groups in terms of time and logistics (Cohen & Sampson 1999) • Group functioning or cohesion may be affected even if only one member is resistant or not committed to the process of collaboration
Clinical educators	
• There may be greater efficiency in planning and orientation phases of placements where administrative and orientation tasks can be covered without the need for repetition with individual students • If more than one student, clinical educators are thus freed from having to have a "social host" role (McAllister 1997) • As the placement progresses students may be managing a greater clinical caseload than is possible by a single clinician – clinical educators may then have more free time to attend to non-client responsibilities • Student groups may also allow a workplace to implement specific projects or changes to service delivery • Students can be assigned joint responsibility for a range of clinical and non-clinical tasks that can assist the clinical educator with other workload demands	• Clinical educators may find managing some of the logistical demands of having groups of students a disadvantage, e.g. needing to schedule time for peer or group feedback/reflection sessions • If there are interpersonal conflicts within the group, it may take significant time and energy to address these

continued over

Universities

- Being able to facilitate a more relevant and current educational approach for their off-campus clinical education programmes
- May help to ease the burden of finding sufficient placements for students

- May initially need to invest time in providing training for clinical educators
- Time or logistical demands may be increased due to increased need for collaboration with and support for clinical educators
- Peer or group placements may provide less face-to-face individual contact hours for students
- May need to take on facilitator or mediator role if problems arise with groups

Challenges of collaborative student learning in clinical education contexts

There are some areas of caution that clinical educators need to consider when planning or implementing peer collaboration. The dependency level and competence of students should be fairly close for the relationship to be equal. Peer-learning situations may accentuate differences between students and lead to competition, which may result in inappropriate expectations (for example, too high for students with weaker skills or too low for students with very strong skills). Additionally, clinical educators need to be alert to the possibility of conflict or personality clash (Lincoln et al 1997a), which is difficult to predict until the group is operating.

Other logistical considerations for the clinical educator involve managing two or more students working in different physical areas, retaining and maintaining a sense of patient control, managing the paperwork and picking up their caseload after the students leave (Best & Rose 1996). There should ideally be good collaboration for planning between university and workplace staff to ensure there is sufficient support for clinical educators, and that they have access to updated theory and practical skills for structuring placements to maximise the benefits for all concerned.

Other challenges are associated with those inherent in managing group situations in general. Managing group dynamics can be difficult if there are negative elements like tension, adversity or frustration. It can be useful to ensure students are aware of normal group development, stages and roles, to establish what is normal and make explicit the expectations and accountabilities involved. This may help alleviate students' anxiety, especially at the start of groups (Cohen & Sampson 1999).

Facilitation of groups is crucial and the role of the clinical educator as moderator or manager includes helping the group stay on task, observing group processes and dynamics, being aware of levels of individual group members and varying their own behaviour to suit the needs of the group. Not all peer groups are helpful or supportive, some may be overly supportive or competitive, members may be prone to giving advice or may have difficulty staying on task. A systematic approach may be needed so that the following goals are targeted: all group members are involved in the supervision process, members are encouraged to provide focused and objective feedback, self-monitoring and reflective skills are encouraged and group activities are adapted according to skill level (Borders 1991).

Despite these challenges, collaborative learning contexts involving two or more students have great potential for all stakeholders in clinical education, with successful models providing good examples of the wide range of possible applications.

SHARED CLINICAL EDUCATION – COLLABORATION BETWEEN CLINICAL EDUCATORS

Description

Shared clinical education occurs when two or more professionals from the same discipline supervise students simultaneously. A pair or team of clinical educators may supervise students on clinical placement together. This may occur when:

- several part-time staff members supervise full-time clinical placements
- clinicians working in specialised areas "share" the students to ensure the students gain a broad range of experiences
- staff workloads mean that no one person is able to provide full-time supervision
- experienced clinical educators share clinical education responsibilities with inexperienced clinical educators in order to model behaviours and approaches and to provide mentoring to inexperienced clinical educators
- clinical educators deliberately "share" student supervision to extend their own learning by creating opportunities for peer observation, feedback and discussion of the clinical education process
- students are simultaneously placed at physically separate placement sites or different organisations.

To be successful, shared clinical education experiences need to be managed carefully. Often, placement sites will call on the expertise of the clinical education staff at universities to advise them on how best to prepare for, organise and evaluate this way of providing clinical education. Shared clinical education arrangements also require close collaboration between the clinical educators involved and the students. In order for the share arrangement to be successful in terms of student learning, clinical educators need to collaborate about timetabling, performance expectations, workload, student learning goals, provision of feedback and the assessment process. The more clinical educators involved in the "share" arrangement, the more important the collaborative process will be. Students will also need to collaborate with their clinical educators to ensure that their learning needs are met, workload is manageable, feedback is consistent and the assessment process is fair. Table 14.3 summarises some of the issues that need to be considered when setting up shared clinical education placements.

Table 14.3 Issues for consideration in shared clinical placements

Issue	Things to consider
Orientation	Who will orient the student to the services? Will individual orientations need to be provided? Does everyone know what will be covered in the orientation?
Expectations	Do we all share the same expectations regarding the level of skill and knowledge that needs to be achieved? Do we all share the same expectations regarding the amount of supervision we should/can provide? Do we share similar expectations regarding the students' attitudes and interpersonal skills? Are our expectations regarding how, what and in what form students will plan for their clinical work consistent?
Rules	Have we agreed on deadlines for submission of paperwork that are consistent? Have we agreed on the minimum and maximum workload for students? Do we agree on the hours of attendance?
Assessment	Who will coordinate the students' assessment? How will we ensure that all clinical educators' assessments are taken into account? What will we do if we disagree about students' assessments? How will we involve the student in the assessment process?
Role modelling	How best can we model collaboration and teamwork? What are some of our own behaviours that we need to be mindful of in the presence of students?
Communication	How will we ensure excellent communication between the clinical educators involved? How will we encourage constructive and timely feedback from the students about the supervisory arrangements?
Privacy and confidentiality	How will we know when it is OK to pass information about the students between us and when it is not? How will we manage if the students disclose information about a clinical educator to another clinical educator? How do we ensure everyone's privacy and confidentiality is maintained?

Examples of successful models of shared clinical education

There are many examples of the successful use of shared supervision models among our allied health colleagues. However, few, if any, of these are ever reported in the literature. Below are two examples of shared supervisory arrangements.

Job sharing

In job sharing two clinical educators share one full-time position. The clinical educators accept groups of three to four students for full-time placements on a regular basis. One clinical educator supervises the students on two days of the week and the other on three days of the week. The roles of the two clinical educators are negotiated ahead of time, for example one provides orientation and tutorials while the other completes the assessment process. Three techniques that have been found to work well are:

1. clinical educators working consecutive days so the students are not constantly changing between people
2. as their working days do not overlap, at the change-over point each week a brief tape recording of comments, feedback and information relating to the students is made and left for the other clinical educator to listen to
3. for the assessment one supervisor leaves a draft of the student's assessment and the second supervisor completes the final version; if there is a discrepancy in their marking, this is discussed over the phone and with the student.

Mixed placements

In mixed placements two clinical educators work in different areas of service delivery in one organisation. One clinical educator works only with children the other with adult in-patients. The students spend two days per week with each clinical educator. Four things the clinical educators learned from this arrangement were:

1. a student could have different levels of skills simultaneously in both areas depending on aptitude and previous experience
2. generic skills, for example communication, clinical reasoning, professional behaviour and learning skills (Engel 1995), impacted on performance with both types of services
3. the support and input from a colleague added a different dimension to the experience of being a clinical educator (McAllister 2001)
4. it was helpful if one person liaised with the university regarding questions, concerns and advice and took responsibility for communicating this to the other clinical educator and students.

Advantages and disadvantages of shared clinical education

Table 14.4 lists the advantages and disadvantages of shared clinical education for students, clinical educators and universities.

Challenges of shared clinical education contexts

Clinical educators involved in shared supervisory arrangements will be challenged to have excellent organisational and communication skills in regard to both their colleagues and students. Some may be challenged to be open to learning from and receiving feedback from their peers. Students will be challenged to establish rapport with several clinical educators and to adapt to each person's professional style and workplace idiosyncrasies. Students will also need to develop their communication skills and flexibility.

Shared clinical education experiences have many advantages and disadvantages for all involved. In our experience the risk of an unsatisfactory experience occurring is increased exponentially in line with the number of

Table 14.4 Advantages and disadvantages of shared clinical education

Advantages	Disadvantages
Students	
<ul><li>Exposure to more professional role models</li><li>Benefit from observing different clinicians working, discussing theoretical background, treatment approaches and personal philosophies with multiple clinical educators</li><li>Exposure to a range of interpersonal communication styles, management styles and learning styles</li><li>A wider variety of clinical experiences may be attained</li><li>May enjoy increased feelings of being "part of a team"</li><li>Student will benefit from being "immersed in a rich and productive learning environment" (Best & Rose 1996, p. 126)</li><li>Learning that there are multiple ways of achieving similar outcomes in some cases</li><li>Students may gain more confidence in their "professional persona" (Lincoln et al 1997b) by experiencing multiple ways of doing, knowing and communicating about clinical work</li><li>May facilitate the development of good time management skills</li></ul>	<ul><li>May lead to increased student stress and reduced learning if not managed appropriately (Best & Rose 1996)</li><li>Differing opinions between clinical educators may lead to the student adopting a "strategic approach to learning" (Boud 2000) rather than a deep approach (Martin & Säljö 1984) in order to keep both clinical educators "happy"</li><li>Students with weak interpersonal skills may find it difficult establishing and maintaining rapport with multiple clinical educators</li><li>Students needing to consolidate theoretical knowledge or clinical skills may have difficulty achieving this across multiple supervisors</li><li>There is a potential for an increased and possibly unrealistic workload. This, combined with dealing closely with multiple people across a week, could lead to exhaustion</li></ul>
Clinical educators	
<ul><li>Increased support from other clinical educators</li><li>Time away from students when they are with other clinical educators, allowing the clinical educator to complete other work</li><li>Sick leave or annual leave can be accommodated more easily</li><li>Skill development in clinical education through discussion and observation of peers (McAllister & Lincoln 2004)</li><li>Provides an opportunity for formal mentoring of beginning clinical educators</li><li>Confidence in managing difficult situations with students may be higher when input from several others is available that supports your view or decision</li><li>Productive, collaborative working relationships may be established that benefit the service or department in other areas</li><li>Individual clinical educators have a reduced commitment to providing clinical education compared with supervising a full-time placement on their own</li></ul>	<ul><li>Failure to work as a team of clinical educators may lead to high dissatisfaction with the clinical education role (Best & Rose 1996)</li><li>Increased time needed to liaise with other clinical educators regarding students</li><li>Scheduling difficulties may require flexibility or a temporary change in work practices during the placement to accommodate colleagues and students</li></ul>
Universities	
<ul><li>Students' learning experiences meet the goals of their courses</li><li>Increased numbers of placements may be available</li><li>Feedback about student performance and the curriculum in general is available from a larger group of people</li></ul>	<ul><li>There is a potential for the shared supervision model to be unsuccessful and result in reduced student learning and dissatisfaction</li><li>Disagreements in the assessment process may challenge the validity and reliability of assessment tools</li></ul>

clinical educators involved. However, when shared clinical education experiences are managed well, students benefit enormously and clinical educators and universities can also reap rewards. It is also likely that shared clinical education placements will increase in the future and therefore we need those who are already working this way to share their experiences.

INTERPROFESSIONAL COLLABORATION – CLINICAL EDUCATION ACROSS HEALTH PROFESSIONS

Description of interprofessional collaboration in clinical education

Interprofessional collaboration refers to situations where there is collaboration between two or more clinical educators from different health professional areas. It could also refer to situations where students have placements or discrete experiences with one or more students from a different professional area. For example, workplaces that function primarily in terms of multidisciplinary teams, where students may be in a number of clinical situations with educators of different professions to their own, or where there is not currently a clinician of the student's profession but clearly a need for one. Additionally, collaboration in workplaces is increasingly recognised as central to coordinated client care and some organisational structures have a focus on multidisciplinary units or teams rather than professional departments.

Examples of successful models of interprofessional collaboration

Joint student educational activities

One example of interprofessional collaboration arose at the Children's Hospital at Westmead, Sydney where a group of allied health clinical educators planned and conducted a number of joint student educational activities. The clinical educators from five allied health departments (physiotherapy, occupational therapy, social work, dietetics and speech pathology) set up regular meetings to enhance their own learning and provide reciprocal support and collaboration. Short workshops were offered to all allied health students on placement at specific times. Topics included confidentiality, ethics, multidisciplinary team functioning and multidisciplinary case management.

Formats of the workshops varied but generally included small group work where students of different professions were asked to collaborate on a task. Some workshops were largely case-based and included role play; others focused more on discussion and sharing information and perspectives from own professional backgrounds. The workshops were evaluated through the use of short surveys and generally reflected very positive experiences for the students, particularly in terms of gaining understanding of different professionals and their roles, and the opportunity to work with multidisciplinary groups on specific tasks or problems.

Shared supervision of students

A further example is shared supervision of students by clinical educators from different professional groups. In this scenario a clinical educator provides feedback to students and their discipline-specific clinical educator about student performance in related areas. For example, a physiotherapy clinical educator may provide feedback to students from nursing, medicine, occupational therapy, dietetics or speech pathology regarding the positioning of patients during eating and drinking. Similarly, a speech pathology clinical educator could provide feedback to students from other disciplines regarding their communication with elderly, communicatively disordered or hearing-impaired patients. These types of experiences will enrich the learning of both the students and the discipline-specific clinical educator – and of course will lead to better patient management.

Advantages and disadvantages of interprofessional collaboration in clinical education

Table 14.5 summarises the possible advantages and disadvantages of interprofessional collaboration in clinical education contexts for students, clinical educators and universities.

Challenges of interprofessional collaboration in clinical education

Clearly, interprofessional collaboration situations need to be carefully planned so that the needs of the clients and students are fully acknowledged and met, and so that means are available for individual students' professional competence to be evaluated. This sort of collaboration may not be appropriate for all students or for all workplace contexts. Students may need to be at a certain level of their training (for example, final year) and should have the demonstrated ability to work in an interdependent way by taking responsibility for their own learning, engaging in regular reflection, seeking support when needed and having organisational skills to work within a structured but less directive clinical education approach.

MULTIPLE LAYERS OF COLLABORATION

Multiple layers of collaboration involve a cycle of collaborative learning between clients, students, clinical educators and university staff.

Description of the cycle of collaboration in clinical education

One potential way of conceptualising clinical education is as a cycle of collaborative learning that encompasses clients, students, clinical educators and university staff. Figure 14.1 represents the collaborative clinical education learning cycle.

Students, clinical educators and clients learning collaboratively

At the centre of the diagram (Fig. 14.1) are the clients of allied health professionals. Students and clinical educators are constantly learning from their interactions with clients or, in the case of clinical educators, sometimes through their students' interactions with clients. Reflection on practice with clients

Table 14.5   Advantages and disadvantages of interprofessional collaboration

Advantages	Disadvantages
Students	
• Students can obtain a holistic and broad view of the client, health care contexts and an understanding of their own and others' roles and responsibilities • Working with different professionals (either peers or clinical educators) can help students strengthen their own profession-specific knowledge and skills, and practise and refine their communication skills with others who are not operating from the same background • Focus on the skills needed for effective team functioning (communication, negotiation, respect, collaboration) invaluable for beginning graduate professional experience • Situations of interprofessional conflict or difficulties may provide useful opportunities to address such issues which can occur in many workplaces, and to give students experience with situations where conflict resolution skills are needed	• The student may require supervision or support directly related to profession-specific practice • Professional rivalries, unclear professional boundaries or comparisons between professions may also occur, which may impact on the success of such a programme for the student or client
Clinical educators	
• May benefit from the support of other team members and other professional perspectives • May help to assess students' generic or professional competencies in a broader workplace context	• May have difficulties assessing students in all areas of competency • May need to rely on other professionals' opinions (which may not provide sufficient detail) • May be disagreements with other professionals regarding standards or criteria of performance
Universities	
• May provide a wider range of possible placements or workplace contexts • Allows students to experience multidisciplinary contexts and to deal with other professionals (hard to provide these things in an academic context)	• Requires significant time for planning, coordination and collaboration • May need to intervene if disagreements or difficulties, or with marginal students • May need to provide further profession-specific placements for students if more clinical situations are needed to cover all competencies for assessment

Figure 14.1   The cycle of collaborative learning between clients, students, clinical educators and university staff

(Fish & Coles 1998) promotes deep learning and careful clinical reasoning (Higgs & Jones 2000) for both students and clinical educators (McAllister & Lincoln 2004). Each client is often a "first-time" experience for students and consequently there is much to learn. For clinical educators often unusual or complex clients precipitate learning. As the client, the student and clinical educator are learning, then true collaboration is occurring. However, collaboration with clients does not occur automatically. Students need to learn how to collaborate with clients to set appropriate, meaningful goals for treatment, to adapt treatments to suit individual clients and evaluate the impact of treatments sensitively.

Students and clinical educators learning collaboratively

Anderson's continuum of supervision (1988) suggests that the middle stage (the longest stage) of a clinical placement is about increasing collaborative interactions between students and their clinical educators. In this stage it is expected that students will do more of the talking during supervisory discussions and they will bring to the discussion their ideas, plans, interpretations and concerns. The clinical educator collaborates with students to expand or modify their thoughts and integrate new knowledge. At the same time clinical educators are developing their skills in clinical education as well as refining more generic skills in areas such as clinical reasoning, interpersonal communication, conflict resolution, teaching and time management. McAllister & Lincoln (2004) argue that the clinical education process is an important professional development tool for allied health professionals. A number of studies have documented the benefits of clinical education in terms of professional development for allied health professionals (Adams & Kilburn-Watt 2000, Short et al 2001).

Students, clinical educators and university staff learning collaboratively

The flow of information from students and clinical educators to and from university staff also promotes collaborative learning. University staff assist students to learn about the latest assessment tools or treatment approaches and students give this information to their clinical educators. Students also often have access to the latest technology, references and texts that they can share with their clinical educators. University staff also may provide professional development activities for clinical educators such as presentations and seminars as a way of "thanking" them for supervising students on placement. Just as importantly, information provided to university staff by students and clinical educators about the context and challenges of the contemporary workplace helps university staff to keep courses and their content up to date and relevant for the workplace. Interactions about unusual or complex clients can also lead to learning for clinical educators, students and university staff members. In our experience collaborative learning between students, clinical educators and university staff can also lead to collaborative research projects as all parties involved seek to find an answer to a question.

Feedback from clinical educators to university staff can also facilitate university staff learning about curriculum design. After all, the success of a health science curriculum can only really be assessed fully by the students' performance on clinical placement and in the workplace after graduation.

Examples of successful models reflecting the cycle of collaboration in clinical education

Below are two examples of successful models that actively promote the cycle of collaborative learning between clients, students, clinical educators and university staff.

1. The clinical affiliate programme of The School of Communication Sciences and Disorders, the University of Sydney, is designed to promote collaboration between clinical placement sites that are consistently and actively involved in the clinical education programme of the school. In return for accepting students on placement, academic and clinical staff of the school present on-site in services for the placement sites and staff of the sites are encouraged to consult university staff about clients or projects. Additionally, small collaborative research grants are made available to establish joint research projects between staff of the site and the university.
2. Kersener & Parker (2001) describe a collaborative project between a university based speech and language therapy programme and local speech and language therapy services. The aim of the project was to develop long-term approaches to addressing shortages in the number of clinical placements available for students. All of the stakeholders were invited to participate in focus groups which sought to determine what the underlying issues were that prevented departments offering clinical placements. A strategic plan that addressed the issues was developed as a result and a subsequent increase in the number of clinical placements offered occurred.

Advantages and disadvantages of multiple layers of collaboration

The collaborative learning cycle between students, clinical educators and universities:

- promotes greater understanding of each other's context
- provides mutual support for each other
- extends and enhances the learning opportunities available to individuals.

As with all collaborative endeavours there are also some disadvantages to this approach. Table 14.6 summarises the advantages and disadvantages.

Challenges of implementing multiple layers of collaboration

Implementing a cycle of collaborative learning between clients, students, clinical educators and university staff requires commitment and time from all involved. Universities and clinical placement sites may have different goals, objectives and areas of core business and these may be in conflict. However, the possibility of professional development for all involved makes this type of approach a worthwhile one in which to invest time and resources.

Table 14.6 Advantages and disadvantages of multiple layers of collaboration

Advantages	Disadvantages
Students	
• Increases integration of academic and clinical work • Learning is relevant to the workplace	• None
Clinical educators	
• Promotes applied research that addresses clinical problems • Increases professional development opportunities for clinical educators • May provide opportunity to participate in and increase skills in research	• May not feel they are an equal partner/contributor to the collaborative process • Need to be mindful of client confidentiality issues • University goals may not be compatible with their organisation's goals • Time commitment required to liaise with universities
Universities	
• Promotes up-to-date and contemporary curriculum content • Provides valuable feedback on the curriculum and learning approaches used • Promotes opportunities for applied research • May facilitate access to participants required for research projects	• Reduced autonomy to decide on course content and structure • Liaison and commitment to outside organisations take time and resources from other academic activities

SUMMARY

It would seem that isolated learning is becoming a thing of the past in both universities and workplaces for good educational and practical reasons. The challenge for students, clinical educators and university staff is to develop innovative and effective ways of facilitating and evaluating collaborative learning approaches. Ultimately a commitment to facilitating collaborative learning approaches by universities and clinical educators will benefit students, their employers and the clients they serve.

REFERENCES

Adams E, Kilburn-Watt E 2000 Clinical supervision, is it mutually beneficial? Radiographer 47:115–119

Anderson J 1988 The supervisory process in speech-language pathology and audiology. College Hill, Boston

Baxter S, Gray C 2001 The application of student-centred learning approaches to clinical education. International Journal of Language and Communication Disorders 36(Suppl):396–400

Best D, Rose M 1996 Quality supervision. Theory and practice for clinical supervisors. W B Saunders, London

Borders L D 1991 A systematic approach to peer group supervision. Journal of Counselling and Development 69:248–252

Boud D 2000 Sustainable assessment: rethinking assessment for the learning societies. Studies in Continuing Education 22:151–167

Bruce C, Parker A, Herbert R 2001 The development of a self-directed and peer-based clinical training programme. International Journal of Language and Communication Disorders 36(Suppl):401–405

Cohen R, Sampson J 1999 Working together: students learning collaboratively. In: Higgs J, Edwards H (eds) Educating beginning practitioners. Challenges for health professional education. Butterworth-Heinemann, Oxford, p 204–211

Dowling S 1979 The teaching clinic: a supervisory alternative. ASHA 21:646–649

Engel C 1995 Medical education in the 21st century: the need for a capability approach. Capability 1:23–30

Fish D, Coles C 1998 Developing professional judgement in health care: learning through the critical appreciation of practice. Butterworth-Heinemann, Oxford

Goodfellow J, McAllister L, Best D et al 2001 Students and educators learning within relationships. In: Higgs J, Titchen A (eds) Professional practice in health, education and the creative arts. Blackwell Science, Oxford, p 161–174

Hart G, Ryan Y 2000 Teaching clinical reasoning to nurses during clinical education. In: Higgs J, Jones M (eds) Clinical reasoning in the health professions, 2nd edn. Butterworth-Heinemann, Oxford, p 276–282

Higgs J, Edwards H 1999 Educating beginning practitioners in the health professions. In: Higgs J, Edwards H (eds) Educating beginning practitioners. Challenges for health professional education. Butterworth-Heinemann, Oxford, p 3–9

Higgs J, Jones M (eds) 2000 Clinical reasoning in the health professions, 2nd edn. Butterworth-Heinemann, Oxford

Hillerbrand E 1989 Cognitive differences between experts and novices: implications for group supervision. Journal of Counselling and Development 67:293–296

Hunt A, Adamson B, Harris L 1999 Community and workplace expectations of health science graduates. In: Higgs J, Edwards H (eds) Educating beginning practitioners. Challenges for health professional education. Butterworth-Heinemann, Oxford, p 38–45

Johnson D W et al 1992 Cooperative learning: increasing college faculty instructional productivity. ERIC (Educational Resources Information Centre), Washington DC

Kersener M, Parker A 2001 A strategic approach to clinical placement learning. International Journal of Language and Communication Disorders 36(Suppl):150–155

Lincoln M, McAllister L 1993 Facilitating peer learning in clinical education. Medical Teacher 15:17–25

Lincoln M, Stockhausen L, Maloney D 1997a Learning processes in clinical education. In: McAllister L, Lincoln M, McLeod S, Maloney D (eds) Facilitating learning in clinical settings. Stanley Thornes, Cheltenham, p 99–129

Lincoln M, Carmody D, Maloney D 1997b Professional development of students and clinical educators. In: McAllister L, Lincoln M, McLeod S, Maloney D (eds) Facilitating learning in clinical settings. Stanley Thornes, Cheltenham, p 65–98

Martin F, Säljö R, 1984 Approaches to learning. In: Marton F, Hounsell D, Entwhistle N (eds) The experience of learning. Scottish Academic Press, Edinburgh

McAllister L 1997 An adult learning framework for clinical education. In: McAllister L, Lincoln M, McLeod S, Maloney D (eds) Facilitating learning in clinical settings. Stanley Thornes, Cheltenham, p 1–26

McAllister L 2001 The experience of being a clinical educator. Unpublished PhD thesis, University of Sydney

McAllister L, Lincoln M 2004 Clinical education in speech-language pathology. Whurr Publishing, London

McLeod S, Romanini J, Cohn E, Higgs J 1997 Models and roles in clinical education. In: McAllister L, Lincoln M, McLeod S, Maloney D (eds). Facilitating learning in clinical settings. Stanley Thornes, Cheltenham, p 27–64

Murphy B, Watson J 2002 Enhancing stuttering clinical teaching through blended individual-group supervision. Fluency and Fluency Disorders December:18–24

Parker A, Emanuel R 2001 Active learning in service delivery: an approach to initial clinical placements. International Journal of Language and Communication Disorders 36(Suppl):162–166

Short K, Gilsenan K, Lincoln M 2001 The evaluation of the impact of student placements on a large area health service. In: Wilson L, Hewat S (eds) Evidence and innovation: proceedings of the national conference of the Speech Pathology Association of Australia, Melbourne, 21–23 May, 2001. The Speech Pathology Association of Australia, Melbourne

Tuckman B, Jensen N 1977 Stages of small group development revisited. Group and Organisation Studies 2:419–427

Chapter **15**

Contract learning

Mary Kennedy-Jones

INTRODUCTION

In this chapter a definition of a learning contract and a rationale for its use are provided. In addition, the challenges of using learning contracts to facilitate adult learning are identified. Finally, some recommendations for the successful use of learning contracts as a teaching and learning tool are proposed.

WHAT ARE LEARNING CONTRACTS?

Learning contracts, otherwise known as negotiated learning agreements, are widely used in adult learning programmes. Learners take control of their own learning through a process of:

- determining their own learning needs
- creating a strategy and determining resources necessary to achieve the learning need
- implementing the learning strategy and using the learning resources
- evaluating the achievement or otherwise of the learning goal and the process by which it was achieved (Knowles et al 1998).

WHY USE LEARNING CONTRACTS?

One of the most significant findings from adult learning research is that, when adults go about learning something naturally, rather then being taught, they are highly self-directing. Evidence also exists that what adults learn on their own initiative, they learn more deeply and permanently than what they learn by being taught (Knowles et al 1998).

In traditional pedagogical education the teacher structures the learning, the learner is told what the objectives are, what resources she/he is to use and what outcome will be evaluated. This imposed structure conflicts with an adult's psychological need for self-direction and may induce resistance, apathy and withdrawal (Knowles et al 1998). Learning contracts provide a medium for planning learning experiences as a mutual undertaking. The learner obtains a sense of ownership and commitment to the plan. In particular, Knowles et al (1998, p. 212) argue that:

> in field-based learning there is a strong possibility that what is to be learned from the experience is less clear to the learner and the supervisor than what work is to be done … the learning contract is a means for making the learning objectives of the field experience clear and explicit for both the learner and the supervisor.

Outlined below are some examples of learning contract templates. Table 15.1 is a template suitable for use in undergraduate clinical education programmes when the learners require additional instruction. The template in Table 15.2 may be used for professional development purposes for graduate therapists, including clinical supervisors.

CHALLENGES IN USING LEARNING CONTRACTS IN THE CLINICAL EDUCATION SETTING

Preparation for introducing learning contracts

The learning culture

The learning culture within the organisation where learning contracts are to be used needs to be sympathetic to the self-directed approach implicit in their use. Specifically, the relationship between the learner and the teacher needs to reflect a respect and value for the learner's ways of knowing and an appreciation of the need for a transaction to occur between the learner and the teacher about how the learning will occur:

> In order for the relationship to flourish effective communication between the learner and the teacher is necessary. Further, the learning environment needs to promote a climate of trust and open and honest communication.

(Earnshaw et al 1996, p. 16).

The key features of a learning environment suited to the use of learning contracts are:

- Teachers and learners need to feel that they can communicate their thoughts, feelings, knowledge and experience. Hence the environment must facilitate a sense of safety for the parties involved.
- Trust is required as the teacher allows learners to learn from their own experience and to make decisions for themselves. The teacher is required

Table 15.1 Undergraduate clinical education learning contract template (from Gaiptman & Anthony 1989)

Learning objective	Learning resource(s)	Evidence	Criteria	Target date	Signature
What do you want to learn or develop?	What will you utilise to achieve your learning objectives? Where can you find information?	How can you show to yourself and your therapist that you have met your learning objectives? What proof will you offer? What product, process, intervention? What is the outcome?	How do you want the evidence to be evaluated? By whom? When? What are the criteria for evaluation?	The date you will offer the evidence	Signature of the clinical supervisor and student once the learning objective has been achieved
Consider your own competency levels and opportunities available in the facility	May include a range of resources, such as observation, demonstration, practice, etc.				

Table 15.2 Professional development for clinical supervisors learning contract template (adapted from Knowles 1990). Deakin University, La Trobe University, Monash University Quality supervision: learning contract

Learner(s): _____ Project title: _____

What are you going to learn? (objective)	How are you going to learn it? (strategies and resources)	How are you going to know you have learnt it? (evidence)	How are you going to prove you have learnt it? (verification)

Signature of the learner: _____

Name of the advisor: _____ Signature of the advisor: _____

to let go of the need to control the learning process, to permit learners to choose their own learning method.

■ An awareness of hidden, covert communication that may undermine the respectful, self-directed, trusting teacher–learner relationship.

■ The teacher can be relied upon to provide the learner with the correct type of advice and the right amount of support to enable the learner to take control effectively.

The settings in which the learners undertake fieldwork or professional development may not provide optimal learning conditions, as described above. For example, in the clinical setting the goals of the organisation are both service-oriented and educational. The need for structure and control of the everyday activities of therapists and students usually stems from a need to manage the high volume of tasks associated with the large, complex organisations in which our students undertake their fieldwork. It is possible, however, to work towards creation of a positive learning environment within the settings described above. Within an allied health department or university department, an open, trusting, learner–teacher relationship, which permits the learner to assume responsibility, can be sufficient for effective, self-directed learning.

Timing of introduction

Another consideration in preparing for the use of learning contracts is the issue of the timing of the introduction of a learner-managed approach. In all allied health educational programmes graduates are required to attain an expected level of competency prior to graduation. Achievement of a range of competencies at a basic level might be better approached using other teaching learning approaches, for example a competency-based learning model. Learning contracts suit a deep-learning approach where the learner is seeking to understand, "to reconstruct meaning through a process of exchange and discovery" (Earnshaw et al 1996, p. 16). Hence, in a programme at La Trobe University, the learning contract approach is used in the final fieldwork placement after basic competencies have been achieved.

Education about learning contracts

Finally, in preparing for the introduction of learning contracts, the need for education of both learners and teachers about the approach should not be underestimated. It is not uncommon for the concepts of collaboration, open dialogue and trust to be unfamiliar to students and teachers, particularly those who have been taught using traditional didactic learning methods. Sessions about adult learning, self-direction, learner-controlled learning and the roles of the teacher and the learner within the approach need to be provided at the outset.

It is easy to fall into the trap of assuming that learners have a basic understanding of the concepts of learner-managed learning and some basic commitment to it. There is a temptation to give less than adequate information about what it is and how it will affect the individual. Even with some knowledge of the approach, people will seek additional structure. Facilitators need to be clear about what it is and able to convey the expectations to the learners.

There is also a need for ongoing peer supervision of teachers as they struggle from time to time with the difficult implementation issue of contract learning, in particular, the letting go described earlier. Further, students who have previously focused on the attainment of grades and meeting teacher expectations within a didactic curriculum are encouraged to consider the benefits of adopting a more empowering, proactive and life-long learning approach.

Setting up a learning contract

In the planning phase determining learning needs can be difficult. Learners who have tended to be passive and accepting in their learning approach may not have undertaken the reflective processing necessary to be able to evaluate their prior learning and determine the gaps in their understanding. In addition learners may consider what they *want* rather than what they *need* when considering the gaps. A process to assist learners to formulate their learning needs in a stepwise manner is outlined in Box 15.1.

Box 15.1 Steps in developing a learning contract	
1. Relevant prior learning	Where have I been?
2. Present knowledge and skills	Where am I now?
3. Learning aims and objectives	Where do I want to go next?
4. Proposed programme of study	How will I get there?
5. Resource implications	What will I need to help me?
6. Assessment scheme	How will I show that I have reached my goals?

When clinicians or clinical educators use a learning contract as a tool for professional development in the domain of supervisory skills, the following self-appraisal checklist (Fig. 15.1) may be helpful in assisting them to reflect upon their competence in a range of areas. Sections include knowledge (of supervision), supervision management skills, supervision intervention skills, traits or qualities, commitment to ongoing training and development, for group supervisors, for organisational supervisors.

On occasions learning objectives proposed by a learner might be unrealistic. Students may "overstate what can be accomplished in the time available" (Anderson et al 1996, p. 33). Other preparation issues include the evaluation outcomes chosen by learner. The outcomes may be reliable but not valid, that is, the relationship between what they want to learn and the achievement criteria is not specific.

Finally, there is often considerable difficulty for learners determining the difference between the evidence and validation components of a formal learning contract. The evidence is the tangible, observable product, skill or behaviour that will be demonstrated once the learning objective has been achieved. The validation component of the learning contract is concerned with how the evidence is to be judged, that is, the features, the quality of the product, skill or behaviour and by whom and when the evidence will be judged.

Implementation issues

Learner differences

Pratt (1988) identified two core dimensions within which adults vary in each learning situation – direction and support. Learners have different needs for assistance from the adult learning facilitator. Some students need direction in the mechanics or logistics of learning while others need emotional support and encouragement.

Direction refers to the learner's need for assistance from other people in the learning process and is a function of an adult's competence in the subject matter and general need for dependence. Adults who have competence in subject matter and low general need for dependence will be much more independent learners. Where students have little competence in the subject

	Learning need		Competent		Expert need
1. Knowledge					
1.1 Understand the purpose of supervision	1	2	3	4	5
1.2 Clear about the boundaries of supervision	1	2	3	4	5
1.3 Understand the following elements: managerial, educator–instructor assessor, provider of feedback, counsellor	1	2	3	4	5
2. Supervision management skills					
2.1 Can explain to supervisees the purpose of supervision	1	2	3	4	5
2.2 Can negotiate a mutually agreed and clear contract	1	2	3	4	5
2.3 Can maintain appropriate boundaries	1	2	3	4	5
2.4 Can set a supervision climate that is: empathetic genuine congruent trustworthy immediate	1	2	3	4	5
2.5 Can maintain a balance between the managerial, educative and supportive functions	1	2	3	4	5
2.6 Can end a session on time and appropriately	1	2	3	4	5
3. Supervision intervention skills					
3.1 Can use the following types of intervention: prescriptive – give advice informative – be didactic confrontative – be challenging catalytic – be reflective, encourage self-directed problem-solving cathartic – release tension supportive – be approving	1	2	3	4	5
3.2 Can give feedback in a way that is: clear owned balanced specific	1	2	3	4	5
3.3 Can usefully focus on: reported content supervisee's interventions supervisee–client relations the wider context	1	2	3	4	5
3.4 Can describe own way of working	1	2	3	4	5
3.5 Can offer own experience appropriately	1	2	3	4	5
3.6 Can develop self-supervision skills in supervisees	1	2	3	4	5
4. Traits or qualities					
4.1 Commitment to the role of supervisor	1	2	3	4	5
4.2 Comfortable with the authority inherent in the role of supervisor	1	2	3	4	5
4.3 Can encourage, motivate and carry appropriate optimism	1	2	3	4	5
4.4 Sensitive to the supervisee's needs	1	2	3	4	5
4.5 Aware of, and able to adapt to, individual difference due to: gender age cultural and ethnic background class sexual orientation personality professional training	1	2	3	4	5
4.6 Sense of humour	1	2	3	4	5
5. Commitment to own ongoing development					
5.1 Have ensured own appropriate supervision	1	2	3	4	5
5.2 Committed to updating own practitioner and supervisory skills and knowledge	1	2	3	4	5
5.3 Recognise own limits and identify own strengths and weaknesses as supervisor	1	2	3	4	5
5.4 Get regular feedback from: supervisees peers own supervisor/senior	1	2	3	4	5
6. For group supervisors					
6.1 Have knowledge of group dynamics	1	2	3	4	5
6.2 Can use the process of the group to aid the supervision process	1	2	3	4	5
6.3 Can handle competitiveness in groups	1	2	3	4	5
7. For senior organisational supervisors					
7.1 Can supervise interprofessional issues	1	2	3	4	5
7.2 Can supervise organisational issues	1	2	3	4	5
7.3 Have knowledge of stages in team and organisational development	1	2	3	4	5
7.4 Can "surface" the underlying team or organisational culture	1	2	3	4	5
7.5 Can facilitate organisational change	1	2	3	4	5
7.6 Can create a learning culture in which supervision flourishes	1	2	3	4	5

Figure 15.1   Self-assessment questionnaire for supervisors (reproduced from Hawkins & Shohet 2000, with kind permission of the Open University Press/McGraw-Hill Publishing Company)

area, even those with low general dependence needs, assistance may be required from the facilitator.

Support refers to the affective encouragement the learner needs from others. It is a product of two factors – the learner's commitment to the learning process and the learner's confidence about his/her learning ability. Learners who are highly committed and confident will need less support (Pratt 1988). Such a model of understanding learner differences is useful when working with students using a learning contract. The need to take control of learning is anxiety-provoking for some students and they frequently seek direction.

Student experience of using learning contracts

Students frequently report that using learning contracts is a time-intensive process. As with any negotiated, democratic, process-oriented approach, time is required to develop and refine the learning contract. Students also state that learning contracts are sometimes confusing to use. In a study by Whitcombe (2001), success of the learning contract depended on the attitude of the fieldwork educators. Half of the fieldwork educators and a third of the students believed that the fieldwork educator's role as a facilitator of learning was the most important characteristic when using the learning contract. Further, the importance of the educator being a good communicator was also rated highly by both educators and students (Whitcombe 2001).

Finally, cultural issues may have an impact on the learner's experience of using a learning contract, e.g. learning behaviours and approaches in one culture do not necessarily make an effective transition into another (Tsang et al 2002). They argue that some Asian students find it difficult to disagree with their supervisor and that they are more likely to be passive learners compared with western students. Traditional Confucian beliefs value hard work and the mastery of knowledge first by memorising the facts. The memorising leads to understanding, which is then followed by reflection and questioning, i.e. "memorising is a step in the process of deep learning" (Tsang et al 2002, p. 184).

Supervisor experience of using learning contracts

Supervisors also report that working with learning contracts is a time-consuming task. Whilst they provide a helpful structure for the working relationship between supervisor and student, they also require considerable communication and negotiation activity. In a study by Solomon (1992), 51% of supervisors reported that they spent between 30 and 60 minutes on the initial negotiation of the learning contract and 10.2% spent longer than 60 minutes. Supervisors regarded the focus on the learner's specific educational needs positively. They welcomed the opportunity to focus their feedback on specific, relevant issues in a more objective manner.

Some supervisors find the transition to the role of facilitator of learning rather than imparter of knowledge quite challenging. As mentioned previously, the need to let go and trust the learner sometimes creates anxiety for educators.

RECOMMENDATIONS

At organisational level

It is necessary for the learning culture within the organisation to be consistent with a learner-focused self-directed philosophy of learning. Staff may require education about how to draft a learning contract and how to act as facilitators of learning rather than didactic teachers. Learners may also need preparation for working with a learning contract. Expectations about the role of the learner and the facilitator need to be explicated.

At planning level

Following the decision to use an adult learning approach in the form of a learning contract, the role of the facilitator/advisor requires clarification. Learners frequently need assistance to clarify expectations.

In one particular undergraduate health professional programme at La Trobe University, the learners spend eight weeks in the term preceding the final-year clinical placement undertaking reflective activities, examining assumptions about clinical practice and using the process model outlined in Table 15.1 to draw up a draft of the learning contract for use on the placement. The subject structure also facilitates a peer-review process where students are able to identify their learning needs in consultation with others.

Further, learners are also encouraged to select a range of evaluation measures. For example, if a learning need relates to the experience of considerable personal embarrassment when conducting a particular task, it may be appropriate that learners themselves determine by a self-rating measure if their embarrassment is diminishing. Alternatively, if the learning need is concerned with mastery of a practical skill, it may be appropriate for an experienced practitioner to judge the performance. In summary, it is necessary for the evaluation measure to suit the type of learning expected.

During implementation

In the implementation phase the facilitator may be required to adapt the instruction style using the direction and support variables discussed earlier in the chapter in order to accommodate the learning-style differences amongst students.

Facilitators may be required to provide additional opportunities for learners to reflect on their existing knowledge so that the gaps in their knowledge become clearer to them. It is important, however, not to take control in this process, instead providing a model for reflection and inquiry that will prepare learners for the life-long activity of determining learning goals and setting out to achieve them.

CONCLUSION

The benefits of using a learning contract approach to shaping adult learning experiences are as follows:

- The self-directed nature of the process ensures that the learning is relevant and that the learner is active in pursuit of the self-determined learning goals.

- Learning contracts require both the facilitator and the learner to be in constant, mutually respectful communication. As with any learning method, communication is probably the single most important ingredient in the teaching and learning process.
- Contract learning is useful not only for student learning but also for teacher development.
- Learning from peers is a learning strategy that is encouraged within the self-directed adult learning approach.
- A learning contract may assist to clarify goals, in particular in relation to fieldwork learning. As mentioned previously, it is possible that what is to be learned from the fieldwork experience is less clear to the learner and the supervisor than what work is to be done.

As Kember et al (2001) argue, the major benefit of a learning contract appears not to emerge directly from the contract itself but from the communication, negotiation and discussion between the teacher and the student (Kember et al 2001). In summary, the key factors to ensure the success of learning contracts within an educational programme include:

- the method fits within the existing educational approach taken by the institution
- the ongoing provision of education and supervision to both staff and students
- enduring resource allocation to develop and maintain the learner-focused approach within the organisation.

REFERENCES

Anderson G, Boud D, Sampson J 1996 The effective use of learning contracts: a guide for teaching staff in higher education. University of Technology, Sydney

Earnshaw L, West D, Dale P (eds) 1996 Making sense of learning contracts. Macmillan, London

Gaiptman B, Anthony A 1989 Contracting in fieldwork education: the model of self directed learning. Canadian Journal of Occupational Therapy 56(1):10–14

Hawkins P, Shohet R 2000 Supervision in the helping professions, 2nd edn. Open University Press, Buckingham

Kember D, Jones A, Loke Y A et al 2001 Reflective teaching and learning in the health professions: action research in professional education. Blackwell Science, Oxford

Knowles M 1990 The adult learner: a neglected species, 4th edn. Gulf Publishing, Houston

Knowles M, Holton III E, Swanson R (eds) 1998 The adult learner, 5th edn. Gulf Publishing, Houston

Pratt D D 1988 Andragogy as a relational construct. Adult Education Quarterly 38:160–181

Solomon P 1992 Learning contracts in clinical education: evaluation by clinical supervisors. Medical Teacher 14(2/3):205–210

Tsang H W H, Paterson M, Packer T 2002 Self-directed learning in fieldwork education with learning contracts. British Journal of Therapy and Rehabilitation 9(9):184–189

Whitcombe S 2001 Using learning contracts in fieldwork education: the views of occupational therapy students and those responsible for their supervision. British Journal of Occupational Therapy 64(11):552–558

SECTION 4

The self in supervision

Chapter **16**

Gods, myths and supervisors

Bernie Neville

INTRODUCTION

We generally use the word "myth" to refer to a story that isn't true. I want to use the word differently here. I want to follow the lead of Carl Jung in suggesting that the myths of pre-scientific civilisations represent the deep truth about the universe as it was experienced by human beings before they learned the laws of logic, and that these myths still richly represent human experience. Jung introduced the word "archetype" into psychology. His experience as a therapist persuaded him that we have deeply embedded patterns of thinking, imagining and behaving which have changed little in the past few thousand years. He suggested that a good way of exploring and understanding these patterns is through the study of the myths of ancient cultures.

The use of the Greco-Roman gods and their stories as metaphors for different perspectives on life, different patterns of behaviour, different constellations of values, needs, instincts and habits has been conventional in most of European history. Each of the god-images personifies a "mode of apprehension" (Jung's term), which gives a distinct and observable shape to our encounter with the world.

Zeus and Aphrodite and the rest represent a plural vision of the world, a way of holding in balance and tension a number of conflicting and competing values, energies, viewpoints, notions of what is what. The key images that have shaped mainstream Australian culture are European, and the key images that shaped European culture, and which still shape it, have their source in ancient Greece.

When we analyse the ways we relate to each other, we may now talk the language of psychology rather than the language of mythology, but the same squabbling gods whom Homer described are still present in our personalities and in our institutions. They are most definitely present in our approaches to supervision.

THE GODS OF ANCIENT GREECE

The people we call Greeks entered the Balkan Peninsula in successive migratory waves between about 2000 and 900 BC. They were a nomadic, cattle-driving, horse-riding people who worshipped a family of sky-gods. The society of the gods, like their own tribal society, was dominated by the most powerful male – Dan or Zdan, the Thunder-god.

When they entered Greece they found the land inhabited by a peaceful, agricultural people who worshipped the Great Goddess, in her various manifestations. In particular they worshipped her as the Earth-mother, who gave them birth, fed them and took them back to herself. With her they worshipped her divine boy-child, who died each winter and was born again each spring. Their social and political system, like their religion, was centred on a powerful female.

These people were no match for the invaders, and the society that emerged from the conquest was a strongly patriarchal one. However, the Greeks did not suppress the indigenous religion, but incorporated the old nature-gods into the family of their sky-gods. The Greeks felt the power of all these gods in their experience of parenthood, of falling in love, of devotion to a craft, of panic, depression and rage. The gods became images of psychological patterns as well as cosmic ones. They have remained so for us.

Panic, depression and rage are not emotions that we *have*; rather they are emotions that have us. Falling in love, or falling into panic, is not something we do; it is something that happens to us. The Greeks had no doubt that such phenomena represented the takeover of our personality by a god. Jung used the word "inflation" to represent this experience of being totally enmeshed in a particular energy, a particular way of seeing things, a particular way of thinking and feeling.

The Greeks saw pathology to be an essential part of the way things are, in the gods as well as in humans. They did not have good gods and bad gods: all the gods have nasty aspects as well as nice ones. Good and bad, creative and destructive, are mingled in their personalities. They are mingled also in the archetypal patterns that shape our thinking, feeling and acting.

I want to argue here that a glance at the Greek pantheon can give us some insight into the patterns that shape the supervision relationship. A brief summary of the gods in supervision is provided in Table 16.1 and explained in more detail in the following text.

Zeus, father of all

Zeus is father of the divine family. He was originally the Thunderer, the ancient and powerful weather-god who ruled the sky. He was the personification of power. More exactly, he was the personification of male power, and he ruled the heavens the way the Indo-European warlord ruled his clan. Over the centuries he gradually became more benevolent. However, behind his benevolence, he does exactly what he wants.

Table 16.1   The gods of supervision

God	Type of supervision
Aphrodite	Supervision that focuses on beauty and pleasure
Apollo	Supervision that seeks clarity, understanding and meaning
Ares	Supervision in which people challenge and are challenged, in which energy is expressed through activity
Artemis	Supervision that focuses on achieving harmony with nature, an environment characterised by affirmation and the protection of "feminine" values
Athena	Supervision characterised by cooperation, the sharing of power, the manifestation of balanced and practical wisdom in the search of excellence
Demeter	Supervision that offers nourishment to the supervisee
Dionysus	Supervision that values growth and emotional excitement, and rewards creativity and spontaneity
Eros	Supervision that focuses on intimacy and community, in which people can express their need to love and be loved
Hades	Supervision characterised by indifference and apathy
Hephaistos	Supervision devoted to the values of work, skill and craft excellence
Hera	Supervision that demands great commitment, in which people give organisational loyalty precedence over their individual needs
Herakles	Supervision that is involved in a constant struggle for achievement
Hermes	Supervision focused on communication, process, flexibility and transformation
Hestia	Supervision characterised by quiet, focused, centred and receptive activity
Prometheus	Supervision that pursues a mission to save humanity through the application of technology
Zeus	Supervision based on centralised power

Zeus does not have to answer to anyone. He makes all the decisions, sometimes after a show of consultation with the other gods in council. He punishes those who offend him but rewards with great generosity those who please him. But his rewards are as unpredictable as his punishments. He acts according to whim rather than according to reason. He is just, but he is the one who makes the laws anyway.

Examining the Zeus archetype in supervision seems to come down to the examination of the personality of the supervisor and how he (almost invariably *he*) operates. This is the nature of the Zeus relationship, where the boss is everywhere present and his power is effectively absolute. He is not anybody's agent, is beholden to nobody, makes the laws and sees that they are carried out. It is difficult to escape the presence of the all-knowing, all-seeing, all-powerful one who hands out his bounty with one hand and hurls his thunderbolts with the other.

The Zeus supervisor may be benevolent and generous. Yet he is outraged when people block his schemes. He may have some difficulty relating to women, yet a female supervisee may flourish in the relationship if she accepts the daughter role and does not try to assert her independence.

There are lots of benefits in being part of a Zeus relationship, as long as you know how to carry out instructions and show adequate respect. Generally speaking, you know what is what. You know what counts for right and wrong. If you like having a strong leader, if you like to be respected for the power you share in, you may relate very well to Zeus. Zeus can be very efficient in producing results, and in handling crisis situations.

Zeus has his pathological aspects, and the Zeus-inflated supervisor is likely to manifest this pathology. Zeus' omniscience can be a problem to his subordinates. Because he knows everything, he does not readily take advice. What is more, he is inclined to become impatient with people who cannot anticipate his directives. The Zeus supervisor may not get the best out of his supervisees. A smiling paternalism can be as great an obstacle to individual talent as a ruthless dictatorship, and the requirement to follow orders – even to guess accurately what the unspoken orders are – does not help supervisees to become creative and responsible professionals. The inability of the Zeus personality to take women seriously is another serious limitation. Zeus may expend a deal of energy chasing women, but he tends either to oppress or patronise them.

If we evaluate supervision from a Zeus perspective, we will focus on the way the directives of the supervisor get to be put into action. The model supervision relationship will be one in which the supervisor makes decisions on the best available knowledge and gives instructions accordingly, ensuring that the supervisee carries out these instructions with the minimum of delay, inhibition or distortion. From this perspective, good supervisees are those who are content to do what they are told.

Glorious Hera

Hera is queen of the gods, and reigns with her husband Zeus on Mount Olympus. In the Greek imagination, Hera represents social stability. She is goddess of family, of social obligations, of the bonds of blood and the bonds of commitment, loyalty and fidelity that unite people.

"Lady" is a fitting title for her. On the one hand it denotes her dignity and the honour due to her as queen of the gods. On the other, it has an old-fashioned feel to it, with connotations of old-fashioned values and "proper" behaviour and keeping up appearances. She is a great and glorious goddess who is capable of extraordinary pettiness and spite. She sometimes appears as an old woman, for she represents the wisdom of the old ways. She is more often represented as a mature and fulfilled woman, who can occasionally bend even Zeus to her will.

For the supervisor whose personality is dominated by the Hera image, the institution and profession are "family" and command complete loyalty. She will happily work long hours for little or no remuneration rather than let the institution down. Supervisees are expected to give the institution the same loyalty. There is no place in Hera's world for individuals who give priority to their own satisfaction and personal fulfilment. Every member must put commitment and loyalty to the organisation ahead of personal whims and satisfactions. It is important to the stability of the organisation that all its members know their roles and responsibilities and carry them out. In this vision, supervisees have a particular role and will do well to stick to it.

The supervisee who knows how to "fit in" may flourish in the Hera style of supervision, because "fitting in" is an essential aspect of it. She or he will be expected to act in the best interests of the ward or clinic rather than out of personal ambition. She will treat senior members of the "family" with great respect. She will not criticise the organisation to outsiders. She will appreciate that there is an established and "proper" way of doing things. She may be made to feel that she is disloyal if she insists on her right to leave work at the official closing time. If she has any ideas that challenge the established way of doing things she will be wise to keep quiet about it.

Hera obviously has a strong connection with Zeus. She accepts and supports the patriarchal political status quo. Supervisees are expected to do the same.

If we evaluate supervision from a Hera perspective we will focus on those aspects of supervision that contribute to the stability of the organisation. From this perspective, it is important that the supervision relationship "fits in" functionally with the organisation's systems. Not much value will be placed on supervision as a context for the personal and professional development of the supervisee. The best supervisee is the one who "knows her place" and keeps to it.

Golden-haired Aphrodite

Aphrodite, for the Greeks of classical times, and for European culture ever since, is the goddess of beauty and sensuality. She is overtly and unselfconsciously sexual, the only goddess who appears naked to mortals. She believes in fun, in immediate gratification, in the ultimate power of beauty. She has none of Hera's concern for respectability and social obligations. She is irresponsible and self-indulgent, careless of the consequences of her actions.

People living in an environment dominated by Aphrodite may pay a lot of attention to personal appearance; they may be obsessed with the need to be attractive; they may be more interested in the elegance of what they do than with its usefulness or efficiency; they may not have much interest in doing anything at all if it is not fun. In the helping professions we do not expect to find very many individuals who are driven entirely by the pursuit of beauty, but it is a drive experienced by individuals in every profession. In writing a report, attacking a problem, conducting a meeting, they may, consciously or not, be seeking the most elegant and beautiful solution rather than the most efficient, useful or economical one. Clearly this applies in the supervision relationship as much as anywhere. Supervisors who are under the influence of Aphrodite see themselves as engaged in an art rather than a job, and will not stay in the profession unless they can find beauty and pleasure in their work. Supervisees whose interest in the profession is based on different expectations may find them difficult to understand.

Aphrodite's approach to dealing with personal and institutional problems is via seduction. We find Aphrodite exercising her charm in the supervision relationship through the attractiveness of the supervisor's personality and her ability to find fun in what she does. The Aphrodite style of supervision provides a stimulating and satisfying context for professional enrichment. Unfortunately, it may have to cope with the pathology of the most beautiful of the gods: sexual seduction, bitchiness, vindictiveness, superficiality, self-obsession and self-indulgence, inability to tolerate the grittiness of reality.

If we look at supervision from an Aphrodite perspective we will focus on the experience of supervisor and supervisee. Are they enlivened rather than deadened by their participation? Are they having fun? From this perspective the strength of the supervision relationship is to be found in the delight people find in the work they share and the elegance with which they do it. The ideal supervisee will be the one who carries out his or her task with grace and charm.

Crooked Hephaistos

Two things distinguish Hephaistos from the other gods. He is the only ugly god among the 12 Olympians. And he is the only god who actually works. Hephaistos is obsessed by beauty. He slaves in his workshop making beautiful ornaments for Aphrodite, his wife, hoping by this means to win her love. She accepts them somewhat contemptuously and hops into bed with Ares, the war-god. Hephaistos has little understanding of relationships.

Hephaistos represents the paradoxical relationship that exists between pain and beauty. He personifies the agonies that people are willing to endure for beauty, the years of boring practice which go into seeking perfect form in any craft, the aching muscles and the calluses which accompany the pursuit of beauty in many professions. Hephaistos identifies entirely with his work, but he does not seem to be entirely happy in it. Many of his stories show him as resentful of the low status given him by the other gods, who actually regard him as a bit of a joke.

Many workers in the health sector seem to worship Hephaistos. They perceive work to be a moral good. To get aches in your bones, blisters on your hands, sweat on your brow gives you satisfaction and distinguishes you as a person of worth. Worshippers of Hephaistos are proud of their craft but have little interest in being slick and fashionable. Service professions like nursing often have strong Hephaistos cultures, with their members convinced that they work inordinately hard, feeling resentful that no one really appreciates them, yet remaining dedicated to their task just the same.

Hephaistos' obsession with Aphrodite represents an aspect of supervision culture that is often overlooked. However, when an organisation allows people to do their work with an eye to beauty and a consciousness of crafting, so that they get aesthetic satisfaction out of what they do, Hephaistos is being truly honoured. Besides, people will often pursue aesthetic goals in their work irrespective of whether these goals are acknowledged by management, simply because human beings have an appetite for (or drive to) beauty, which has to be satisfied somewhere.

Hephaistos is not very good at looking at the big picture. Students whose skilling comes through a relationship dominated by Hephaistos may be so focused on the craft that they fail to notice what is going on more widely in the institution or profession or in the political and social context that shapes it. Hephaistos rightly resents the power of Zeus but he carries out his orders without reflection. However, once he starts reflecting on his oppression he may not be averse to attempting a bit of sabotage.

If we look at supervision from the perspective of Hephaistos, we will be interested in the quality of the work. We will expect supervision to contribute to the ethos of a profession in which members see themselves as engaged in a work worth doing, are proud of their part in it and appreciate their work as craft. From this perspective the best supervisee will be the one who understands this and is prepared to put in the work required to achieve this kind of excellence.

Grey-eyed Athena

Athena is the goddess of civilisation, of household arts and crafts, and of the defence of civilisation against those who would destroy it. More than any other god, she represents a point of balance between the male-dominated and autocratic culture of the Greek invaders and the concrete, matricentric culture of the people they conquered and assimilated. She represents normality, consensus, balance. In political terms she is democracy.

Athena is a goddess who has many attributes that we stereotypically call masculine. She is, like her half-brother Ares, a war-god. Not crude, brutal warfare, waged for the thrill and glory of it, but cool, intelligent, calculating, strategic warfare, waged to defend one's city and citizens. She is not easily fussed. She is the goddess of practical wisdom, of common sense. She has little interest in relationships, except in so far as they have strategic value.

Supervisors who are committed to the values of Athena give a great deal of attention to the sharing of power. Decisions about practice are perceived as decisions to be made cooperatively. Supervisees' technical and professional skills are acknowledged and respected. The preferred way of developing strategies or dealing with problems is a collaborative approach that recognises and utilises people's different kinds of expertise. The preference for group-based decision-making comes from a sense that this is the best way of making decisions, not from any desire for intimacy. In the Athena style of supervision decisions are made coolly and sensibly, after full debate, with full attention to practical implications. Too much emotionality is frowned on. Female supervisees who wish to challenge the essentially masculinist assumptions of the institution may not be welcome. Athena may represent the independent, resourceful, clear-sighted feminine, but she accepts the ground-rules laid down by Zeus. She is content to work in a man's world.

If we look at supervision from the perspective of Athena, we will expect to find a collaborative relationship between supervisor and supervisee, a relationship of mutual respect, in which both people own the process and take responsibility for its outcomes. Good supervision, from this perspective, will be marked by common sense, collaboration, balance and an absence of fuss.

Shining Apollo

Apollo is the eldest son of Zeus, the symbol of what the classical Greeks understood by being Greek and civilised. He is reason and moderation personified.

The Greeks were inclined to identify Apollo with the sun. They imagined him as showing clearly what is what, as illuminating the world, bringing light to the darkness, enabling us to make sense of our experience.

Apollo establishes order and the rule of law. Not autocratic do-it-because-I-say-so law (which is the law of Zeus), but rational law, based on a reasoned estimation of what constitutes good and bad behaviour. He is the god who gives mortals the capacity to think clearly, to understand how the world works, to find meaning and beauty, to organise their lives in an ordered way. He demands that we seek moderation in all things and look at the world in a detached and reasonable way, without being carried away by emotion.

Apollonine consciousness has generally been hostile to women, whom it marginalises as trivial, intuitive, emotional, sensual and irrational. In mythology, Apollo appears to be unable to have any sort of satisfactory relationship with a female – goddess, nymph or mortal – except with his mother and sister.

The supervision relationship that is dominated by an Apollonine sensibility will place a high value on a rational approach to its work. Individual whims and impulsive decision-making are strongly discouraged and emotional outbursts are looked on with distaste. It is assumed that all problems can be solved and all crises dealt with through the application of cool intelligence. The power of the supervisor is subject to checks and balances, designed to moderate any excesses. Considerable emphasis is placed on developing and maintaining structures that are truly rational – not based on mere tradition, superstition or personal taste. People are expected to behave rationally and there is some surprise when they do not. There is an assumption that if matters are clearly explained to people, they will understand and act on that understanding.

The pathology of Apollo emerges in a tendency to dogmatism and rigidity. Once the Apollonine supervisor sees the way things are, he or she has little tolerance for those who cannot. He (usually he) wants things to be obvious, and has little patience with ambiguity and illusion. He is inclined to insist that the supervisee accept his assessment of a situation, because its reasonableness is perfectly clear to him and those who can't see this must be stupid or bloody-minded. He is blind to the critical influence of emotions, relationships and unconscious drives on people's behaviour, and sometimes makes bad decisions because his perspective prevents him from taking in certain kinds of information. The Apollo-dominated supervisor may pride himself on the excellence of its theory, but he may treat people very badly.

Science and medicine are the province of Apollo, and organisations made up of scientists and pursuing scientific goals are inclined to bring both the good and the bad qualities of Apollo into the way they organise themselves. The god of scientific healing is particularly powerful in the culture of medical institutions.

When we approach supervision from the Apollo perspective, we will examine the relationship in as detached and objective a way as possible. This will enable an accurate diagnosis of its effectiveness. We may, of course, have a tendency to simplify complex situations, to reduce them to basic principles that are held up as obviously true. Nevertheless, we will have enormous faith in the ability of people to follow a rational course of behaviour as soon as it is pointed out to them.

Artemis the huntress

Artemis was originally an Asian goddess of wild animals, who was worshipped on mountain tops. When the Greeks made her part of their Olympian family she became the virgin daughter of Zeus and twin sister of Apollo. As a young girl she begged Zeus to let her remain a virgin, avoiding the male-dominated world and going off to live in the wilderness with her girlfriends. Zeus assented, and Artemis tries to protect the virgin forest and her virgin followers from male exploitation and oppression.

The picture of Artemis and her girlfriends living in the forest tells us something about the particular sensibility of Artemis-dominated supervision. It is based on an ideal of companionship rather than hierarchy, natural rhythms rather than abstract order. It values its difference, sees itself not only as special but as constantly under threat from an outside world, which would destroy it. The bonds between people, which are very important in such an arrangement, are based on the sharing of an ideology rather than on intimacy. Supervisees in such a relationship are expected to be passionate about their mission, which is generally concerned with the protection of the fragile, the natural or the oppressed. There is often an attempt to do away with formal management structures in order to engage in more "organic" decision-making. Intuition is highly valued, and there is some distrust of conventional structures.

Artemis has her negative side. She is very easily offended, and responds to offence with a degree of violence which sometimes seems out of proportion to the transgression. Artemis-dominated supervisors can be paranoid, assuming hostility or betrayal where these do not exist. Supervisees, female as well as male, may need to exercise a great deal of care if they want the relationship to remain harmonious.

If we approach the supervision relationship from the Artemis perspective we will be predisposed to see the way that supervisor and supervisee share common values and a common purpose as its greatest asset. We will not be much fussed by the fact that they tend to ignore formal management structures – their concern to protect the fragile and their capacity for intuitive decision-making more than compensate for it.

Fierce Ares

Ares is the god of war, a much simpler god than most of the others. The myths indicate that he is not very smart. However, we would be wrong to over-simplify him by reducing him to the pathology of warfare. The positive side of Ares must not be overlooked. Ares is the god of energy, of vehemence, of conflict, of activism, of challenge, of fire in the belly and fire in the eyes. He may be emotionally immature and inclined to act without thinking. When he gets too carried away he can be enormously destructive. Yet we cannot live a human life without him.

Some institutions are completely dominated by Ares. They operate within a macho ideology in which conflict is relished for its own sake, any sign of subtlety or sensitivity is viewed with suspicion or contempt and relationships are entirely competitive. The "manly" virtues of toughness and courage are extolled. The organisation's heroes are those who crash through obstacles rather than negotiate their way around them. Supervision within such a culture is inclined to reflect the macho values of the organisation.

A supervision relationship dominated by Ares will be difficult for supervisees who worship gentler gods. Ares has no concern for the values and feelings of others. Nevertheless, living with Ares does not have to be a wholly negative experience. At its best, Ares supervision is full of challenge and excitement. Conflict is not suppressed or avoided but is welcomed and even enjoyed. Arguments are valued. Supervisor and supervisee revel in each other's energy. The supervisor acknowledges the supervisee's need to resist, to assert the right not to be pushed around. They both know that they don't have to concern themselves about offending sensitive personalities, because people who can't take the heat don't stay around. Intellectual subtleties may be neglected, and the delight in fighting for fighting's sake may lead to some unfortunate decisions, but there is real engagement in what is going on. Ares is often mistaken, but never boring. Women are not necessarily excluded from an Ares culture and many women enjoy working in such an environment.

At his best, Ares is a mover and energiser who makes things happen. At his worst he is a bully and blusterer for whom the obvious solution to any problem is the random application of violence. The Ares supervision relationship may manifest the best and worst of him together.

If we approach supervision from the Ares perspective will see competition as an end in itself. From this perspective the best way to make an institution competitive in the marketplace is to force its members to compete with each other. We will be pleased to see supervisors and supervisees cheerfully battling each other, and have little sympathy for those who can't handle it. There is no place for subtle theorising; energy and passion are what count.

Dionysus, the loosener

Dionysus personifies impulse and ecstasy. His presence is felt in drunkenness as well as in religious experience. He is the god of the flow of life, the god of the sprouting seed, the god of feeling, of joy, of tragedy, of spontaneity, of newness, of creativity, of growth. He is also the god of fragmentation, of uncontrollable emotions, of tearing apart and devouring. The Athenians knew the dangers of ignoring him, and attempted to civilise him by dedicating their theatre to his honour.

A supervision relationship may be dominated by Dionysus. From Apollo's or Athena's point of view, such relationships are deeply flawed, because they seem to lack structure, rules, agreed procedures. Yet they have their own kind of structure, based on feeling rather than rationality, on satisfying individuals' need to do their own thing rather than on serving group needs or causes. Patriarchal (Zeus/Apollo/Hera) organisations rightly regard Dionysus as subverting their values. Where Dionysus rules, people are encouraged to be spontaneous, to be totally engaged, to immerse themselves in the flow of life, to put more value on personal growth than on role or status. Eccentric or bizarre behaviour is tolerated. The ability to improvise is highly valued. The criteria of effectiveness in Dionysian supervision are criteria of personal satisfaction, not of service or productivity.

The Dionysian supervisor believes in letting his or her supervisees set their own goals, make their own choices, create their own environment. Supervision in such a relationship has the capacity to be a continuing, flowing process, where experience constantly enriches the individual. However, an excessive attachment to Dionysian values can lead into Dionysian pathology.

The Dionysian sensibility is not given to reflection, and Dionysian types do not have much capacity for self-criticism. They sometimes give an inordinate amount of power to a charismatic leader, whom they then follow blindly. Dionysian organisations have a tendency to collapse into self-indulgence and chaos. If Dionysus is the only god worshipped in the supervision relationship, there will be an absence of those qualities that bind members of a group together and enable them to act effectively.

If we approach supervision from the perspective of Dionysus, we will value the free flow of energy and ideas, the emergence of people's full potential, the engagement of all concerned in the creation of something new. In the criteria defining good supervision, efficiency will rank much lower than creativity. Abstract structures will be seen as inhibiting rather than facilitating the learning of the supervisees.

Mother Demeter

There is clearly a pattern in human affairs that we call mothering, and Demeter personifies it. She gives birth, she suckles, she provides, she is anxious for her child, she grieves. This is a psychological pattern as well as a biological one, and men as well as women share in it.

Supervisors with strong Demeter values take mothering seriously. Central to their image of themselves is their task of providing a safe and supportive environment for their supervisees. They take responsibility for the care of their supervisees, exercising the power of the carer and nourisher. Rather than, "Do what I say because I say so", which is the message of Father Zeus, Mother Demeter says, "Trust me. I know what is best for you." For their part the supervisees may be content to be looked after; they may even take it for granted, seeing it as the supervisor's duty.

Efficiency is not usually a central concern of the Demeter supervisor. Demeter is not interested in consultation or participative decision-making, nor in rational management structures. The demands she makes are different. If you accept the notion that mother is always right, if you love mother as mother loves you, she will take care of your every need. If you are not a good child, if you bite the breast that feeds you, she will withdraw it. There is plenty of room for the pathology of dependence in supervision dominated by Demeter. Supervisees may be unwilling to grow into adults, and the supervisor may be reluctant to let them.

If we approach supervision from the perspective of Demeter we will be most impressed by the way supervisors look after the interests of their supervisees, giving them the personal and professional support they need. After all, the mother–child relationship is the best place to grow.

Winged Eros

The power of Eros is felt by humans and gods alike, in their propensity to fall obsessively in love. It is felt in the delight and anguish of intimacy. Eros is singularly the god of relationship, and of the creativity that is generated by relationship.

In an organisation dominated by Eros, the highest value is intimacy. The ideal emotional climate is positive, supportive, free of risk. Notions of hierarchy, or even of authority, have no place in Eros' value system.

In supervision dominated by Eros values, the central element is the quality (and intensity) of the relationship between supervisor and supervisee. They may have a sense of common purpose, may be productive in many ways, may have established ways of going about their work, but these are secondary to the satisfactions of relationship. It is love that makes supervision creative and productive.

Eros pathology readily appears when Eros is the only god being honoured. If intimacy and openness are good, we might suppose that more intimacy and openness are better, and that still more openness and intimacy are better still. However, experience of closeness is not always as unambiguously positive as this. Sometimes, relationship maintains its intensity while reversing its meaning. Love turns to hatred or contempt. Sometimes the relationship-focused organisation slides into self-indulgence and bitchiness. Sometimes people are simply so involved with relating to each other that they forget that their purpose in being together was to achieve something. Unless Eros is accompanied by more responsible gods like Hera and Apollo he may become destructive.

If we take the Eros perspective we will see relationship as the core element in effective supervision. Good supervision starts with a good relationship. To improve the quality of relationships is to improve the quality of communication, and better communication will lead to more effective practice.

Hermes the cowboy

Hermes was the most popular of the gods. He was the god of travellers and messengers, heralds and liars, shepherds, merchants and scholars. He is a very slippery god, an opportunist without any respect for conventional morality, a trickster, a con man and a thief. He is elusive, unpredictable and mischievous, and cannot resist any opportunity to make a profit on a deal. He is also very charming.

In a Hermes style of supervision there is a great deal of attention to looking good, but not so much concern whether the image bears any relationship to reality. Hermes-inflated supervisors are not particularly concerned if they lack specific knowledge and experience in the particular areas in which they are training their supervisees, as long as they can "facilitate" the supervisees' learning. Often they have advanced in the profession through smooth talking rather than through loyalty or hard work. They place a lot of emphasis on mobility and flexibility. They are not bothered by ambiguity and paradox. They are imaginative and inventive. They are not much constrained by tradition or ethics. Supervisees in such a relationship will find basic assumptions undermined, will cease to be sure of all the things they used to be sure of, and (hopefully) will learn to respond spontaneously and flexibly to the challenges of the task. Their supervisor will be a companion on their journey, rather than a trainer or instructor.

At its best the Hermes way of being is magical, exhilarating, constantly testing the limits of our inventiveness and flexibility. At its worst, it thrives on deception and trickery. For Hermes, there is no essential difference between truth and lies, between honest and dishonest dealing. A Hermes-dominated supervisor may be pathologically slippery and elusive, not only with regard to moral principles, but also with regard to goals and practices and the treatment of subordinates. It is impossible to pin them down, because they don't actually believe in anything. When something goes wrong, they devote their energy to "damage control" (by which they mean maintaining the appearance that everything is all right) rather than remedying the situation.

As the health professions respond to the current need to market themselves, they become permeated by a Hermes culture and dominated by Hermes personalities. Everything becomes a commodity, whose only value is its market value. This is a source of great stress, as organisations traditionally dedicated to Demeter or Hera or Apollo are suddenly expected to abandon their focus on care or service or research and become slick marketeers. Supervisors and supervisees in such a context can lose their focus on the essentials of their craft and devote their energy to pretending whatever they have to pretend in order to sell themselves.

On the one hand, Hermes is the god of transformation. On the other hand, we can never really trust him. He is the god who subverts the established order of things, who unfreezes what is frozen so as to make change possible. On top of that, he is the god who creates visions (and illusions). He thrives on images. He facilitates, makes things easy. If we approach supervision from the Hermes perspective, this is what we will look for.

THE POLYTHEISTIC SUPERVISOR

There are many more gods in the Greek pantheon than above. There is no space here for major gods like Hestia, Persephone, Hades, Poseidon or the Titan Prometheus, each of which represents a specific energy, a specific way of dealing with the world.

It was obvious to the ancient Greeks that if we give all our devotion to a single god we will find ourselves expressing that god's pathology, not just the god's positive energy. Furthermore, if we give all our attention to a single god, the neglected gods will make sure we suffer for it. When Paris settled the divine beauty contest by declaring that Aphrodite was more beautiful than Hera and Athena, he certainly got his reward from Aphrodite, but he had two vengeful goddesses intent on making his life miserable.

Jung used the image of "inflation" to indicate what happens when a single archetypal energy comes to dominate our lives. When we see someone inflated by power (Zeus), rage (Ares), lust (Aphrodite) or any of the other gods, it's not a pretty sight and it's generally damaging for them and those around them. When we are "inflated" we can only see the world through a narrow window, and only feel it through a narrow range of emotions. Psychological health (and effective supervision) depend on our readiness to worship all the gods.

Supervision is a complex business. It demands authority, stability, crafting, critical intelligence, passion, compassion, creativity, balance, nurturing, emotional engagement, focus, love, a commitment to science, flexibility. All the gods must be included and respected. Obviously there will be tension in this. The gods don't dwell together in harmony; they spend a lot of time squabbling. Some of them – Hera and Dionysus, Hephaistos and Ares, Zeus and Prometheus – actually can't stand each other. The polytheistic supervisor will not try to shut out the squabbling voices, but will acknowledge them all, and find creativity in the tensions between them.

FURTHER READING

Bolen J S 1985 Goddesses in everywoman: a new psychology of women. Perennial
Bolen J S 1990 Gods in everyman: the archetypes that shape men's lives. Quill
Hillman J 1995 Kinds of power: a guide to its intelligent uses. Currency
Miller D 1981 The New Polytheism. Spring
Neville B 2002 Educating psyche: emotion, imagination and the unconscious in learning. Contemporary Arts Media
Richards D 1993 Great Zeus and all his children: Greek mythology for adults. Greyden Press
Tripp E 1970 Dictionary of classical mythology. Collins, Edinburgh

Chapter **17**

Finding meaning and preventing burnout

Lindy McAllister

INTRODUCTION

Have you ever wondered why some clinical educators continue happily to take students year after year? And enjoy it? Whereas others might take one student every few years, or refuse to take any at all? In my years of experience as a clinical educator and as a manager of clinical education programmes I often wonder about these issues. What contributes to some clinical educators finding continued satisfaction and meaning in their role, while others become disenchanted and burned out?

In this chapter I will draw on some of my research with clinical educators to explore how clinical educators derive meaning in their roles, in large part, from being true to themselves by developing authentic relationships, approaching their roles in ways that allow them to live out their values and beliefs about people and education, and by enacting these with confidence and competence. I will discuss how being true to oneself and achieving congruence between plans and actions is achieved through a process of heightened attention to thoughts, feelings and actions. The ability to achieve this dynamic self-congruence is partly developmental but can be enhanced through planned reflection.

Burnout has been described as a cognitive-emotional reaction to chronic stress in human services settings. According to Leiter (1989), contributing factors to burnout appear to be high work demands in the absence of organisational and collegial support, under-utilisation of an employee's potential, and the tactics used by individuals to manage their stress. Burnout is often discussed in terms of three stages:

1. Physical and emotional exhaustion, with perhaps accompanying memory problems, feelings of frustration, blaming others and loss of one's sense of humour.
2. Attitudes that are negative and dehumanising of others, accompanied perhaps by anger, irritability, rigidity, and a sense of powerlessness, hopelessness and overwhelming weariness.
3. Terminal burnout, accompanied by boredom, utter cynicism about all aspects of life, and, sometimes, serious mental health problems. Stages 1 and 2 are unfortunately often observable in health professionals and educators.

In this chapter, burnout will be discussed in terms of a failure to be authentic and true to one's sense of self, to manage one's self and others, and to manage the dilemmas of time, purpose and control (Edwards 1996) inherent in clinical education. Emotional labour (Staden 1998) in humanistic clinical education relationships as a contributor to burnout will also be discussed. Strategies for avoiding burnout and seeking continued growth and development as a clinical educator will be provided.

To seek understanding of some of the questions raised at the start of this chapter, some years ago I undertook a phenomenological study of the lived experiences of five speech pathology clinical educators. I wanted to understand what it was like to be a clinical educator: What did they think? do? feel? And why? I observed and interviewed the clinical educators regularly across the life span of the student placements in which they were routinely engaged at the time of data collection. Three clinical educators had one student, two had three or four students at one time. Three had capable students, two had students who either had previously failed or would subsequently fail placements.

The clinical educators had a range of experience as clinicians and as educators (the names used are pseudonyms chosen or approved by the participants). Jenny had worked for only eight months as a speech pathologist, and was taking her first student at the time of data collection. Emma had worked for about two years and was taking her second cohort of students. Ann had worked for several years and was now a full-time clinical educator, with groups of students. Annette was also a full-time clinical educator with several years of experience. Robin had worked for over 30 years and had countless students in that time. They worked in a range of settings: hospital, community settings, schools, university clinics. The clinical educators were interviewed between eight and 16 times each. All the clinical educators were female, an important fact to consider when thinking about the language and concepts conveyed in the quotes used in this chapter. However, male clinical educators with whom I have workshopped this material, report they can readily relate to the examples used, and the experiences discussed appear from workshopping to apply across national boundaries, genders and disciplines.

The hundreds of pages on interview transcripts and field notes collected in the course of the study were coded and these codes grouped into categories, and later into themes. These themes and categories yielded the six major dimensions and multiple elements in a model of the experience of being a

Table 17.1 Dimensions and elements of the model of the experience of being a clinical educator (reproduced with permission of Lindy McAllister

Dimension 1: A sense of self
Elements
1. Having self-awareness and self-knowledge
2. Having self-acceptance
3. Having a self-identity
4. Choosing a level of control
5. Being a life-long learner

Dimension 2: A sense of relationship with others
Elements
1. Being people-oriented
2. Perceiving others
3. Values in relating to others
4. Seeking to implement values and perceptions in relating to others

Dimension 3: A sense of being a clinical educator
Elements
1. Understanding of role
2. Motivations for becoming a clinical educator
3. Desired approaches to clinical education
4. Affective aspects of being a clinical educator

Dimension 4: A sense of agency as a clinical educator
Elements
1. Perceptions of competence and capacity to act as a clinical educator
2. Creating and maintaining facilitative learning environments
3. Designing, managing and evaluating students' learning programmes
4. Managing self
5. Managing others

Dimension 5: Seeking dynamic self-congruence
Elements
1. Bringing a higher level of attention to the role
2. Drawing the selves together
3. Striving for plan–action congruence

Dimension 6: Growth and development: possible stages and pathways
Elements
1. Embarking on the journey of becoming a clinical educator
2. Moving from novice to advanced beginner
3. Developing competence in the role
4. Pursuing professional artistry
5. Suffering burnout

clinical educator, listed in Table 17.1. These six dimensions as experienced in the lives of clinical educators are not actually separate or linear, as Table 17.1 might suggest. The core phenomenon of the sense of self osmoses through into and influences Dimension 2, a sense of relationship with others. Dimensions 1 and 2 in turn influence Dimension 3 and so on. A better way of portraying the relationship between these six dimensions is to use a visual metaphor of Russian dolls. In a set of Russian dolls, or babushkas, the innermost dolls sit quietly inside, unseen, unheard, but essential to the integrity of the set. Without the invisible inner dolls, the outer doll who shows her face to the world is not whole. The Russian doll metaphor is portrayed graphically in Figure 17.1. Dimensions 1–4 are clearly shown in the nested dolls. The emotional and cognitive energy of Dimension 5, seeking dynamic self-congruence, is portrayed as an "energy field" around the outer doll. Dimension 6, growth and development as a clinical educator, is not captured in this portrayal.

Dimensions 1–5 and their elements will be discussed in this chapter and illustrated with quotes from interviews. It is beyond the scope of this chapter to discuss in detail Dimension 6, but the contributions of actively seeking meaning and avoiding burnout as discussed in Dimensions 1–5 are highlighted

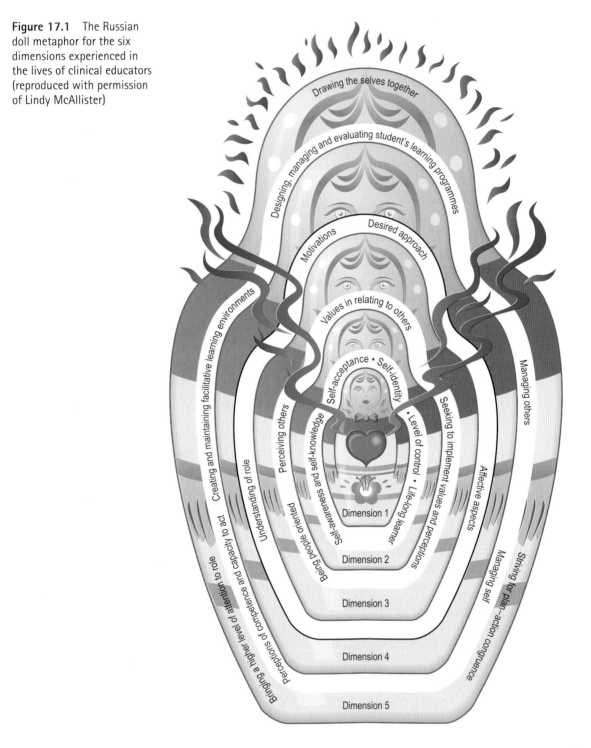

Figure 17.1 The Russian doll metaphor for the six dimensions experienced in the lives of clinical educators (reproduced with permission of Lindy McAllister)

in terms of growth and development opportunities. The quotes used in this chapter are drawn from all participants, although some participants' voices are heard more than others in this text, as they had more to say that is relevant to the two themes of finding meaning and avoiding burnout.

DIMENSION 1: A SENSE OF SELF

The core phenomenon in the model of the experience of being a clinical educator developed in my research was "sense of self", which influenced how clinical educators related to others, approached being a clinical educator and took action in the workplace. One's sense of self develops across the life span, as self-awareness, self-knowledge and self-acceptance grow. One's sense of self is brought into play as a clinical educator. One of my study participants, Ann, expressed this well in saying: "the most important thing you bring into your work is yourself". (Double quotation marks are used to offset quotes from interview transcripts. Single quotation marks are used to signal indirect speech in quotes or for emphasis in the normal text of the chapter.) Another, Annette, echoed this, stating: "it's important to know yourself before you're involved in the helping professions". This sense of self also encompassed knowing how you prefer to learn. For example, Ann described herself as "a very verbal learner – I do learn as I speak. I talk through issues then I come to conclusions", whereas Jenny saw herself as "a learn through observation person". Being self-accepting was an important aspect to satisfaction in the role as clinical educator. Ann and Annette both commented on their "fallibility", Annette acknowledging that "I make my mistakes, as [students] make their mistakes too, and hopefully we both learn from them". (In keeping with conventions involved in presenting interview data, […] brackets are used to indicate that word(s) have been inserted to preserve the participant's intended meaning in a selected quote.) Self-acceptance was more difficult for the less experienced clinical educators like Jenny, who expressed a "fear of the students' knowledge".

The more experienced clinical educators like Robin saw taking on the clinical educator role as an "opportunity to put on a different hat". They could be comfortable in their various life roles, and with multiple self-identities, including that of clinical educator. Less experienced clinical educators like Emma spoke of herself as a "people pleaser", becoming aware that this self-identity needed modification, during the course of a placement with a student who was passively aggressive and non-performing. "Pleasing" this student by not confronting her was not helpful to either the student or the client, and certainly did not serve Emma well in terms of her sense of self-efficacy.

Having a sense of self also embraced being aware of one's level of need to control people, time and events, and seeing oneself as a life-long learner. The clinical education environment is complex and dynamic. Experience tells us that clinical educators who attempt to control every aspect of the clinical education context, including patients, students, interactions, clinical, management and educative interactions and tasks, will not find this a rewarding or successful experience. Novice clinical educators struggle with the issue of control. Emma, for example, often spoke of her feelings of "confusion and not being in control", noting that she could tolerate disorder for short periods of time if it was a "situation you can learn from" but that she liked to either "be in control or know things will be in control [soon]". More experienced clinical educators such as Ann could articulate their aim of "not retaining power and control … [being] a puppet master" and could "go with the flow" more.

Some clinical educators have an ambivalent relationship with control. Annette, who at the time of her participation in the study was experiencing burnout as a clinical educator, was having trouble enacting her self-image as a relaxed and supportive clinical educator who could let students self-direct their learning. One day when we were reviewing a video of Annette giving feedback to her student who was struggling to pass the placement, she commented that she was aware of "an intensity in myself … I thought 'heavens, back off' … I don't think that was characteristic." (In keeping with conventions involved in presenting interview data, the device "…" is used to indicate that phrases or sentences have been omitted that were not essential to conveying the intended point of the selected quote.) Annette was shocked by her attempts to control the interaction and the outcomes. Although she talked of learning and passing being the students' responsibility, she unwillingly found herself "lying awake at night worrying" about how to get the student to pass level. Annette's attempt to control the ultimately uncontrollable was leading her down the road to burnout.

Clinical educators who enjoy their role and stay in it for some time see being a clinical educator as an opportunity for continuing their own learning. Emma described how for her, "learning was a passion", as it was for Robin, who said of herself: "I've always been keen and eager to learn … there's a lot to be enthusiastic about". Annette found that having students "keeps you on your toes" both in terms of learning about clinical practice and about self-development. Clinical education offers meaning beyond the immediate meaning of being an educator. Working with students in clinical education offers many opportunities for both personal and professional growth. Elsewhere, I have described how clinical educators can use their participation in clinical education to promote both their learning and the learning of their students (McAllister & Lincoln 2004).

Clinical educators who find meaning in their work as a educators have a strong sense of self, with heightened self-awareness, a strong self-identity, self-acceptance, a willingness to "let go" of control and go with the flow (whilst, of course, not abrogating client care and student learning responsibilities), and see clinical education as an avenue for life-long learning.

DIMENSION 2: A SENSE OF BEING IN RELATIONSHIP

Who one is as a person – one's sense of self – in turn influences one's sense of relationship with others. This dimension includes perceiving others as they truly are, not as we might wish them to be, being people-oriented rather than self-oriented, holding personal values, and actively seeking to implement those values and perceptions in relating to others. Although Rogers (1969), Titchen (1998) and many other educators in human service professions have argued for the importance of humanistic values and relationship to the outcomes of educative endeavors, Pickering (1984, 1989–1990) commented on the neglect of the interpersonal domain in much of the clinical education literature. The participants in my study who found continued meaning and a future in clinical educator roles were those with a strong sense of "self in relationship". They recognised the importance of "relationship" and constantly sought to improve their interpersonal skills. Like Ann, they had a genuine desire to "relate well with people", to "collaborate", and, like Annette, they "appreciated that people are very important and therefore [I] put them above a lot of other things".

A number of values were discussed, often by the more experienced and/or self-aware clinical educators in my study, including values related to authenticity, trust, empathy, respect, sensitivity, empowerment, mutuality, openness and caring. The more experienced clinical educators – Ann, Annette and Robin – often commented how important it was for them to "know [their students] as people" and to be genuine and authentic in relating to them. Annette expressed values common to humanistically oriented educators (Rogers 1969); that is, that clinical educators should endeavour to help students maintain their "dignity", maintain respect for them at all times, and remain "always optimistic for the potential for change in people". All the clinical educators in my study wanted their students to know they "would be there for them", to encourage and support, and to intervene if necessary. Trusting their students to be responsive and responsible was important, as was having students trust them, so that the clinical educators could "step in" to a problematic situation or interaction with a client, and "step out" if things were going well. Empowering the students to be themselves, to develop their own style and, as Ann said, "not be clones of me" was valued by the clinical educators. Nonetheless, the clinical educators were not selflessly altruistic. They wanted something back from the students: affirmation of a meaningful collaboration, a mutual relationship with some rewards. They wanted their students "to share who we are, what we each know", and to "learn together". Clinical educators are sustained in and find meaning in their roles through such mutual affirmation.

Most of the clinical educators spoke of caring for their students, one in terms of "putting them above other things", some even of their "love and care" for the students. Caring was a standard by which four of the five participants in my study judged themselves. They saw caring as an act of commitment to the wellbeing of others, one that requires time, energy and emotional investment of the self in tasks and interaction. Where caring involves management of emotions, as discussed in a later section, emotional labour can result (Staden 1998). This needs to be carefully managed or burnout can result.

Clinical educators sought to implement their values and perceptions of others in three main ways. Firstly, they developed good communication skills, used "to get to really know people", provide feedback, teaching, debriefs, and support to their students. They believed that "establishing rapport was vital. You can't start working unless you have it." Secondly, they responded to their students' emotional needs as well as learning needs, helping students manage their stress and anxiety, so that it did not interfere with their learning and client care. Finally, the clinical educators were willing to put in extra time and effort, to "go the extra mile", "to take the time to get to know [their students] as people", to be willing "to impart a bit of yourself". Not to put in this time and effort would have, as Emma commented, "taken a lot of the enjoyment out of it [clinical education] for me". It would also have yielded fewer satisfying 'returns' and diminished the sense of meaning found in the work. Where meaning and enjoyment of work are diminished, the risk of burnout is increased.

By responding to the emotional needs of their students, maintaining respect and optimism, and enacting personal values, clinical educators can be true to themselves, work 'authentically', maintain their energy and optimism, and avoid burnout. Clinical educators who are not true to themselves are at risk of burnout.

DIMENSION 3: A SENSE OF BEING A CLINICAL EDUCATOR

How one seeks to relate to others influences one's sense of being in the clinical educator role. This dimension includes how clinical educators understand their role, motivations for being in that role, desired approaches to fulfilling that role and emotional aspects of practice. The desired approaches adopted by clinical educators changed with experience and confidence in the role. It was interesting in my study of clinical educators to discover that theory of clinical education and supervision was only one factor guiding how they approached their work. Their desires to be true to themselves and to maintain empowering relationships with others were equally important. The technical skills of being a clinical educator were but one aspect of their work; the interpersonal and emotional aspects were equally as important to them. The clinical educators in this study were essentially humanistic in focus, not technical-rational or managerial in orientation, despite attempts to impose this orientation on clinicians by health service managements (Fish & Twinn 1997).

The clinical educators in this study discussed their preferred roles in terms of being "consultative and collaborative with students" in establishing learning goals and approaches for the students and their clients, using "joint problem solving", being "supportive" or offering "a shoulder to cry on", and "providing different learning opportunities". They acknowledged the need to be a "directive teacher at the beginning of placements", moving to "collaborator" and "facilitator" of students' learning as things progressed. "Responding to student needs" and "getting the balance of roles, tasks and responsibilities right" were key approaches for the clinical educators. "Juggling" and "balancing" were common metaphors used by the clinical educators to describe how they managed their roles. They saw "learning to be a juggler" as a complex task, but one vital to success and satisfaction in the role and avoiding burnout. Those who tried to maintain simultaneous focus on everything in their work environment were more likely to experience burnout.

Understanding one's motivation for taking on the role was also important to finding meaning in the role over a long period of time. Those who took on the clinical education role as a means of life-long learning, or as a way of "reducing professional isolation" or promoting their own "personal or professional development" found more satisfaction in it than those who felt pushed into taking students.

The approaches taken to being a clinical educator were varied. They included: promoting relevance to the clinical world rather than dwelling on theory only; helping students integrate theory and practice; being collaborative with their students rather than directive and didactic; "having a plan" for the placement to ease students into independence; exercising control or allowing freedom whilst ensuring client care was not jeopardised; being flexible; balancing and juggling; modelling of life-long learning. These approaches are not new to the clinical education literature and will be familiar to readers. In terms of this discussion of finding meaning and avoiding burnout, I want to focus on just a couple of these approaches.

Several of these approaches to being a clinical educator hinge on managing what Edwards (1996) called the dilemmas of control, of people, tasks and time. Clinical educators who understand their relationship with control, as discussed in the earlier dimension of sense of self, can be collaborative and flexible, rather than directive and rigid. Like Emma, they can be "in touch with where the students are at". They can "step in" and "step out" of students' interactions with clients or others, depending on students' preferences and clients' needs. They are better at juggling roles and tasks, and at minimising feeling stressed by lack of time; they may be acutely aware of time pressures but be better at "going with the flow". Clinical educators like Jenny, the novice, who try desperately to "fit it all in" (that is, administrative, client and student-oriented tasks) may ultimately experience burnout. It is not possible to control the clinical education context, or to "fit it all in". Clinical educators who last in the role recognise this, and instead, prioritise maintaining positive relationships with students which give them meaning and satisfaction, and allow them to know when they must "step in" and take action to address what is truly important for student learning or client care.

Clinical educators in this study often spoke of the affective, or emotional, aspects of being a clinical educator. They tried to focus on the "humour", "joy", "enjoyment" and "satisfaction" of interacting with students and clients, as well as acknowledging the "tiredness", "frustration", "confusion", and for novices, the "anxiety" and "fear" of being a clinical educator. Celebrating the positive aspects of "the job" of clinical educator and trying to identify and manage the dilemmas and ambiguities inherent in the role are key survival strategies. Students experiencing problems or failure on placements can present clinical educators with quite ambiguous behaviour that is often confusing and tiring to attempt to understand. Caring clinical educators can over-invest their time and emotions in students, particularly those struggling on placements. Annette, who engaged in prolonged emotional labour in the course of having several failing students in a row, finally became burned out. She could see this happening in herself but was powerless to halt the progress of the burnout. She was "lying awake at night worrying about [her student] and what was going wrong". She was full of self-doubt, exhausted, and had reverted to a more controlling style of interaction with her students. Eventually she left her job as a clinical educator. This was a great loss to the field of clinical education, one which could perhaps have been prevented by seeking peer support early on and outside professional supervision sessions, using planned reflection, setting limits on herself and the university so that she did not always get the weaker students.

DIMENSION 4: A SENSE OF AGENCY

The fourth interlinked dimension arising from my study of clinical educators was a sense of agency. How clinical educators saw themselves, the types of relationships valued, and their sense of being a clinical educator influenced their sense of agency as a clinical educator and the foci of that agency. How clinical educators perceive their competence, capacity and confidence to act is an important aspect of this dimension, one which can be supported through planned reflection, mentoring and professional development. The creation of supportive learning environments was important, as was designing, managing and evaluating learning programmes. Managing self and others were also key elements in this dimension. This self- and other-management was often directed towards containing possibly negative or relationship-damaging emotions and attitudes, as well as fatigue. Management of self and others was also directed at achieving desired learning and development outcomes for self and students.

The clinical educators in my study experienced a sense of competence to take appropriate action as a clinical educator commensurate with their experience and professional education for the role. Robin, by far the most experienced clinician and clinical educator, had no qualms about telling a student: "that it's not working out". Jenny, at the other end of the continuum of experience, did not feel ready to have students: "I'm still trying to consolidate my own skills … and having someone else to try and teach things to is going to be challenging; I don't know what's normal … I haven't got the experience to say what's typical". Emma, also new to the role, described feeling like she "was flying by the seat of her pants; [that she] was going by logic and [her] own experience and also trying to make that up by reading theory about supervision". Emma was working with a challenging student during data collection for my project, and frequently spoke of "feeling out of my depth". Both these novice clinical educators expressed a need for support and sought this from more experienced clinical educators in their workplace. Emma also read about clinical education. Even Annette, an experienced clinical educator, acknowledged there were some areas in which she lacked confidence. She believed her "strengths were more in the interpersonal area and I have to work more on the technical skills … juggling it all, getting it balanced, time management".

Ann captured the feeling of growing empowerment, confidence and comfort in the role, in commenting how "when you start out as a clinical educator you feel like if someone points out an area that's difficult your world's going to fall apart … [Now I know] it's not going to fall to pieces and I can sit there and listen to what students are saying and try and work out what's the issue for them". Becoming and feeling more competent and confident in the role enhances meaning and satisfaction.

Clinical educators need skills in creating and maintaining facilitative learning environments, and in designing, managing and evaluating students' learning programmes. Strategies for doing this are included in many clinical education workshops. The content of these will not be reiterated here, except to stress the importance of interpersonal skills in the creation of facilitative learning environments. Positive learning environments for students are those in which clinical educators have good interpersonal skills, as well as knowledge and skill in the clinical area (Edwards 1996). Good interpersonal skills are crucial for effectiveness and enjoyment of the clinical educator role. Clinical educators who are not prepared, mentored or supported in their roles may not achieve competence or satisfaction. If so, they are at risk of burnout and loss to the field.

Perhaps the most crucial skills for effective clinical education are those related to managing self and managing others. Self-management enables clinical educators to manage their time in order to be available to students, as well as manage their own caseload and administrative tasks, manage their emotions to maintain the desired learning environment and manage their fatigue and stress. Novice clinical educators find self-management difficult. They have not yet learned to predict the range of tasks involved in clinical education, and are not adept at juggling foci of attention, tasks and roles. They are also often poor at managing their fatigue, anxiety and stress. Sometimes they are over-planned, "tightly planning the day to get through". They understandably fear "fitting it all in", as Jenny did. In trying to maintain a positive environment, they may, like Jenny, "put on a calm front" or, like Ann, "put in hours organising themselves". The reality is that the clinical education environment is volatile, and prolonged pretending and the emotional labour of managing or keeping the lid on one's emotions place clinical educators at risk of feeling inauthentic in their role, dissatisfied and questioning the meaning of what they are doing. Putting in too much time jeopardises their other work roles, energy levels, and personal and professional satisfaction, and predisposes clinical educators to burnout.

Managing others is also crucial. Just as clinical educators need to develop skills in managing their own dilemmas of control, tasks and time (Edwards 1996), they need to assist students to recognise and manage their dilemmas, emotions and fatigue. Clinical educators need to be skilled at using their interpersonal skills to "check out if students are okay". Robin was able to do this through using incidental chat with students, clients and colleagues to pick up on cues as to how things were going for the students and their clients. Clinical educators must respond sensitively to students, being firm when called for to achieve learning outcomes and client care, but sensitive to avoid "bursting the bubble" of students' often fragile self-esteem and self-identities as fledgling clinicians. They may, like Emma, need to be prepared to "spend a whole supervision session dealing with [students'] emotions and anxiety" about their clinical performance. This management of others can be incredibly frustrating and tiring, and, if not dealt with through support and opportunities for debriefing, can be a major factor in burnout.

DIMENSION 5: SEEKING DYNAMIC SELF–CONGRUENCE

Enabling one's sense of self to be lived out authentically through relationships, approaches to the role of clinical educator and actions in the workplace requires considerable meta-cognitive and meta-mood monitoring. I talk about this dimension as one of seeking dynamic self-congruence, that is, congruence between who one wants to be and who one actually is in the workplace. This involves bringing into play what Torbert (1978) refers to as a "higher level of awareness" to what one is doing, thinking and feeling, in order to draw the selves together (personal self, self in relationship and self at work), and to seek congruence between what one plans to do and what one actually does. I have deliberately referred to this process as one of 'seeking' and of being 'dynamic' as it is not always possible to achieve congruence, nor is this achievement a steady-state phenomenon. It requires active cognitive as well as emotional awareness (Goleman 1995), and is, I believe, something that develops with experience in a role. Novice clinical educators are often too immersed in the moment and too self-focused as they seek to survive in their new role (Christie et al 1985) to have much spare processing capacity needed to bring a higher level of attention to what they are doing. Emma, for example, spoke of how as a novice clinical educator, her "degree of conscious awareness [of her thoughts and behaviours] during the moment to moment was variable … It wasn't full consciousness but it wasn't totally unconscious … I guess after the event when I would reflect on what was happening, it would come between 90 to 100%". Emma was discussing her difficulty in reflecting-in-action (Argyris & Schön 1974). She could, however, reflect-on-action and integrate these insights into subsequent action. She made regular time for reflection and evaluated her interactions with students. With experience, clinical educators in my study were able to reflect-in-action, and like Emma described, to "let things happen in [their] subconscious" and "allow ideas to come bubbling up". Annette described that she "didn't need always to be involved in close supervision to monitor things – I think I pick up on [subtle] cues as a way of knowing when to 'step in' and 'step back' ".

Drawing the selves together refers to striving for congruence between who one is a person and who one is as a clinical educator, in relationship with others, especially with one's students. Enacting one's values in an empowering interaction is what most clinical educators aspire to. They actively seek, like Emma, to avoid "doing anything that is detrimental to [students'] self-esteem".

Striving for action-plan congruence refers to clinical educators' aspirations to do as planned in order to achieve desired outcomes such as maintaining positive relationships and learning environments, and achieving desired learning goals. Congruence in not always achieved, however, as captured in the famous line: "many a slip 'twixt cup and lip'". For example, despite thoughtful planning of how to deliver a formal evaluation of clinical performance to her student, Emma described being "shocked by her [student's] reaction; I thought 'oh no, what have I done?' ".

Sustained high levels of attention are difficult to achieve, even for expert clinicians, because the complexity of the context, emotions and fatigue interfere with clinical educators' abilities to bring a high level of attention to their thoughts, actions and feelings. Clinical educators may act in ways that run counter to their sense of self. Emma talked of "being annoyed when I'm tired or not totally on the ball". Annette, fatigued, suffering burnout and, working with a challenging student, talked of how "being fully aware" became harder and harder. Clinical educators, despite good intentions, may "panic and be insensitive" in handling a situation. They may, like Annette, "not like what I see myself doing". When this happens, it is helpful to be able to debrief with a colleague, and to be forgiving of one's self.

The clinical educators in my study commented on how experience and practised reflection on that experience assisted them to bring a higher level of attention to their work. Unexpectedly, they particularly valued the data collection interviews, which were conversational in nature. They reported that having permission to talk at length and receive my undivided attention and non-evaluative responses to assist them to think and talk through what they were doing, thinking and feeling proved enormously beneficial for them. It was cathartic, supportive, and the insights they drew for themselves as they talked of their experiences were instructive. Annette commented that the interviews made her "aware of strategies that you do use subconsciously … I think it's clarified some of the things that I haven't analysed in great depth [because] sometimes when you are really busy with three students you might switch into automatic at times". Having what Titchen (1998) calls a critical companion can facilitate clinical educators to bring a higher level of attention to their role. As a result they are better able to draw their selves together, and strive for plan–action congruence. A critical friend would be an invaluable resource for clinical educators seeking meaning and sustenance in their role, and striving to avoid burnout.

DIMENSION 6: GROWTH AND DEVELOPMENT AS A CLINICAL EDUCATOR

As noted earlier, it is beyond the scope of this chapter to discuss this dimension in any detail. However, the illustrative quotes and discussions of Dimensions 1–5 have highlighted many aspects of growth and development in clinical educators. With respect to the theme of this chapter, it is clear that the ability to grow and develop in the role of clinical educator involves actively seeking meaning and consciously using a range of strategies to avoid burnout. Growth and development in the role reciprocally enhance clinical educators' abilities actively to use such strategies.

SUMMARY AND IMPLICATIONS FOR CLINICAL EDUCATOR

A review of the chapter highlights a number of strategies used by clinical educators to find meaning, satisfaction and sustenance in their work, and to avoid burnout. These strategies can be grouped into several major categories:

- See accepting students on clinical placements as an opportunity for parallel personal and professional growth for students and clinical educators. I have provided numerous examples of how to develop personal and professional skills in both clinical educators and students in McAllister & Lincoln (2004).
- Develop your sense of self, as this lies at the core of being a clinical educator. Explore your motivations for a range of life activities, your values, your various selves (person, worker, educator, parent, partner, friend and so on). Identify what matters most to you and how you can express what matters across your life roles. You can do these things in a range of ways – personal growth workshops or courses, developing a critical friendship, finding a mentor, seeking formal supervision outside the workplace, taking time to reflect on your practice.
- Be yourself – be all your "selves"! My work with clinical educators in recent years using storytelling has highlighted the value of seeking authenticity in your work as a clinical educator in finding meaning and sustainability in the role. Not being yourself seems to hasten burnout.
- Develop the meta-mood and meta-cognitive monitoring necessary to strive for congruence between your "selves" and between your intentions and actions. Make time to work alongside your critical friend and obtain his/her feedback on your performance; use reflective journalling; audio- or video-record and review samples of your work with students, with or

without a critical friend present. (See McAllister 2003 for more information on this approach.)

- Learn to juggle! Accept that there are more tasks to do than hours in the day. Accept that you can't be everywhere all the time, and that you can't watch or pick up on everything that's happening. Consciously choose what to focus on when, and know why this is the important focus at this time. Practise multi-focusing and multi-tasking as you gain more experience.

- Affirm with yourself and your students the centrality of the relationship with them in your role as a clinical educator. Resist the time pressures to become task- and outcome-focused, and find meaning and satisfaction in the person- and process-focused aspects of the work. Clearly convey your expectation that it will be a mutually beneficial relationship.

- Explore your relationship with control. If you are by nature "controlling", practise "stepping back"; if you are disinclined to exert control when you should, set yourself challenges to be more assertive when called for; practise "stepping in".

- Be self-accepting; the clinical education environment is complex and volatile; it's not possible to "get it right" all the time; sometimes the best clinical educators "stuff up"; be open with your students when this happens, make amends and rebuild bridges, and then forgive yourself.

- Recognise the warning signs of burnout. If you are engaged in external supervision, or have a critical friend or mentor, these relationships will help both buffer and alert you to the warning signs.

- Manage the emotional labour involved in intense human interactions such as those in clinical education. Find opportunities to let off steam safely, to debrief with colleagues; tell students when you are unhappy or displeased with how things are progressing (in ways that are respectful and preserve their dignity); don't allow yourself to be sucked into 'games' with students. You will need to develop your sense of self and communication skills to communicate confidently about such matters. Take breaks from having students – as Annette's experience tell us, constant runs of failing or challenging students can lead to burnout.

- Insist that your colleagues and managers support you when you have students. Negotiate with colleagues to share the student and the associated workload. If you're the designated student supervisor in your workplace, ask your manager for time and funds for personal development, and/or paid external supervision.

- Hone the various skills required to be a successful clinical educator, so that you can more effectively manage the dilemmas of time, purpose and control. Learn to manage yourself, your time and your tasks; only then can you support this learning in your students.
  And finally:

- Celebrate your achievements as a clinical educator! In taking on the roles and responsibility of being a clinical educator, you are making an invaluable contribution to the continuity of your profession, to quality care of clients, to the standing of your workplace, to the growth and development of your students and to yourself. Those contributions deserve to be recognised, and savoured.

REFERENCES

Argyris C, Schön D 1974 Theory in practice: increasing professional effectiveness. Jossey Bass, San Francisco

Christie B A, Joyce P C, Moeller P L 1985 Fieldwork experience, part II: the supervisor's dilemma. American Journal of Occupational Therapy 39(10):675–681

Edwards H M 1996 Clinical teaching: an exploration in three health professions. Unpublished PhD thesis, University of Melbourne, Melbourne

Fish D, Twinn S 1997 Quality clinical supervision in the health care professions: principled approaches to practice. Butterworth-Heinemann, Oxford

Goleman D 1995 Emotional intelligence. Bantam, New York

Leiter M 1989 Conceptual implications of two models of burnout: a response to Golembiewski. Group and Organizational Studies 14:15–22

McAllister L 2003 Turning a mud map into a curriculum map. In: Edwards H, Baume D (eds) Case studies in staff development. Kogan Page, London, p 29–36

McAllister L, Lincoln M 2004 Clinical education in speech language pathology. Whurr, London

Pickering M 1984 Interpersonal communication in speech-language pathology supervisory conferences: a qualitative study. Journal of Speech and Hearing Disorders 49:189–195

Pickering M 1989–1990 The supervisory process: an experience of interpersonal relationships and personal growth. National Student Speech Language Hearing Association Journal 17:17–28

Rogers C 1969 The characteristics of a helping relationship. In: Bennis W, Benne K, Chin R (eds) The planning of change. Holt, Rinehart & Winston, London, p 153–166

Staden H 1998 Alertness to the needs of others: a study of the emotional labour of caring. Journal of Advanced Nursing 27:140–146

Titchen A 1998 Professional craft knowledge in patient-centred nursing and the facilitation of its development. Unpublished PhD thesis, Oxford University

Torbert W R 1978 Educating toward shared purpose, self-direction and quality work: the theory and practice of liberating structure. Journal of Higher Education 49(2):109–135

SECTION 5

Beyond clinical education

Chapter **18**

Professional supervision

Kerry Ferguson

INTRODUCTION

Professional supervision until the last decade has been largely misunderstood, narrowly defined and predominantly relegated to the "psychologically minded" health professions. In recent times professional supervision has become accepted as a professional development option, although in the broader health professional disciplines (those professions traditionally split between psychological and physical approaches) the practice remains in the domain of the "psych types".

This chapter examines the practice of professional supervision. The chapter addresses what it can provide, who is having it, who is giving it, and what are the rules of engagement. Processes and procedures that frame the practice and their impact are also discussed. Strategies for finding appropriate professional supervision are provided.

The once clearly understood domain of health practice has been dramatically changed. Health services have been integrated into the community, and the professionals that remain in "traditional" institutions experience a much-changed landscape. Staff numbers have been reduced, middle management has been downsized, and information technology and flexible work practices bring an unfamiliar isolation for the health worker. The needs of the individual health professional now, more than ever before, need urgent attention.

Definitions of professional supervision are largely derived from the counseling literature. This is essentially due to professional supervision having been predominantly located in the counselling and psychology-related fields. The practice of professional supervision evolved through professional licensing requirements and from psychodynamic theory, incorporating a need to debrief and make sense of the personal and professional relationship dynamics.

Hart (1982, p. 12) defines supervision as:

> *an ongoing educational process in which one person in the role of supervisor helps another person in the role of supervisee acquire appropriate professional behaviour through an examination of the supervisee's professional activities.*

Boyd (1978, p. 7) defines counsellor supervision as:

> *the purposeful function of overseeing the work of counsellor trainees or practicing counsellors (supervisees) through a set of supervisory activities which include consultation, counseling, training and instruction, and evaluation.*

Bernard & Goodyear (1998, p. 6) define supervision as:

> *An intervention provided by a more senior member of a profession to a more junior member or members of that same profession. This relationship is evaluative, extends over time, and has the simultaneous purposes of enhancing the professional functioning of the more junior person(s), monitoring the quality of professional services offered to the client(s) she, he or they see(s), and serving as a gatekeeper of those who are to enter the particular profession.*

Bordin (1983) views the supervision process as: assisting the supervisee gain mastery of specific skills; enlarging one's knowledge of clients; being aware of process issues; and developing an increasing awareness of self and the impact on process. A definition of professional supervision is proposed as follows (Ferguson 1989):

> *Professional supervision is a process between someone called a supervisor and another referred to as the supervisee. It is usually aimed at enhancing the helping effectiveness of the person supervised. It may include acquisition of practical skills, mastery of theoretical or technical knowledge, personal development at the client/therapist interface and professional development.*

Professional supervision is one option for professional development and, as health professionals, most people make a large commitment to this task. Never before has professional development had to provide so much.

In one study (Ferguson 1998) of allied health professionals in an acute public health sector the change in health professional roles was a major issue for the therapists. The participants reported seven areas of concern: career/professional development, involvement in change management, changes in professional roles, quality of service, organisational values and practices, personal/professional interface, survival of the professions. The participants in this study were asked about their supervisory arrangements and were insistent that some form of supervision was necessary for them to survive in the current health care climate. The kinds of dilemmas that they were facing included being told to provide less than adequate care and to go against their professional judgement.

Professional supervision can meet a variety of goals for the individual, including the management of organisational change, changed expectations, roles, cultures in organisations and structures, diminished resources, including less senior professionals to guide and develop and assist staff with professional development. One of the participants in the study stated: "When you're juggling lots of things I think having an outside perspective can be really helpful" (Ferguson 1998).

Supervision is essentially between two people who meet to form an important relationship. The relationship is essentially a "blind date". In order to decide whether to create a continuing relationship or establish the basis for a good relationship, both need to consider and talk about what they want from the relationship. The supervisors may be motivated to give something back to the profession or make a contribution to the professional development of the supervisee or be recognised for their experience and wisdom. The supervisees may want specific skills, professional development and mentoring support, and even straight information – as well as someone else taking some of the responsibility for doing very complex work.

The relationship is commonly based on an apprenticeship model, common to most professions, in which supported mentored practice is integrated with the knowledge gained in an academic programme. The decisions these two people make about what kind of relationship they want are crucial to the success of that process and define the remainder of the chapter.

This chapter addresses that relationship, its goals and practices, ethical issues, training, and the future and challenges in the field of professional supervision.

CONTRACTING

The contract is an essential component of professional supervision. It constitutes a working agreement between the two parties, who are the supervisor and the supervisee, and it is about both sides. It will monitor the progress and success of supervision and can parallel the process of therapy. As such it provides ongoing material for the supervisory process and can mirror the therapy process (D J List, personal communication, 2004).

Contracting empowers the supervisee in the relationship as both parties have a say in how it will be reached and enacted. It empowers the supervisee in what is otherwise an imbalanced relationship between a senior professional and a less experienced worker. Cutcliffe et al (2001) describe the components and elements of a contract as being personal and particular and can include roles and responsibilities, contextual matters, administrative arrangements, modes of working, goals, frameworks and the resources of both the supervisee and the supervisor.

The negotiation of the contract is a critical aspect of the supervision process and has the potential to establish the basis for a successful relationship. It is a shared process and acknowledges the rights of both parties. There may be non-negotiable elements, including external agency requirements such as registration conditions and the preferred framework of the supervisor. The contract can be a dynamic agreement and should be reviewed and re-appraised at specific intervals. The supervision contract can be addressed by utilising the following 10 components:

1. rights and responsibilities
2. dual roles

3. authority issues
4. boundary issues
5. purposes (goal-setting)
6. context
7. monitoring
8. evaluation
9. termination
10. administrative arrangements.

Rights and responsibilities

Rights and responsibilities are clearly defined in a contract. In supervision, supervisors inform the supervisee of their theoretical model and framework for practice, also indicating their competency to practise and how this competency was attained. Supervisors indicate their ability to include respect for diversity and alternative frames of reference. This embraces cultural differences, including gender, race, sexual orientation and age. Kurpius et al (1991) dictates this ability as a basic competency for the supervisor. If supervisors do not believe they are adequately skilled to address an issue raised in supervision, they declare this to the supervisee and refer to an appropriate source.

Dual roles

There is an array of roles, the most common being:

- *Assessor* – the supervisor is charged with assessing the merit of the supervisee
- *Employer* – either the supervisee or the supervisor holds a higher position in the organisation or has a managerial role or the party is accountable to the other party
- *Friend* – the parties have a social relationship
- *Colleague* – they work or study together
- *Therapist* – the supervisor is also the supervisee's therapist.

This is not to suggest that dual roles are necessarily a problem but the duality needs to be managed and requires clarity. More problematic dual relationships such as sexual or family are addressed later in this chapter.

Authority issues

Two equal individuals are predominantly in an unequal relationship with respect to authority, responsibilities and experience. How a respectful relationship is established will determine the success of the relationship. How they talk to each other and the rules of engagement through the contracting process will assist in ameliorating the power imbalance.

Boundary issues

The supervisee's personal issues in supervision are treated appropriately, making a referral when necessary and delineating therapy and supervision.

Most supervisors include the personal as it applies or relates to the professional activity. The need for any in-depth analysis or treatment usually forms the basis for a referral decision.

Purposes (goal-setting)

The supervisor, bearing in mind contextual and any assessment requirements, determines the goals for supervision and the expected outcomes against these goals. Evaluation intervals are determined. Goals commonly fall into the categories of:

- *Technical* – acquiring specific skills or knowledge
- *Career* – deciding direction, e.g. move into private practice; changing direction; advancing to the next level, e.g. becoming a manager
- *Personal* – feeling in control and separating personal from professional
- *Professional* – e.g. become a better therapist, client welfare.

Supervisors, because of their theoretical model, may see the supervisee at a particular stage of development and may wish to impose a specific goal to promote the supervisee's developmental advancement.

Context

When beginning supervision, a critical task is for the supervisor and the supervisee to understand the context of the supervisee. To a lesser degree the context of the supervisor can also be elucidated. The understanding of context can become a major facilitation task and focus for the supervision and can be undertaken in a variety of ways. Supervisees can map the hierarchy of the organisation and place themselves in that scheme.

It is imperative to understand the contextual parameters of the supervision and the following would all be critical elements in determining the way supervision is undertaken:

- supervisees sent against their will: the employer determined they need supervision and it is a condition of them continuing their employment
- the supervisees don't get along with their boss
- limitations of the supervisees' agency, e.g. they can only see clients for a maximum of three sessions
- they work in a denominational agency, e.g. Catholic agency that is required to report all under-age pregnancies
- they are working predominantly with families and their own marriage is "on the rocks".

The supervisee can chart the communication relationships of the organisation (who talks to whom) and what are the rules of engagement. The supervisee can be asked to articulate the goals or purposes, history and culture of the organisation and, if not known, to undertake this as a homework task. The supervisee can be asked to articulate the current challenges/crises of the organisation. The following quote by a participant in the Ferguson

(1998) study is a prime example of the type of context vacuum that could be addressed in supervision:

> *because we don't understand how the problems are being solved it's really hard to get staff involved. You just feel like the pawn. You feel like, well to fix this problem we know we have to do this, and that means you go there. So you just go there and you don't ask why. Why are you making me do that? Why are you closing a medical ward? How can you afford to build a whole lot of new theatres but we've got no boys in the service room? You know?*

Monitoring

Monitoring is achieved in a variety of manners: regular evaluations, assessing the goals against the outcomes, record-keeping and regular feedback between both parties.

Evaluation

Where there are no professional requirements for registration or qualifications, the supervisor and the supervisee determine the evaluation process; the freedom to include evaluation is at the discretion of the supervisor and/or the supervisee. It may be a standard practice of the supervisor and is part of the way he/she delivers supervision. In my experience it is usually agreed upon between the two parties. Evaluation can take the form of assessing the progress of the goals at regular periods of time. If the supervision was time-defined, a mid-point review is instituted.

If there are external assessment requirements or conditions, these need to be negotiated and the evaluation determined with all involved parties, e.g. promotion, registration, work problems.

Termination

Hoffman (1994, cited in Bernard & Goodyear 1998, p. 88) refers to the common themes of doubt on the part of the supervisor and the supervisee as they reflect on whether they have achieved enough and as to how extensively they have achieved their goals. In particular, this refers to when supervision is time-limited. The goals of supervision will largely determine when supervision will terminate. Supervision can extend over a long period of time and can take the form of a longstanding career development practice. In this case termination may be determined by the personal or professional circumstances of either the supervisee or the supervisor. The loss of the relationship, the transition of the relationship to one of colleague, will have been developed through the final phases of the supervisory process.

Administrative arrangements

Arrangements are to a large extent covered above and in part reflect the circumstances of both the supervisor and the supervisee. However a brief list of such arrangements would include:

- time allocated for each session
- the location of the meeting

- the cost of the sessions
- the time period of the supervision
- the terms of assessment, if any
- the procedures for terminating the contract.

CHOOSING A SUPERVISOR

Choosing a supervisor is a complex process and largely depends on the needs of the supervisor and the reason the supervisee is having supervision. If it is about technical expertise in a specific therapeutic intervention then it is logical to go to an experienced and technically "brilliant" supervisor regardless of discipline. If supervisees are new graduates in the induction phase of their career and establishing their professional identity, it is more appropriate that they select a supervisor from within that profession.

Ekstein & Wallerstein (1972) suggest that in both cases a supervisor from within the profession should apply and technical expertise without professional identity fails the supervisee. Supervisors should be able to appreciate the developmental stage of the supervisee and the associated needs of that stage and meet the desired outcomes of the specific professional goals the supervisee sets for supervision. Supervisees must ultimately have a choice in the selection of the supervisor. Cutcliffe et al (2001, p. 200) believe that:

> it is more important for the supervisor to be competent in and understand the process of supervision, than it is to share the same clinical background as the supervisee.

THE SUPERVISORY RELATIONSHIP

Kaiser (1992) identifies four main elements of the supervisory relationship: accountability, personal awareness, trust, and power and authority.

1. *Accountability* – the act of taking responsibility for one's behavior and for the impact of that behavior on self and others.
2. *Personal awareness* – this assumes the existence of transference and counter transference. It includes an awareness of one's vulnerabilities and potential or actual emotional responses to the client and a willingness to divulge this information; in some cases the colliding of two personal stories. Cultural differences and sexual or romantic attraction can be dealt with through the process of supervision but require a level of awareness of the parties.
3. *Trust* – treating the supervisee with integrity and respect and creating an environment in which the supervisee feels safe to risk disclosure and discuss mistakes is a basis for a trusting relationship. Impartiality is a key element in establishing and keeping the trust of the supervisee. Avoiding demeaning supervisees and encouraging their perception as competent individuals will establish their confidence in the relationship.
4. *Power and authority* – the degree of emphasis on the hierarchical nature of the supervisory relationship and the balance between dependency and autonomy; the emphasis on evaluation can heighten the power of the

supervisor. Noelle (2002) notes that the influence of the supervisor can run deep: supervision can evoke a fear of being found wanting as a professional.

Another key element to a successful supervisory relationship is being able to withstand differences and preparedness to resolve the inevitable conflict that will emerge from time to time. Mueller & Kell (1972) note that conflict is inevitable whenever two people engage in an extended relationship. It can arise from the two parties' perception of right and wrong, opposing goals and their personal approaches to resolving disputes. The essential issue to sustaining the relationship is how the conflict is resolved.

A successful supervisory relationship requires a flexible approach that allows for individual differences and stages of development as well as attending to the needs of the client. Worthington's (1984, p. 74) investigation of supervision suggested that "supervisors do change their behaviour to match the needs of their supervisees". Using a framework/model assists in understanding the relationship.

According to Littrell et al (1979), a developmental framework provides several advantages for supervisors and supervisees. They assert that a framework depicting supervision as a process with sequential and qualitatively distinct stages through which supervisees progress is not only more comprehensive, but it more accurately explains supervision than do descriptions of supervision using only one or two models (e.g. Gurk & Wicas 1979). A second advantage is the description of successful completion of each stage as a benchmark against which to assess supervisees' current skill development. Thirdly, a developmental framework challenges supervisors to change their roles, methods and goals, as supervisees' needs change at each respective stage.

Bernard (1979) similarly calls for a range of approaches. The supervisor needs a range of role alternatives, a framework in which to function and guidelines for determining goals and approaches.

Stenack & Dye (1982) and Littrell et al (1979) use Bernard's (1979) model of supervision to describe the supervision process. Bernard's model includes three roles/models of supervision: teacher, counsellor and consultant. Stenack & Dye emphasise the relationship aspect of the roles, whereas Littrell et al focus on the tasks of the models. Littrell et al (1979) add a fourth role/model, that of self-supervision.

When the models and foci of the three sets of authors are combined, the following description is presented:

1. The *Teacher* model embraces the teacher–student relationship, which includes didactic activities, evaluation, and conceptualisation and implementation of theory. In this model, the goals of the supervisor are to transmit knowledge and help supervisees develop skills (Rappaport et al 1973).
2. The *Counsellor/Therapist* model focuses on the counsellor/therapist–client relationship. The supervisor acts as a therapist to help counsellors understand their own personality dynamics, and resolve personal issues and needs as they affect counselling. The task of this model is to understand and overcome personal and emotional concerns that prevent effective counselling (Kell & Mueller 1966, Kell & Burrow 1970, Ekstein & Wallerstein 1972).

3. The *Consultant* model emphasises the professional relationship and assumes the supervisee has the ability to express his or her own supervision needs. The relationship is more collegial and issues related to implementation and conceptualisation of theory are discussed.

4. The *Self-supervisor* model according to Littrell et al (1979) concentrates on incorporating the attitudes, skills and knowledge of the previous models as a self-supervisor.

A fifth possible model is the *Process* model of supervision. This model includes the "parallel" principle of supervision where it is argued that whatever happens in the client–supervisee relationship may also occur in parallel form in the supervisor–supervisee relationship (Searles 1965, Ekstein & Wallerstein 1972, Mueller & Kell 1972, Mattinson 1975, Doehrman 1976, Loganbill et al 1982). This fifth model could be viewed as an aspect of the counsellor/therapist model.

Gaoni & Neumann (1974) discussed four stages of supervisee development. In the first stage, the supervisee expects the supervisor to assume responsibility for patient care and provide continuous treatment suggestions. In the second stage, the supervisee becomes an apprentice and attempts to learn the "tools of the trade" by imitating the supervisor. At the third stage, the supervisee has developed to the point where he/she looks to the supervisor to help work through patient–therapist relationship issues. The final stage sees the supervisee as skilled and the supervisory relationship as one of mutual consultation about cases.

MODES OF SUPERVISION

Using flexible approaches to modes of delivery of supervision with specific objectives in part driving the style of supervision to be used is recommended by Goldberg (1985). Similarly, Halgin (1986) suggested that allowing supervisees a choice in method of presenting information accommodates their learning and professional styles. However, there are obvious limitations regarding organisational boundaries, equipment restraints, time constraints and how the supervisor wishes to provide supervision. Table 18.1 depicts the range of supervision formats (Inskipp & Proctor 1993, Carroll 1996, Kanz 2001, Locke & McCollum 2001, Noelle 2002).

Live supervision and audio and videotape (delayed review) involve higher levels of scrutiny and may create more anxiety for the supervisee. Live supervision is often recommended for beginning therapists, audio and videotape is somewhat less intrusive, while verbal reports (the least obtrusive method) are suggested for advanced students (Noelle 2002).

The elements that hinder the process of group supervision are discussed by Enyedy et al (2003). They include:

- between-member problems
- the supervisor's lack of supervisory experience
- the supervisor's personal style
- problems in working with a co-supervisor
- supervisee and other negative emotions

Table 18.1   Supervision formats

Supervision mode	Description	Comments
One-to-one supervision	Typically revolves around supervisees' accounts of their work, with the supervisor facilitating reflection, conceptualisation and planning for future sessions. Can include process notes	Allows for very specific objectives (accreditation) and is unobtrusive. Self-report relies heavily on recall and selection of material by the supervisee. The relationship is a core element of the process
Audio or videotape	Partial or complete recording of sessions	Allows direct access to the sessions without being there and not obtrusive for the clients. Requires careful editing, otherwise time-consuming
Group supervision	Supervision is conducted on a collective and/or alternating basis (e.g. common issues discussed with all supervisees and/or some individual turn-taking). The supervisor leads the group	Can maximise learning in the helpful context of peers; efficient use of supervisors' time (one-to-many) and others may also contribute. Provides potentially good balance between personal and vicarious learning for supervisee. Peer rivalry may limit efficiency (and other group processes); requires extra skills of supervisor
Peer-group supervision	Two or more health professionals take turns or elect a group member to supervise one another's work informally; group may be joined occasionally by the formal supervisor (e.g. monthly)	Easy to arrange, though some matching is important (e.g. similar levels of supervisee experience). Inexpensive in terms of formal supervisors' time, but may be inefficient for supervisee (e.g. irrelevant focus, group dynamics)
Co-therapy/ co-working	Supervisor and supervisee carry out some/all work together	Can be particularly efficient, providing opportunity to graduate roles and to offer immediate feedback. More common in training facilities where the supervisor is also an employee
Live supervision	Direct observation of the supervisee's work. Includes a variety of delivery options: the most common is the use of the one-way mirror, and may also include a reflecting team, phone calls to the supervisee during the session, the supervisor entering the room to assist the supervisee during the session and/or supervisees taking a break during the session when they indicate they need it, after a specified period of time, or when instructed by the supervisor. The purpose of this is to consult with the supervisor and/or the reflecting team and for the team and supervisor to give feedback	Provides the client with the best treatment possible while training supervisee to be a competent professional. Supervisors actually see what the supervisee is doing and have closer control if necessary. More intrusive method of supervision for the supervisee and the clients
E-mail/ computer supervision	Provides immediate feedback online, computer screen can be seen in the session	E-mail is not private, confidentiality is not ensured. Can meet needs for under-resourced areas, e.g. no supervisors available in immediate vicinity

- logistical constraints, e.g. room size, time to meet
- poor group time management
- inability to manage the group dynamics.

Essentially the success of group supervision relies heavily on the group leadership skills of the supervisor, who requires in-depth knowledge and experience in group process and dynamics.

Whilst one-to-one supervision relies heavily on the recall and conceptualisation skills of the supervisee and supervisee, it allows for a greater exploration of the supervisee's experiences and self-awareness, and allows for the process-centred style of supervision to be utilised fully. Process notes require the supervisee, preferably immediately after a particular session, to write an account of the session detailing communication patterns and a meta-analysis of the content.

In summarising the literature, Walter & Young (1999) assert that individual or one-to-one supervision remains the most frequently used format or modality for providing supervision.

As discussed, decisions on selection of modality and the supervisory theoretical framework can be addressed through the contracting process and will depend on a variety of reasons, including the supervisee's goals, level of experience and developmental stage, the supervisee's preferred learning style, the goals of the supervisee and the supervisor.

ETHICAL ISSUES IN SUPERVISION

Ethics is about the supervisory relationship itself and starts with a basic respect for both parties, including frames of reference, personal belief systems and professional respect. Three aspects require specific attention: confidentiality, duty of care, and disclosure to clients.

Confidentiality issues need to be explained, as do the limits of the confidentiality agreement. The supervisory relationship is confidential with the proviso of supervisors' duty to disclose if they have knowledge that the supervisees are acting in a way that could cause harm either to their clients or themselves.

Duty of care – Responsibility for the care of the client must be established; if the supervisee is in a trainee relationship this is a critical issue to be resolved before the commencement of supervision. Notwithstanding the issue of responsibility, the supervisor must adequately respond to ethical violations, ensuring that any risks to a third party by the professional practices of the supervisee are handled and any risks to the supervisee are also addressed expeditiously. The supervisor is also obliged to disclose to the supervisee when the supervisor believes the supervisee is not competent in the execution of therapeutic practices.

Disclosure to clients – the supervisor needs to determine that any clients potentially discussed in supervision are aware of the supervision arrangements, including the limitations of supervisory confidentiality.

A list of supervisor ethical guidelines was developed by Ladany et al (1999), based on the 1995 Association for Counselor Education and Supervision guidelines. Their guidelines and definitions include the above and also elements noted in the contracting section, such as evaluation procedures, defining roles and responsibilities, and boundary concerns.

Harrar et al (1990) report on the various American Psychologists' ethical and legal standards for supervision, including dual relationships, client consent, and third-party payments. These latter two issues are more fundamental to the supervisor–trainee supervisee relationship. They also refer to the supervisor's legal liability – both direct and vicarious liability – confidentiality, the duty to protect and standard of care.

Addressing the topic of professional boundaries, Lamb (1999) asserts that boundaries mark the limits, rules, activities and/or parameters of appropriate and ethical practice. The elements of professional boundaries identified are roles such as therapist–client, supervisee–supervisor, gifts, and dual relationships, e.g. sexual contact, social contact and business relationships.

Kurpius et al (1991) raise the dilemma of the standards as put forward by the Association for Counselor Education and Supervision that states supervisors should interact in such a way to assist the supervisees' self-exploration. Yet the same organisation's ethical standard states that, when self-disclosure is part of the programme, the supervisor should have no administrative, evaluative or supervisory authority over the supervisee. The dilemmas between issues to be addressed and issues that are potentially unethical practices is far from straightforward – as discussed in the contracting section, most dual relationships can be addressed through that process. However, given the inherent power imbalance, sexual relationships between the parties or direct family relationships would be deemed an ethical problem.

Supervisor qualifications are included as an ethical issue by Harrar et al (1990). An ethical principle for psychologists is that they only provide services and use the techniques for which they are qualified by training and expertise. This principle suggests that psychologists must receive training and develop competence in supervision before offering the service.

PREPARATION FOR SUPERVISION

Supervision has elements in common with therapy, teaching and consultation, but it also has unique aspects – and as such demands its own unique training (Bernard & Goodyear 1998).

There is scant, if any, consensus on what should be included in a supervisor-training programme. Geron & Malkinson (2000) refer to necessary supervision skills in family therapy, such as establishing a contract, evaluation, parallel processes, resistance, transference and counter transference. Kaiser & Barretta-Herman (1999) also suggest that a supervisor training programme should include addressing transference and counter transference; ethics; the supervisory relationship, including process, purpose and function of supervision; the relationship between supervisor and supervisee being the medium through which supervision occurs; power and authority; power differential between supervisee and supervisor; cross-cultural supervision; work with diverse staff; and the associated cultural differences, e.g. communication and evaluation. Kurpius & Baker (1977) noted that practice of supervision requires the supervisor to be skilled in various counselling theories and techniques and to be able to adapt to various role options.

Exploring the issues of supervisor qualifications and preparation, Christie et al (1985) found that current supervisory practices were "inadequate". As health professionals continuously strive to improve their professional skills, so must supervisors in parallel strive to develop their skills as supervisors (Christie et al 1985, p. 679):

> *Supervisors felt a need for and asked for initial, as well as additional, formalised training in developing their supervisory skills.*

Supervisors need to ensure competency and ethical standards of practice by engaging in some form of assessment of their practice. Boyd (1978) suggests that supervision should be performed by experienced supervisors who have been prepared in the methodology of supervision.

Success of supervision is directly related to the competency of the supervisor; training is a crucial aspect of the success of supervision. Supervision training, as Cutcliffe et al (2001) report, is varied and there is a shortage of empirical studies validating the efficacy of the technique. Training courses vary from half-day programmes to year-long certified courses. There is no consensus on content, framework or experiential practice, nor are there prerequisites for becoming a supervisor or entering training. To state the obvious, this area is currently delivered via ad hoc arrangements, unless specified by a registration authority.

THE FUTURE OF PROFESSIONAL SUPERVISION

As Bernard & Goodyear (1998) note, there is a corpus of knowledge in the professions that is larger than any one discipline. They again acknowledge "pysch"-related professions but, whilst the statement is partially true, they fail to recognise the broader health professional groups who are also creating a body of knowledge in the field of professional supervision. There is an urgent need to consolidate the entire field to establish a field of knowledge for health professionals.

Besides the licensing requirements, many agencies now require new graduates to engage in supervision, particularly where there are no in-house provisions of any substantial professional supervision or the therapist is working independently. The organisation regards this imperative as quality service delivery initiative and a survival tactic for the clinician. However, as there are generally no feedback loops and no regulation of the practice of supervision, the attainment of these goals may be entirely serendipitous.

As noted earlier, most practitioners in psychologically related fields – and many in health fields – would like to have supervision as part of their professional development and survival as a health professional; it is essential that approved courses be developed to provide a bank of qualified supervisors to undertake this highly specialised professional activity.

Clinical education has been largely developed by academic institutions whilst professional supervision has been largely developed by the professional groups – drawing on the expertise of both groups could result in gains for all and the establishment of common competencies and standards.

Professional supervision is here to stay and never before has it been in such demand across all the health professional groups. It will be a worthwhile and fulfilling undertaking to consolidate the already huge wealth of knowledge and expertise in the related fields of clinical education, professional supervision and mentoring, in order to provide a comprehensive professional activity to all health professionals.

REFERENCES

Association for Counselor Education and Supervision 1995 Ethical guidelines for counseling supervisors. Counselor Education and Supervision 34:270–276

Bernard J M 1979 Supervisor training: a discrimination model. Counselor Education and Supervision 19(1):60–68

Bernard J M, Goodyear R K 1998 Fundamentals of clinical supervision, 2nd edn. Allyn and Bacon, Boston

Bordin E S 1983 A working alliance based model of supervision. Counseling Psychologist 11(1):35–42

Boyd J 1978 Counselor supervision: approaches preparation practices. Accelerated Development, Muncie

Carroll M 1996 Counselling supervision: theory, skills and practice. Cassell, London

Christie B A, Joyce P C, Moeller P L 1985 Fieldwork experience part II: the supervisor's dilemma. American Journal of Occupational Therapy 39(10):675–681

Cutcliffe J, Butterworth T, Proctor B 2001 Fundamental themes in clinical supervision. Routledge, London

Doehrman M 1976 Parallel processes in supervision and psychotherapy. Bulletin of the Menninger Clinic 40(1):9–104

Ekstein R, Wallerstein R S 1972 The teaching and learning of psychotherapy, 2nd edn. International Universities Press, New York

Enyedy K, Arcine F, Puri N et al 2003 Hindering phenomena in group supervision: implications for practice. Professional Psychology: Research and Practice 34(3):312–317

Ferguson K 1989 Post-graduate clinical supervision: attitudes and practices. Master's thesis, La Trobe University, Melbourne

Ferguson K 1998 The nexus of health reform and health professional practice: narratives of health professionals in times of change. Doctoral thesis, La Trobe University, Melbourne

Gaoni B, Neumann M 1974 Supervision from the point of view of the supervisee. American Journal of Psychotherapy 23:108–114

Geron Y, Malkinson R 2000 On becoming a supervisor in family therapy. Clinical Supervisor 19(1):61–75

Goldberg D 1985 Process notes, audio, and videotape: modes of presentation in psychotherapy training. Clinical Supervisor 3(3):3–13

Gurk M D, Wicas E A 1979 Generic models of counselling supervision: counselling/instruction dichotomy and consultation metamodel. Personnel and Guidance Journal 57(8):402–407

Halgin R 1986 Pragmatic blending of clinical models in the supervisory relationship. Clinical Supervisor 3(4):23–46

Harrar W, VandeCreek L, Knapp S 1990 Ethical and legal aspects of clinical supervision. Professional Psychology: Research and Practice 21(1):37–41

Hart G M 1982 The process of clinical supervision. University Park Press, Baltimore

Inskipp F, Proctor B 1993 Making the most of supervision. Cascade, Twickenham

Kaiser T 1992 The supervisory relationship: an identification of the primary elements in the relationship and an application of two theories of ethical relationships. Journal of Marital and Family Therapy 18(3):283–296

Kaiser T, Barretta-Herman A 1999 The supervision institute: a model for supervisory training. Clinical Supervisor 18(1):33–46

Kanz J 2001 Clinical-Supervision.com: issues in the provision of online supervision. Professional Psychology: Research and Practice 32(4):415–420

Kell B L, Burrow J M 1970 Developmental counseling and therapy. Houghton Mifflin, Boston

Kell B L, Mueller W J 1966 Impact and change: a study of counseling relationships. Appleton-Century-Crofts, New York

Kurpius D J, Baker R D 1977 The supervisory process. In: Kurpius D, Baker R, Thomas I (eds) Supervision of applied training. Greenwood Press, Westport

Kurpius D, Gibson G, Lewis J et al 1991 Ethical issues in supervising counseling practitioners. Counselor Education and Supervision 31:48–57

Ladany N, Lehrman-Waterman D, Molinaro M et al 1999 Psychotherapy supervisor ethical practices: adherence to guidelines, the supervisory working alliance, and supervisee satisfaction. Counseling Psychologist 27(3):443–475

Lamb D H 1999 Addressing impairment and its relationship to professional boundary issues: a response to Forrest, Elman, Gizara, and Vacha-Haase. Counseling Psychologist 27(5):702–711

Littrell J M, Lee-Borden N, Lorenz J R 1979 A developmental framework for counseling supervision. Counselor Education and Supervision 19(2):129–136

Locke D, McCollum E 2001 Clients' views of live supervision and satisfaction with therapy. Journal of Marital and Family Therapy 27(1):129–133

Loganbill C, Hardy E, Delworth U 1982 Supervision: a conceptual model. Counseling Psychologist 10(1):3–68

Mattinson J 1975 The reflective process in casework supervision. Tavistock, London

Mueller W J, Kell B L 1972 Coping with conflict: supervising counselors and psychotherapists. Prentice Hall, New Jersey

Noelle M 2002 Self-report in supervision: positive and negative slants. Clinical Supervisor 21(1):125–134

Rappaport J, Gross T, Lepper C 1973 Modeling sensitivity training and instruction: implications for the training of college students, volunteers and for outcome research. Journal of Consulting and Clinical Psychology 40(1):99–107

Searles H 1965 The informational value of the supervisor's emotional experiences. In: Searles H (ed) Collected papers on schizophrenia and related subjects. Hogarth Press, London

Stenack R J, Dye H A 1982 Behavioural descriptions of counseling supervision roles. Counselor Education and Supervision 21(4):295–303

Walter C, Young T 1999 Combining individual and group supervision in educating for the social work profession. Clinical Supervisor 18(2):73–89

Worthington E L 1984 Empirical investigation of supervision of counselors as they gain experience. Journal of Counseling Psychology 31(1):63–75

FURTHER READING

Campbell J M 2000 Becoming an effective supervisor: a workbook for counselors and psychotherapists. Accelerated Development, Philadelphia

Ferguson K, Edwards H 1999 Providing clinical education: the relationship between health and education. In: Higgs J, Edwards H (eds) Educating beginning practitioners. Butterworth-Heinemann, Oxford

Kaslow F W (ed) 1986 Supervision and training: models, dilemmas, and challenges. Haworth Press, New York

Langs R 1979 The supervisory experience. Jason Aronson, New York

Langs R 1994 Doing supervision and being supervised. Karnac, London

McMahon M, Patton W (eds) 2002 Supervision in the helping professions: a practical approach. Pearson Education, Frenchs Forest

Shipton G (ed) 1997 Supervision of psychotherapy and counseling. Open University Press, Bristol

West J, Bubenzer D, Pinsoneault T et al 1993 Three supervision modalities for training marital and family counselors. Counselor Education and Supervision 33:127–138

Whiffen R L, Bing-Hall J 1982 Family supervision: recent developments in practice. Academic Press, London

Williams A 1995 Visual and active supervision. W W Norton, New York

Chapter 19

Mentoring in the health professions

Miranda Rose

CHAPTER CONTENTS

INTRODUCTION

This chapter discusses mentoring relationships in the allied health professions. It aims to provide a framework for practitioners to utilise in examining the mentoring relationships they are currently in, have been in or wish to experience. The chapter begins with an explanation of mentoring practice and describes the origins and developments of mentoring in the business and health communities. The benefits and pitfalls of mentoring are discussed, along with the empirical evidence about the efficacy and outcomes of mentoring programmes. The major functions and activities associated with mentoring practice are elucidated and resources for developing mentoring programmes are highlighted. Finally, the overlap between the three complementary but distinct fields of clinical education, professional supervision and mentoring is reviewed and suggestions are offered on ways of enhancing mentoring practices.

In the foreword to a detailed and practical text on mentoring (Zachary 2000) Parks Deloz wrote:

> *Great mentors extend the human activity of care beyond the bounds of family. They see us in ways that we have not been seen before. And at their best they inspire us to reach beyond ourselves; they show us how to make a positive difference in the wider world.*

To be seen as we have not been seen before and to be shown how to manifest potential are indeed wonderful opportunities for growth. When coupled with wisdom willingly imparted, the ingredients needed for personal transformation become available.

WHAT IS MENTORING?

Mentoring has reached such widescale acceptance in the community that the term has made it to colloquial status. However, as with the field of professional supervision (see Chapter 1), it has been extremely difficult to achieve a consistent definition of mentoring. Across the business, education, psychology and health literature, definitions of mentoring vary in their inclusion and emphasis of various psychosocial and career functions. Psychosocial functions include developing a sense of competence, identity and effectiveness in professional life, while career functions are primarily concerned with career advancement (Kram 1988). Thus, as in the case of professional supervision, poor definitions have created opportunities for misinterpretation and confusion in the literature on mentoring. Writing from a nursing perspective, Morton-Cooper & Palmer (2000, p. 189) defined a mentor as:

> *someone who provides an enabling relationship that facilitates another's personal growth and development. The relationship is dynamic, reciprocal and can be emotionally intense. Within such a relationship the mentor assists with career development and guides the mentee through the organisational, social and political networks.*

The term mentor originates from Greek classical literature, where in Homer's Odyssey, Ulysses (or Odysseus as he is sometimes called) appointed his friend *Mentor,* to care for his home and his son, Telemachus, while Ulysses was away at war for a decade. In the story, Mentor became more than a teacher, assuming considerable personal responsibility for Telemachus' development. In the modern version of the classic or natural mentoring relationship, the mentee seeks a supportive and socially well-networked individual, usually a member of the same profession, who is more experienced than the mentee (the second person in the mentoring dyad). Mentors and mentees (sometimes referred to as protégés) interact frequently, either in person or in some cases (for example, the Speech Pathology Australia Mentor Programme) by telephone, to discuss issues of specific and personal interest to the mentee.

Issues of career development and enhancement are often central to the mentoring relationship. In classic versions of the relationship, mentors are not part of the mentees' workplace but rather are sought through one's professional organisation or informal contacts. In more recent corporate and formal versions of mentoring programmes, mentors might be on site and even in the same department as the mentee. These latter formal relationships are frequently organised by a third party, such as human resources personnel, a continuing education coordinator employed within the organisation, or the department head.

Several functions of formal mentoring have been described in the literature and were succinctly summarised by Hajzler (2001):

- Career functions
    - sponsorship and advocacy
    - exposure and visibility/social status
    - coaching, training, instruction and information
    - protection
    - providing challenging or "plum" assignments
    - bypassing bureaucracy/access to resources
    - socialisation/host/guide
- Psychosocial functions
    - role modelling
    - acceptance and confirmation, support and encouragement
    - counselling, advice and guidance.

Subtle distinctions can be drawn between in-house formal and organisationally led/sponsored mentoring and the natural informal mentoring obtained outside the workplace and perhaps facilitated by one's professional organisation. Rolfe-Flett (2002) suggested that organisation mentoring has the following organisation and personal objectives:

- reduce staff turnover
- provide support in difficult environments
- develop targeted staff
- support career planning
- manage knowledge by sharing tacit information
- extend staff leadership abilities
- build relationships and improve communication in the organisation
- develop a learning and coaching culture
- become an employer of choice.

Formal mentoring relationships may take many forms (Douglas & McCauley 1999), including:

- one-on-one mentoring – a junior person assigned to a more senior person outside the direct reporting line
- apprenticeships – junior person assigned to senior person in direct line of management
- team coaching – a group of junior staff are assigned to one senior staff outside the reporting line
- peer coaching – a staff member is assigned to another staff member at the same level
- executive coaching – a senior staff member is assigned to an external consultant
- action learning – a group of staff members are brought together to work and learn from each other
- structured networks – a group of managers meet to support each other.

The objectives of non-workplace or informal mentoring relationships may place greater emphasis on the psychosocial functions. In addition to the objectives previously mentioned for formal mentoring programmes, informal mentoring may include:

- introducing the mentee to significant players in the local community or profession
- providing links to national and international contacts
- offering strategic advice about promotion or job opportunities beyond the current employer or organisation
- ensuring the emotional and social welfare of mentees as they undergo the transitional phases of a new job or location.

The culture of the society or organisation where the mentoring takes place may be an important determiner in the specific activities included in the mentoring relationships. Differences between European and North American organisational mentoring relationships have been suggested (Clutterbuck 2001, as cited in Rolfe-Flett 2002). North American relationships tend to emphasise sponsorship and advancing the career of the mentee, while European relationships emphasise learning and self-reliance and discourage notions of sponsorship. Rolfe-Flett suggested that the Australian version of corporate mentoring is a hybrid of both the sponsorship model and the learning and development models. In Australia, notions of favouritism for elite groups are not consistent with the equity policies of the public sector and would therefore not be publicly encouraged.

THE RISE OF MENTORING PRACTICES

Mentoring practice has exploded in popularity over the past few decades, particularly in the business world. It is estimated that one in five organisations worldwide has formalised mentoring programmes (McKenzie 1995, as cited in Hajzler 2001) so that mentoring appears to have become an expected activity in business culture (McCauley & Douglas 1998). However, mentoring has not been restricted to business relationships. Any search on the world wide web using "mentoring" as the search term locates a plethora of organisations with mentoring activities. These activities extend to dyads of older citizens and school students, peers in high school or universities, citizens and at-risk young people who may experience drug abuse, family breakdown or unemployment, and citizens and pre-release prisoners (Golden 2000).

In line with the rise in mentoring activity in the general and business communities has been an increase in mentoring practice in the health sector.

As described in Chapter 1 of this text, the recent rise in the popularity and adoption of mentoring programmes in allied health and nursing across the globe may well be in response to the changing contexts of and pressures on professional practice. Certainly there is an increased recognition of the difficult transition that is undertaken by health professionals from final-year student to newly qualified professional. A study of new graduates in the field of occupational therapy identified that the new practitioners felt inadequate when confronted with novel situations, and found time management and supporting co-workers a significant source of stress (Atkinson & Steward

1997). A similar study in speech pathology echoed the transitional difficulties experienced by the occupational therapy graduates, identifying time management, organisational tasks and implementing modes of service delivery according to caseload demands as areas of concern (Ferguson 2000).

Increased complexity in the workplace has led to higher levels of job-related stress (Brockner et al 1992). Workplaces concerned about rising employee attrition rates argue strongly for mentoring programmes. Similarly, the rise in mandatory continuing education programmes for the professions has led practitioners to seek out mentoring relationships at higher rates than ever before. However, a search for literature concerning mentoring in allied health locates few specific references. It appears that the mentoring practices undertaken in the health sector have relied heavily on the business literature for direction, with Kram's (1988) seminal research project on mentoring in a business context being frequently quoted.

PHASES IN MENTORING RELATIONSHIPS

Mentoring relationships have been found to pass through a series of stages, building on each other to form a developmental sequence (Kram 1988, Zachary 2000). An awareness of the phases can help both mentor and mentee to reflect on their relationships. Zachary (2000) defined four phases:

1. preparing
2. negotiating
3. enabling
4. closure.

During the *preparation* phase, the mentor and mentee reflect on their personal motivations for mentoring, their readiness for mentoring and the expectations they have of the roles. In the initial contacts, the parties are assessing the viability of the relationship. The may ask themselves the following questions:

- Will this person be able to give me what I think I need (mentee)?
- Is this person open to my ideas (mentor)?
- Is this the kind of person I want to spend time and energy with? (mentor and mentee)
- Is it physically possible for us to meet/have regular contact?

Thus, in the preparing phase the tone of the relationship is set.

The *negotiating* phase involves laying the important groundwork for the relationship and is vital in terms of what *fruit* (products) the relationship may eventually produce. During the negotiating phase the mentor and mentee come to agreement about:

- the goals of the relationship and the processes for working on the goals
- deciding how confidentiality will be maintained
- the boundaries and limits for the relationship
- the frequency and nature of contact
- what will happen when conflict arises
- how the relationship will be closed/adjourned.

Agreement between: _____ (mentor) and _____ (mentee)

Date: _____

Purpose: _____

Activities: _____

_____

_____

_____

Communication methods and frequency: _____

_____

_____

_____

Review: _____

_____

_____

_____

Problems/help: _____

_____

_____

_____

Figure 19.1   Sample mentoring contract/agreement (adapted from Rolfe-Flett 2002)

The negotiating discussions can be difficult for some people. Dealing with some of the *softer* issues such as relationship boundaries and limitations can be confronting and may require several attempts and revisions before a shared understanding is reached. In many mentoring partnerships, a written agreement is constructed that details the former issues. An example of an agreement is presented in Figure 19.1.

The *enabling* phase is the implementation phase where a firm foundation of trust is required in order to develop the necessary challenges for growth. This is *the work* of mentoring. Here the myriad of individual partnerships play out their natural courses, with some reaching the heights of grace, beauty and transformation, while others may derail and end in dissatisfaction. During the enabling phase, there may be the need to return to the negotiating phase, as new or unexpected events emerge, requiring a renegotiating of the roles or processes. Perhaps the relationship hits a period where there appears to be nothing left to gain; the parties may return to negotiating, and having reviewed progress come to a realisation that they are approaching the closure phase.

Finally, the *closure* phase involves evaluating, acknowledging and celebrating the relationship and its achievements. Several other authors discuss an extension to the closure phase where the relationship is renegotiated, perhaps emerging as friendship or one whereby the parties become two peers. For some pairs, this final stage may be fraught and untimely, leading to a sense of abandonment, anger or resentment (Kram 1988). Setting up the agreement at the outset during the negotiating phase can do much to prevent such outcomes but human relationships are complex and dynamic and there is always some risk that the closure phase will be unsatisfactory. In many mentoring relationships the stages are not strictly linear and as challenges occur or circumstances alter there will be movement back from the enabling phase to the negotiating phase and a new direction or process commenced (Zachary 2000).

ESSENTIAL COMPETENCIES AND STYLES OF MENTORING

Effective mentors require a broad range of skills and it is useful in the preparatory stages for mentors to review their competencies in order to ascertain their readiness for the task. Mentors might consider how they rate on the following set of skills:

- establishing relationships
- building and maintaining relationships
- developing trust
- coaching
- communicating
- encouraging
- facilitating learning
- setting realistic goals
- guiding
- managing conflict
- problem-solving
- providing and receiving feedback
- reflecting
- ending relationships (Zachary 2000, Rolfe-Flett 2002).

Experienced clinical educators may be well placed to act as mentors (although probably not with their current students due to possible role conflicts) given their educational and relationship expertise. The list of competencies articulated by Zachary (2000) and Rolfe-Flett (2002) closely matches those described for clinical educators. Clinical educators who embody the principles of facilitation of student learning will find the practices of mentee-centred mentoring relationships familiar and comfortable. An exploration of the literature addressing *styles* of mentoring reveals similar language and constructs to those described in the area of *supervisory styles* (see Chapter 6). Sosik & Godshalk (2000) investigated three types of leadership styles – transformational, transactional and laissez-faire – in terms of their presence and effectiveness in mentoring relationships. They surveyed 230 adults enrolled in masters of management programmes in a university in the USA. The transformational style of mentoring was the most favourable and was strongly associated with reduced mentee job-related stress. The transformational style has four major characteristics (Bass & Avolio 1994):

1. individualised consideration – giving personal attention to mentees to promote their development and achievements
2. intellectual stimulation – enabling mentees to think of old problems in new ways
3. inspirational motivation – communicating high performance expectations to mentees through the projection of a powerful, confident, dynamic presence
4. idealised influence – displaying role-model behaviours to mentees through exemplary personal achievements, character and/or behaviour.

BENEFITS AND LIMITATIONS OF MENTORING

The literature addressing the benefits and limitations of formal mentoring relationships was eloquently summarised by Hajzler (2001) in his doctoral thesis. An adapted version of his table summarising the benefits and limitations (representing work from Douglas 1997, McKenzie 1995, and Murray & Owen 1991 – all as cited in Hajzler 2001) is represented in Table 19.1. The benefits of mentoring have strong intuitive appeal and are certainly well documented in the literature. The organisational benefits of development of managers, increased commitment and productivity from members of the organisation and improved organisational communication speak for themselves. Similarly, the potential for career advancement, personal support, increased confidence and greater personal fulfilment is an enormously beneficial and attractive outcome of mentoring.

A study of the development of physiotherapy expertise captured the importance and benefits of mentoring. One clinician reflected on her mentor as follows (Martin et al 1999, p. 238):

> with great theoretical and practical knowledge she was critical of her own practice, dared to try new things, to 'play' with new solutions, to use her fantasy, enjoy the patients and her work. Her attitudes helped [me] develop critical thinking, the courage to try new ways and to listen.

While there has been widespread support for mentoring programmes – with a somewhat religious zeal expressed in some business publications on mentoring – little has been written about the potential pitfalls. Being conscious of potential pitfalls may help to avert problems that could be encountered in mentoring relationships. Undertaking mentoring programmes without considerable thought, awareness and planning could easily land well-meaning individuals in difficult and potentially damaging situations. It is my contention, gleaned from observation of some health organisations and conference papers on mentoring programmes, that well-meaning allied health managers may set up formalised in-house mentoring programmes

Table 19.1   Potential benefits and limitations of mentoring relationships (adapted from Hajzler 2001, p. 57)

	Benefits	Limitations
Organisation	Development of managers Reduced turnover Increased commitment Low cost of programmes Improved organisational communication Increased productivity	Lack of organisational support Creation of a climate of favouritism Difficulties in coordinating programmes with other organisational initiatives Costs of programme Frustration in upward mobility
Mentee	Career advancement Personal support Learning and development Increased confidence Assistance and feedback Professional networking Increased awareness of organisation	Neglect of core job Negative experiences Unrealistic expectations Over-dependence on relationship Role conflict between manager and mentor Not taking responsibility for own development Inept mentor Being object of jealousy and gossip Having a mentor who takes credit for mentee's work
Mentor	Personal fulfilment Assistance on projects Financial rewards Increased self-confidence Revitalised interest in work Professional assistance on work projects Close relationship with mentee	Lack of time Lack of perceived benefit Lack of mentoring skills Pressure to take on role Resentment/possessiveness of mentee

without sufficient attention to the complexities of role boundary and overlap. An inadequate approach to the preparation of mentors and mentees in mentoring programmes can lead to role confusion, and development of hostile and destructive relationships where the power imbalances and complexities of confidentiality inside the workplace are compromised. Thus, the *naïve* mentoring programme may paradoxically lead to a reduction in productivity and increased work-related stress.

EVIDENCE OF THE EFFICACY OF MENTORING

One research study that was specifically conducted in the context of the health sector provides an understanding of the factors that might influence mentoring outcomes. Koberg et al (1998) surveyed 585 health care workers in a large metropolitan private hospital in the United States of America. Of the 387 participants (60.2% of the 585 people surveyed) who identified that they had experienced a mentoring relationship, 66% were registered nurses, dietitians, therapists, pharmacists and other professionals; the remaining 34% were hospital administrators, directors or physicians. Thus, the sample investigated is likely to be relevant to the readers of this text. Utilising bivariate correlations, analysis of covariance and multivariate analysis of covariance techniques, Koberg et al revealed that several participant variables were related to positive mentoring outcomes. Mentoring activity increased as the mentee's education levels increased and was higher for white employees as compared to Hispanic- or African-Americans.

Further, mentoring was higher between same-sex and same-race mentoring dyads than among opposite-sex and cross-race dyads. However, there was no significant difference between men and women in the amount of mentoring they each received. Mentoring also increased as the levels of trust in the working group and the perceived leader approachability increased but was not found to relate to the organisation ranking of the participants. Importantly, mentoring was significantly associated with greater levels of self-esteem and involvement of the participants in the workplace and with a reduced sense of staff wanting to leave the organisation. Koberg et al's data certainly have limitations in terms of the fact that the analyses were largely co-relational and therefore a causal relationship between mentoring and self-esteem or reduced desire to leave the workplace cannot be inferred. However, the strong relationships found in the study are encouraging and certainly warrant further investigations that aim to explore the predictive capacities of mentoring on these latter desirable outcomes.

A small-sample, Australian study examined the effects of a mentoring programme for newly qualified speech pathologists and occupational therapists (Holland et al 2001). The study demonstrated the effectiveness of a specific mentoring programme and highlighted the benefits for staff and the organisation beyond the mentoring dyads. The mentees reported that the support they received from their mentors had a positive influence on their clinical reasoning and increased their overall confidence as professionals. The mentoring relationship provided opportunities to discuss their fears and anxieties about departmental roles and responsibilities and allowed them the opportunity to raise issues honestly without fear of recrimination. The mentees reported feeling less isolated and more secure. The mentors reported becoming more aware of the transitional needs of new graduates and gaining enhanced clinical skills through discussion of complex cases. The mentors reported being more aware of their clinical protocols and rationales by having to help mentees with them and that such awareness led to more informed practice.

ENHANCING MENTORING RELATIONSHIPS

Most authors writing about mentoring advocate reflecting on the mentoring experience. How best to reflect is a highly personal matter (see Chapter 7) but Zachary (2000) suggested the following stems as a trigger to effective reflection on mentoring:

- About my mentee:
    - what am I thinking?
    - what am I wondering?
- My most difficult mentoring challenge so far is:
    - what is working well?
    - what could be working better?
- A new learning that has affected me:
    - reflecting on the phase of the mentoring.

ALLIED HEALTH MENTORING PROGRAMMES IN AUSTRALIA

A brief informal survey of professional associations in Australia revealed that many professions have made considerable recent progress in the development of formal mentoring opportunities for their members. The professions differ in how organised these programmes are, whether they are coordinated by national or state-level organisations and whether they target particular mentee groups such as new graduates or rural practitioners. A summary of the programmes available through professional organisations in Australia in 2004 is provided in Table 19.2. Interested readers should contact the relevant professional organisation for further details.

An innovative and well-coordinated mentoring programme has recently been established for professionals working in private or public practice in Melbourne or rural Victoria. With the assistance of government funding from the Department of Human Services (Victoria), the MentorLink-Allied Health Program offers mentoring education, mentor–mentee matching,

Table 19.2 Summary of formal mentoring programmes coordinated by Australian allied health and nursing professional groups

	State or national	Emphasis	Costs	Formal evaluation	Training provided
Dietetics	National; and * from 2004	Recent graduates	Included in DAA membership	Yes	Yes, but not mandatory
Nursing	Various	Aged care, rural and remote	Nil	Yes	Yes
Occupational therapy	State*	Rural and recent graduates	$50 once-off	Yes	Yes
Pharmacy	Nil				
Physiotherapy	State*	Rural and recent graduates	$50 once-off	Yes	Yes
Podiatry	State*	Rural and recent graduates	$50 once-off	Yes	Yes
Prosthetics and orthotics	Nil				
Radiography	Nil				
Speech pathology	State by state with national coordinator; and * from 2004	New graduates	Nil	Yes	Yes

*Victoria served by MentorLink-Allied Health (see text)
DAA, Dietetics Association of Australia.

programme evaluation services and, if required, conflict support to recent graduates in the occupational therapy, physiotherapy and podiatry professions. There is an objective to expand the programme to include seven health professions over the next few years. The programme is organised through a user-friendly website (http://mentorlinklounge.com) with helpful self-assessment, partnership agreement, development plan and programme evaluation forms. In addition, programme project officers monitor the mentoring partnerships regularly. The aim to reach out to rural and recent graduates and support them in their early transitional years appears to be being met, with recent rural occupational therapists reporting an increase in professional confidence of 43% after 12 months' participation in Mentorlink (Rural Health Services, Education and Training report 2001, as cited on http://mentorlinklounge.com).

ESTABLISHING MENTORING PROGRAMMES

Having located individuals who wish to be mentors (with competencies as previously discussed) or mentees, there is a need to consider what preparation the individuals require for their roles. Preparing practitioners for successful mentoring relationships has much in common with preparing them for successful clinical education relationships (see Rose & McAllister 1999). The knowledge, skills and attitudes needed for effective mentoring are largely encompassed by those utilised by clinical educators. The mentor and mentee need to become aware of:

- their motivations and expectations of the relationship
- the context where their relationship will take place and the demands on the relationship imposed by the context
- the functions and roles of the mentee and mentor
- styles of mentoring
- phases of mentoring relationships
- the need for an agreement at the outset (whether written or verbal) that sets out the roles, boundaries, methods of operating, confidentiality safeguards and ways that potential conflict and inevitable closure will be handled
- the need for ongoing reflection about the mentoring relationship and its benefits and possible limitations.

Much of these preparatory needs could be achieved through workshop experiences with individual reading and reflection tasks.

MATCHING DYADS

Research investigating formal workplace mentoring suggested that cross-cultural and cross-gender mentoring was less successful than same-gender and same-culture dyads. This was explained in terms of the potential for such pairings being susceptible to ineffective power imbalances and stereotyping (Noe 1988). In business culture, mentoring dyads are frequently highly selected. Selection can begin by gathering biographical data about the mentors and mentees in terms of their areas of expertise and interests and this can be circulated to potential mentees for short-listing. Alternatively,

Rolfe-Flett (2002) suggested arranging an interactive workshop where the pool of mentors and mentees come together and establish rapport before moving to a selection process. In health-related mentoring programmes it is more common for the participants to complete an expression of interest form and for a coordinator to match the mentors and mentees on the basis of their identified needs, goals, capabilities and experience levels. Arranging a mentoring programme on personality types or learning styles may in fact create a situation where the initial attraction of being alike wears off and reveals pairings of people with insufficient difference to be of interest or support.

MAINTAINING AND EVALUATING MENTORING PROGRAMMES

Mentoring programmes can be evaluated from a number of perspectives and dimensions. Positive and negative outcomes for the organisation, the individuals and the clients/patients can all be sources of information. A number of evaluation options for formal mentoring programmes have been identified by Rolfe-Flett as follows:

- Participants keep a journal of their experiences and use this as a guide in order to take part in interviews or surveys.
- Mentors and mentees formally review each contact by completing a reflection sheet and supply these to the evaluation procedures.
- Workshops are held where mentors and mentees discuss their experiences and these are recorded and coded.
- Questionnaires are sent to mentors and mentees asking them to reflect on the objectives they set at the outset, the processes undertaken and their sense of achievement/progress.
- One-to-one interviews are held with the participants and feedback about the programme is recorded.
- Focus groups of mentors are run separately from mentees and the participants are asked to reflect on what could be done differently in the next programme.
- Supervisors or managers could be surveyed on their perceptions of the programme and workplace productivity/client satisfaction/staff harmony etc.

In informal mentoring relationships, the participants need to reflect on their experiences and consider ways to assist in enhancing the relationship. The use of personal journals and debriefing sessions can be of great value in the reflection process (see Chapter 7).

THE FUTURE OF MENTORING IN HEALTH PRACTICE IN AUSTRALIA AND THE NEED FOR RESEARCH IN MENTORING IN ALLIED HEALTH

In today's increasingly competitive health care environment, which is characterised by consolidations, mergers, ownership changes, and managed health-care programmes that have altered the way patients get care (Iverson, Deery, and Erwin, 1995), mentoring can facilitate organizational socialisation by helping workers adopt appropriate role behaviour, learn work skills and abilities, and acquire the norms and values of the work group (Clawson, 1980). Mentoring also can reduce turnover among valued young professionals (Kram, 1985) and promote transfer of knowledge and values (Kram, 1996) that support a hospital's mission

(Koberg et al, 1998 p. 70).

Mentoring is here to stay. Our complex, cluttered and rapidly changing workplaces and professional lives will increasingly place supportive, facilitative and enabling relationships such as mentoring in high demand. There is a need, however, for research and direction on the specific nature of mentoring within the cultures and practices of the health sector. The business world has offered much in terms of describing and researching key factors that operate in mentoring relationships within the corporate domain. However, it would be foolish to assume a one-to-one translation of knowledge and practice from the corporate world to the health sector. I therefore look forward to a burgeoning research base in mentoring in the health professions in the next decade and to discover the gems and wisdoms that make it succeed in our special places of work.

REFERENCES

Atkinson K, Steward B 1997 A longitudinal study of occupational therapy by practitioners in their first year of professional practice: preliminary findings. British Journal of Occupational Therapy 60:338–342

Bass B, Avolio B 1994 Improving organisational effectiveness through transformational leadership. Sage, Thousand Oaks, California

Brockner J, Grover S, Reed T, DeWitt R 1992 Layoffs, job insecurity, and survivors' work effort: evidence of an inverted-U relationship. Academy of Management Journal 35:413–425

Douglas C, McCauley C 1999 Formal developmental relationships: a survey of organisational practices. Human Resource Development Quarterly 10:203–220

Ferguson A 2000 Feedback from Newcastle graduates. Australian Communication Quarterly 2:11–13

Golden S 2000 The impact and outcomes of mentoring. National Foundation for Educational Research, Slough

Hajzler D 2001 A phenomenological investigation and comparison of the experience of "good" clinical supervision and "good" mentoring. Unpublished thesis, La Trobe University, Melbourne

Holland K, McMahon S, Copley J et al 2001 The effectiveness of a mentoring program for new graduate allied health professionals. Focus on Health Professional Education 3:42–58

Koberg C, Boss R, Goodman E 1998 Factors and outcomes associated with mentoring among health-care professionals. Journal of Vocational Behavior 53:58–72

Kram K 1988 Mentoring at work: developmental relationships in organisational life. University Press of America, Lanham

Martin C, Siosteen A, Shephard K 1999 The professional development of expert physical therapists in four areas of clinical practice. In: Jensen G, Gwyer J, Hack L, Shephard K (eds) Expertise in physical therapy practice. Butterworth-Heinemann, Boston, p 231–244

McCauley C, Douglas C 1998 Developmental relationships. In: McCauley C, Moxley R, Velsor E (eds) The centre for creative leadership handbook of leadership development. Jossey-Bass, San Francisco, p 160–193

Noe R 1988 Women and mentoring: a review and research agenda. Academy of Management Review 13:65–78

Rolfe-Flett A 2002 Mentoring in Australia. A practical guide. Prentice Hall, Frenchs Forest, NSW

Rose M, McAllister M 1999 Becoming a clinical educator In: Higgs J, Edwards E (eds) Educating beginning practitioners. Challenges for health professional education. Butterworth-Heinemann, Boston, p 271–278

Sosik J, Godshalk V 2000 Leadership styles, mentoring functions received, and job-related stress: a conceptual model and preliminary study. Journal of Organisational Behaviour 21:365–390

Zachary L 2000 The mentor's guide: facilitating effective learning relationships. Jossey-Bass, San Francisco

RESOURCES

www.mentorlinklounge.com The website for the Victoria mentoring programme for Allied Health (currently serving the occupational therapy, physiotherapy and podiatry professions with aims to expand in near future).

www.mentoring.org The website for the National Mentoring Partnership organisation of the United States of America. Their "Learn to mentor toolkit" may be of interest, although aimed at adult–child mentoring dyads.

www.nmn.org.au The website for the National Mentoring Network of the United Kingdom. The paper "Running a mentoring programme: key considerations" by David Sims, Jim Jamison, Sarah Olden and Anne Lines (2000) may be of particular interest, although aimed at school student–adult dyads.

SECTION 6

Evaluation and future directions in clinical education and supervision

Chapter 20

The anatomy of educational evaluation in clinical education, mentoring and professional supervision

Della Fish

INTRODUCTION

How one conceives of clinical supervision (clinical education, mentoring and professional supervision) will shape how one seeks to evaluate it. But much of the current literature shows that evaluators often start a long way down the road from this point. As a result, I would argue, their work rests on unexpressed, undefended and sometimes unwarranted assumptions. These assumptions are about the nature of clinical supervision itself. And these then shape what should be evaluated, who should engage in it, when it should occur, how it should be done and what should count as evidence. These tacit assumptions have been imposed upon an uncritical professional world by bureaucrats and managers. They treat everything about developing professional practice as if it were simple, when in fact (education being values-based), it is problematic. This means that there is no one correct general way of seeing education, and educators must engage in practical reasoning in order to choose the best way of thinking about it for the given context, or must develop principles of procedure whose provenance is transparent.

The usefulness of proceeding as if evaluation is a simple technical process is that it provides managers with the sort of evidence *they* need. Its downside is that it reinforces *their* view of professionalism and it does not provide the real evidence that will help professionals to improve clinical supervision and their own practice.

For example, where clinical supervision is seen as just another task in the round of health care duties of a nurse, then the evaluative role is taken by nursing researchers who seek to generate and weigh the evidence about whether clinical supervision is "value for money" and "improves patient care". The assumption here is that, to be credible, clinical supervision should be evaluated (audited) in much the way that all other health care activities now are. It follows, then, that all that is needed are instruments that can measure (preferably on a large scale) the elements necessary to respond to these questions. It is further believed that these ultimately need to be, and can be, "standardised across the country". Thus, what is evaluated is that which can be measured in respect of the efficacy of the supervision. The evidence is collected by researchers brought in to the clinical setting, and must be able to be couched in quantitative terms and presented in charts.

The search is then on for instruments which will measure outcomes. Examples of this are: the effects of receiving clinical supervision (the Manchester Clinical Supervision Scale: Butterworth 1998); "whether it is a good thing" (Winstanley 2001); whether it is cost-effective and impacts positively on patient care (The Nurse Stress Index: Harris 1989). Whether or not clinical supervision "is a good thing" will depend on the kind of thing one thinks clinical supervision is! Of course, such instruments are hard to find (see, for example the Clinical Supervision Evaluation Project: Butterworth 1998) and are – for obvious reasons – difficult to create, pilot, field-test, validate and make reliable. Further, for the professional audience, they tend to leave an aftertaste of disappointment, because after all that work the scientific evidence provided is fairly superficial. For example, "trials of the Manchester Clinical Supervision Scale have shown that clinical supervision is addressing improvement in skills, encourages reflective practice, and attends to personal development" (Winstanley 2001, p. 222). But what does it offer the supervisor seeking to improve practice?

A very different starting point takes us down a very different road, placing the responsibilities for evaluation in the hands of practitioners.

Clinical supervision as an educational enterprise

At the base of all the terms used for clinical supervision lies the concept of the *education of professionals in clinical settings.* And this is so, whether their emphasis is centred on *enabling* (facilitating a professional's personal growth) or *ensuring* that professionals adjust to their new roles in a workplace setting; whether the focus of education is an individual post or "broad professional functioning"; whether the education is carried out in an undergraduate or postgraduate context; and whether assessment is a part of the activity or not (see Chapter 1). That is, the central intentions and main activities of clinical supervision are educational, its processes are enacted in the practice context and its quality depends on its educational achievements. Its processes and products are therefore best appreciated through *educational* evaluation, the anatomy of which will be the main focus of this chapter.

It is the case that many writers, following Proctor (1986), have argued that clinical supervision has a management (normative) and a therapeutic (restorative) intention, as well as an educational (formative) role (see, for example, Bowles & Young 1999). However, I am more sympathetic to the view of Cutcliffe et al (2001) that "clinical supervision should not be confused with or amalgamated with managerial supervision or personal therapy/counseling" (see Chapter 1).

Clearly, a form of supervisory overview may be used in the health care workplace, for management purposes, by those who wish to audit professional activities as a means of costing and controlling them and who often proliferate protocols as a result, in order to defend and protect the system they manage (see Cotton 2001). But because of its complex human character, the true *value* of professional practice (including supervisory practice) is not really susceptible to crude forms of measurement. As writers are beginning to point out, there has been an audit explosion (Power 1997, O'Neill 2002), which has affected the daily lives of professionals who "have to work to ever more exacting – if changing – standards of good practice and due process", the new demands of which "damage their real work" (O'Neill 2002, p. 49).

I would argue that resources might be better channelled into educational supervision and its evaluation, as the real key to improved patient care – including improved risk management (see also de Cossart 2004). Audit (at systems level) is not sufficient alone to register quality in professional practice. However, as Bishop (1998) points out, the results of such auditing can be drawn upon as one small evaluative element in the illumination of clinical supervision. For these reasons, this chapter will advocate the use in educational evaluation of all relevant data-collecting processes and all relevant evidence which is already available, but it will not discuss in detail ways of systems-auditing the work of clinical supervisors (though it will provide a further reading list of texts that do).

Supervision in a clinical setting may also be reshaped to a therapeutic end for the practitioner, and its success can then be tested by monitoring the health of the practitioner, although not all professionals subscribe to this view (Yegdich 1999). Such reshaping thus brings with it a reshaped means of evaluation, which it is beyond this chapter to explore in detail, though it will offer references for pursuing such approaches, from the numerous texts that deal with the evaluation of therapeutic supervision (see further reading).

Rationale and intentions for this chapter

At the heart of the term "evaluation" lies the term "values". Values are at the base of all educational activities, whether we recognise this or not. The presence of underlying values is what renders education and all its concepts problematic rather than simple. There is, for example, no one simple definition of an educated person with which everyone will concur. Thus, what we value about both professional practice and education in clinical settings, how we express their guiding principles, and articulate (understand) their nature, will shape the choices made about how to evaluate them. Such choices relate to the aims and processes of evaluation as well as the character of the end-product of that evaluation.

The intention in this chapter, then, is to provide a basis from which readers can stand back, recognise their own values, and (re-)construct their own understanding and critique of the principles, processes and products of educational evaluation in the context of clinical supervision (its underlying bones, muscles, tissue and organs). In highlighting both the nature of professional and educational practices and the central role in them of professional judgement (the brain which directs the intelligent life of such practices), it also seeks to show readers why protocols handed on by others will not exactly fit their individual context and thus why they need to construct their own evaluative processes. This chapter does not advocate revolution despite its provocative stance. Rather, it hopes to influence evolution from a technical rational view of evaluation (which currently at least may be a required necessity but which I am arguing is not sufficient) to a broader one that is more sympathetic to the nature of professional practice and ways of developing it (see Chapter 6).

It is hoped first, then, to provoke readers to give consideration to how *they* conceive of the nature of professional practice generally and educational practice specifically, and the values that underlie their vision. Such an understanding should then inform their own practice as clinical supervisors as they seek to engage in educational evaluation: that is, as they seek to investigate, diagnose and manage the care and development of their own individual educational work *in its particular situation and context*, and *as they reconsider the ends they believe they are seeking in their work*.

This chapter therefore seeks to:

1. explain the values and beliefs which inform my own thinking about education and professional practice and their implications for educational evaluation (as an illustration of how educational evaluation is driven by our understanding of the nature of professional practice and education)
2. explore the intentions and nature of educational evaluation (which, I shall argue, is a form of educational research and is separate from both assessment and appraisal) and show how it relates to quality assurance and professional standards
3. show what, consequently, can be said about the evaluation of clinical education, mentoring and professional supervision and how such evaluation might be carried out, and offer some principles which will enable readers to create their own means of evaluating the clinical supervision in which they are engaged.

Critical review of some key current texts on clinical supervision and its evaluation will be found embedded in the text at relevant points.

THE NATURE OF PROFESSIONAL PRACTICE IN HEALTH CARE AND EDUCATION

Our values and beliefs create a lens through which we look. How and what we value shapes the very way we describe and discuss professional matters. I offer here my own credo. I shall offer my beliefs (and highlight their underlying values) about professional practice and education in two subsections. I shall indicate the implications for evaluation at the end of this section.

Readers are invited to use this section to help them to explore their own values and beliefs, in order to understand and critique the rest of this chapter, consider critically the literature on clinical supervision and its evaluation and construct their own approach to clinical education and its evaluation.

Beliefs and values in relation to the nature of professional practice

I have elsewhere (Fish & Coles 1998, Chapter 3) set out in detail the arguments for my current position in respect of professional practice, and there is only room here to sketch the key details.

I see professional practice as complex, uncertain and unpredictable. I value artistry as well as technical competence in professional practitioners. I do not share the notion that practice can adequately be described under the headings of knowledge, skills and attitudes (which we use in the UK to shape a National Curriculum for schoolchildren, who have no moral responsibilities to vulnerable patients and who are not seeking to develop professional judgement and intelligent conduct!). *Knowledge* is too easily regarded as referring only to formal (book) theory, which does not do justice to the knowledge that is constructed (in various ways) during practice; *skills* is not a wide enough category to attend to the complexity of professional procedures, and important professional capacities (like acting with professionalism, and exercising professional judgement); and *attitudes*, being concerned with visible behaviour, does not highlight the moral significance of the way we conduct ourselves.

I would argue that professional practice is driven by and rests upon intelligent conduct. Behaviour is a surface feature and cannot be relied upon to guarantee probity. Our behaviour may be feigned to demonstrate expected characteristics when required, but may well hide a lack of commitment to underlying ideas and values. Intelligent conduct has a moral thrust. Here our activities are shaped by commitment to our beliefs and values and do not vary according to who is watching us (see Michael Oakeshott's 1966 essays).

I do not regard professional practice as "master-able", but only as able to be developed endlessly. Such development is a life-long enterprise and comes from a willingness to improve through change that gains its thrust from inner conviction. I hold that the quality of professional practice (and life itself) is degraded if we believe that we can measure everything that matters and that what we cannot measure does not matter. The nature of professional practice is best understood holistically, not by trying to atomise it into all its component parts. Indeed, it is more than the sum of its parts. At its heart lies professional judgement, which cannot be replaced by the production of protocols – a fact that civil servants and administrators do not understand because they follow a rule book. Professional judgement I regard as a central and defining characteristic of professional practice (whether that practice is in health care or education). I value good judgement highly (see Fish 1998, Fish & Coles 1998).

For me this means that it is important that professional practice is recognised as discretionary. It follows that professionals need good education to help them to exercise their judgement, and understand and improve their practice in making sound judgements. They cannot simply be trained to follow templates. Risk management is a prime example of this. Risk is endemic to life and cannot be eliminated. We delude ourselves if we think that prescribing and proscribing all the practitioner's activities will eliminate the risks incurred where professionals make more of their own decisions. Indeed, protocols have been shown to increase rather than reduce the danger of making a mistake (see Schön 1987). Thus, practitioners must remain broadly autonomous, making their own decisions about their actions and the moral bases of those actions (for which, of course, they must be fully accountable). That accountability by the professional should involve far more than technical accountability (demonstrating that in their performance they have followed the rules via protocols). O'Neill makes the point that this approach often obstructs or distorts the proper aims of professional practice, and makes professionals not more accountable but less so (O'Neill 2002, p. 49–52). Rather, I would argue, we should require of professionals *answerability* (the need to be able to give an account of, and to be accountable for, conduct as well as just skills – for those values, beliefs, theories, principles and moral and ethical matters that underpin the professional's decision-making, judgement and consequent activities).

Professional practice gains its meaning from being theorised. The processes it draws upon include the analytical, interpretative and appreciative viewing and "re-viewing" of the actions of the practitioner in the wider context of the history and traditions of professional practice and in terms of the political, social and moral dimensions of the actions taken. This permits us to make more sense of practice than appears on the surface. The ability to theorise practice is essential to improving practice. This is because it involves revealing the depth of thought and feeling which lies beneath our actions, recognising the wellsprings of our judgements, decisions, reasoning and actions (our beliefs, assumptions, values and theories). It includes recognising honestly the *results* within our practice of our assumptions, our reasoning, values, beliefs, judgements and action, and it involves identifying the problematic, the contestable and the dilemmas endemic to our practice. Reflective practice is a significant means of theorising and understanding our experience and turning it with rigour into practical wisdom.

Practitioners need to share their theorising about practice, because their "knowledge out of practice" becomes formal and coherent "theory", by being tested in practice, and publicly justified and sustained through debate in the public sphere. Theorising thus establishes agreements and disagreements between the new knowledge and what others know, and reconciliation with what others have already contributed to the common stock of knowledge. By this means it is given a place in the public realm of knowledge (Kemmis 1995, p. 15). Theory and practice thus develop reflexively together and the so-called theory/practice gap is a myth and a product of the technical rational view of professionalism.

Clearly, in holding these views I also have concomitant beliefs about what and how to facilitate the learning of such practice, and how it should be assessed (at undergraduate and postgraduate level) and how the educational provision should be evaluated.

The aims of education in professional contexts

Again, it is possible to see clearly the values that lie beneath the following statements about what we should be trying to achieve in education within professional contexts.

Learning to become a professional is "a matter of coming ever more fully into membership of a tradition of practice" and, "at its maturity it is a matter of taking part in shaping practice more fully for the future" (Golby 1993, p. 8). This involves understanding the inherited traditions of a profession, and considering critically and practically their present relevance (see Fish 1995, p. 73–74). The educator's task, therefore is:

- to equip professionals with the ideas, vision and language to offer a critique of present ways of operating (challenge the given and re-view the taken-for-granted) and with the ability to deliberate about the choices available to us as practitioners by considering their moral and ethical dimensions
- to present the profession as theoretically based and morally informed
- to recognise that in professional practice the importance of professional know-how is balanced by the importance of practical wisdom and that theoretical knowledge (often derived from practice) provides the understanding out of which good practice is shaped and reshaped
- to open up to aspiring professionals the means of investigating, refining, extending and reshaping their own practice
- to initiate professionals into a tradition of educational *thought*, which exposes the taken-for-granted political assumptions and educational values of contemporary practice, rather than socialising them into the unexamined values and taken-for-granted assumptions of the present system
- to facilitate critical debate about which values should inform professional practice
- to develop reflective practitioners who examine the extent to which their practice is actually shaped by their best ideas, values and ideals *and* who at the same time are prepared to challenge those ideas and values
- to uncover the moral and intellectual touchstones in relation to which the educational quality of learning in a professional context and the practice of those in a particular profession can be critically appraised and appreciated – and then judged.

Good education (clinical supervision) and improved patient care

So how does the educational development of health care professionals improve the care of patients? And where is the evidence that it can?

Arguably, professionals who are more knowledgeable *and therefore more articulate* about themselves, about how they conduct themselves in clinical settings, about their skills and procedures, about their professional judgements, and about their responsibilities in relation to the traditions of their profession, and who have learnt to keep these under review through reflection and investigation of their practice, will be better at caring for patients. But education rarely cashes out into immediate visible change. It is not, like training, a quick-fix enterprise, aimed at making a cosmetic change to behaviour.

Rather, in changing professionals' understanding, education guarantees the development of their conduct.

But, argue the cynics, you cannot measure most of those things, so you have no means of proving that all the resources put into clinical supervision will be worth continuing. As we shall see below, measurement is not the only means of proof.

Further, improved patient care is not the simple, clear-cut matter that is pretended either. It too is not easily measurable. It too is a values-based concept. There is no template for it. Patients are all individuals, with differing needs; what is required is emphatically *not* a new protocol that applies to all, but rather improved judgement about how to adapt what is known to the individual case.

The implications of these values and beliefs

Rich complexity such as that described above is three-dimensional. The nature of practitioners' work might be justly described as requiring artistry rather than mere technical competence (which arguably is two-dimensional). The ever-present networks of actions and interactions of life in professional practice are underpinned by multiple levels of intentions, motives and sensitivities that affect the way we conduct ourselves as professionals. About these matters there is no absolute truth to be pinned down and crystallised, only a range of interpretations, which need to be pieced together into a mosaic of probability. These "truths-to-life" are more akin to what is found within the humanistic and artistic disciplines rather than through the exact sciences and are the subject matter of the arts (novel; drama; music; visual art). We can either simplify professional practice and weigh, as significant, only its surface and quantifiable elements, or we can recognise these as surface features and seek to take soundings from beneath them, in an attempt to understand better and develop our practice *as a whole*.

What then might this involve?

THE INTENTIONS AND NATURE OF EDUCATIONAL EVALUATION

This main section will chart the emergence of evaluation in professional practice, by considering the meaning of quality in professional practice, and tracing the relationship of evaluation to accountability and to quality assurance. It will then explore the nature of educational evaluation and educational research.

The emergence of evaluation in professional practice

Quality in professional practice (health care and education)

If professional practice is as described above, then quality in such practice comes from deepening insight into one's own values, priorities and actions, and not from the imposition of quality inspection and control mechanisms, with their emphasis on testing and visible performance and their belief that change can be imposed from outside the profession and that quality is measurable. Quality cannot be *inspected* into a professional organisation, cannot be externally imposed and will never come from tight prescription. Quality control and inspection have the effect of demotivating the professional by reducing the challenge that autonomy offers, and turning practice into a factory-like monotony and the practitioner into a delivery agent. (The ubiquity of this notion is evident in our acceptance of the language of the post-person as applied to health care and education!) I would argue that quality comes from inside people and groups, as a result of a shared commitment to improvement *through understanding.* As part of this, practitioners have a responsibility to bring criticality to bear on all aspects of their practice and on the literature associated with it.

Educational evaluation, accountability and quality control

What we mean by "quality" is rarely asked. It is often left to rest on shared assumption, and such assumptions arise by default from the consumerist view of life and its inevitable requirement for quality control. Quality control is an industrial term used to cover all the inspectorial procedures necessary to ensure the production of goods to a minimum standard of acceptability. The notion that this makes for quality is somewhat risible, even in this context. However, it does "assure" the customer that a *basic* standard was established before the goods left the factory. Quality here is linked to measurement because goods are tangible and measurable. Simple measurements of visible outcomes are thus an inevitable requirement of quality in such a context. This might be characterised as a technical-rational way of thinking. (Though, in a final irony, it is being replaced in some parts of industry by a more collective and sophisticated approach to quality that involves the entire workforce.)

In the 1980s, in the consumerist society of most of the western world, the call for professionals to be publicly accountable became inevitable, for a variety of reasons (see Fish & Coles 1998, Chapter 1). The language in which this was discussed was softened slightly (quality *assurance* replacing *control*), but it was the only concession to the professional context. The problem arose with the automatic imposition of production-line (technical-rational) thinking that *how* professionals should be accountable for the effectiveness of their work was through "measurable outcomes". As a result, the quality of health care and education is now "measured" in much of the western world by league tables, which professionals know and the public is beginning to see reward mendacity (people soon learn to "massage" the figures and this very metaphor indicates how acceptable this idea has become). What is ignored here is the lived experience of both parties in the professional relationship. It is for this reason that I do not concur with Driscoll's (2000, p. 179) comment that "clinical supervision will not be sustainable without some form of measurable outcome". Arguably, instead of accepting this, we should ask:

- Given the nature of professional practice (which is complex and which provides a service rather than goods), what is it for *professionals to be accountable?*
- What makes for quality in *professional* work (what kind of evidence would assure us of the effectiveness of their work)?

There may be some enlightenment to be gained from measuring outcomes on professional practice, but this alone is nowhere near sufficient to illuminate our understanding of professional practice, to develop it and to provide adequate *accountability* about its quality to the public and to individual patients. Other evidence must balance this. To give depth to this process, it must involve practitioners being expected *to account for* their actions as well as *give an account of* them. It is the second of these that enables the complexities of practice to be given proper weight. If done properly it is as valid as any other form of data (though the way of validating it may be different and less well understood in our current society).

Quality assurance and standards

The establishment of standards is endemic to the technical-rational approach to quality control. (Inspection of goods requires a *basic* standard against which to judge them). Again, we have automatically taken this as the way forward in professional practice too. We now try (in most professions) to write "baseline performance indicators". And books on clinical supervision advocate this approach. For example, Driscoll (2000, p. 188) argues: "Devising and writing standards in clinical supervision practice using a structure–process–outcome model allows each element to be examined independently."

In other words this is the routine approach to evaluation. He offers the following questions to guide the setting of explicit standards:

- What do you want to achieve? (the outcome)
- How do all involved intend to achieve this outcome?
- What sorts of things will help you?

Driscoll provides a (long) list of advantages of standard-setting when implementing clinical supervision, many of which I would challenge. He argues, for example, that:

- "it provides a forum for implementing quality supervision" (this assertion is not based on an in-depth examination of quality in professional practice, nor does it take account of the complexity of how professionals learn in practice)
- "it encourages the development of knowledge" (pre-setting objectives often blinkers the learner to knowledge that arises in practice)
- "specific elements related to local needs are addressed" (you do not need to set baseline standards for this to happen and different learners need different things).

The only disadvantages he lists are "time consuming; more paperwork; alterations to standards need to be communicated to everyone; initial disputes in devising agreed content; after completion may be filed away until a few days before audit". This critique comes from within the technical-rational paradigm rather than standing back from it.

He also reminds us, by reference to Fowler (1998, p. 57), that when writing standards we should be SMART about it and that such statements should be:

S Specific
M Measurable
A Achievable
R Realistic
T Timed.

Again, I would argue that this is a very technical-rational approach and is insufficient to support good-quality evaluation of the work of professionals in health care and education. It excludes a focus on the real elements of professional practice and treats them as simple rather than complex and problematic. It covers up the real growth points that need to emerge from practice. It might bring the short-term advantage of providing an easy and simple approach to quality assurance, but in the longer term it sells professionalism short and encourages the public to believe that there is very little to it. It is about monitoring and providing evidence of effectiveness in an extremely narrow way.

A new (and rather different) standard for professional practice for the 21st century might be to invite professionals to work CREATIVELY, rather than SMART-ly and thus in ways that seek to be:

C Contributory to a Culture in which professionals are more in Control of their practice
R Reflective practice-focused
E Educationally focused and Enquiry-based rather than management-driven
A Accountable, giving rich accounts of practice to the profession and the public
T Transformative of the practitioner's understanding of practice
I Interprofessionally agreed
V Values-based
E Evaluable by humanistic enquiry
L Linked to quality of care through staff development
Y Yielding of high motivation to busy professional.

This is about the process rather than the product of professional work. It would shape the work of the clinical supervisor and supervisee, without foreclosing on what will be learnt (by both) in the practice setting. It requires certain desirable conduct at the level of principle, without prescribing the outcome. And it fits the character of professional practice.

Quality (the effectiveness of clinical supervision) would be evaluated then, on the basis of evidence that these principles had informed practice *and* the richness of the accounts of that practice, and of what both supervisor and supervisee had learnt. Increasing richness of understanding would almost inevitably characterise practitioners' development through their careers. Appraisal would take account of this, and set comments about such development on record.

Having argued for the educational nature of clinical supervision, and set the context for evaluation in the professions, what then can we say about educational evaluation itself?

The nature of educational evaluation and educational research

The nature of educational evaluation

Educational evaluation is a form of educational research. Educational evaluation seeks to investigate and understand the processes that have taken place in an educational programme or educational provision, with a view to developing or refining them. It is to be distinguished from *assessment* (which is concerned with learner progress) and *appraisal* (which is concerned with staff performance).

The recognition that educational evaluation is one form of educational research is the key to understanding the approaches, methods and instruments that are appropriate for the enterprise of assuring quality in teaching and learning. And the approaches to enquiry here are not the same as those appropriate for research in medical science. (And processes to gain validity, proof and truth, and how evidence is utilised, are all different.)

Decisions about the design of educational evaluation

Decisions about the design of educational evaluation are shaped by how we construe three areas:

1. the nature of the educational practice to be enquired into
2. the nature of knowledge within that practice
3. the nature of enquiry itself.

Researchers do not always make their views about them explicit, but in fact, any research design is based upon assumptions (explicit or implicit; appropriate or inappropriate) about each. Further, the probity of the enquiry, and its success, depend on the logical connection between these three.

The nature of educational practice

As we have seen above, the nature of educational practice is that it is a values-based, complex, human activity, which requires to be investigated and understood from a range of perspectives. It is an activity where the whole is greater than the sum of the parts. Subjective meanings are also part of its reality and *mind is as real as matter*. Further, what is invisible is more important than what is visible. This contrasts with the nature of practice in the sciences where empirical evidence is central, and where objectivity is eternally striven for.

Most particularly, the enterprise of understanding professional practice, and of recognising the artistry in it, involves focusing upon one's own professional judgements and seeing one's individual practice within the broader context of the traditions of the practice of one's profession.

The nature of educational knowledge

The nature of educational knowledge is that it is time-bounded, context-bounded, and constructed between people on the spot and never static. There are many different ways to know, and there is no such thing as an objective fact, free of theory and free of values. This contrasts with scientific enterprises where knowledge is believed to be absolute, universal, quantifiable; where abstract and context-free generalisations can apparently be made; where "facts" are sought which confirm (or render null) theories and hypotheses; where the knower is separate from what is known.

The nature of enquiry

Enquiry (research) can be located in a range of different ways of seeing the world, and according to the nature of the practice enquired into and the focus of understanding of the enquiry. The approaches and methods then follow. The choice of paradigm needs to be appropriate to the nature of what is to be enquired into. For example, the scientific/positivistic paradigm is appropriate for those for whom the foundation of their professional practice is predominantly their propositional (factual) knowledge, and who see research as having the duty to extend that kind of knowledge. They rely upon this paradigm to produce more and more up-to-date information, which they can acquire and then put into practice. Here the approach is exclusively quantitative.

Alternatively, enquiry can be situated in qualitative research (which does not eschew quantitative evidence). Within the qualitative approach lie three paradigms:

1. interpretative
2. critical
3. artistic/holistic.

The interpretative paradigm is where the complexities of human interaction are explored. This paradigm seeks to enlighten practice and aid decision-making about its complex moral basis. Equally, for those interested in the emancipation of practitioners and the political dimensions of practice, enquiry can be conducted from within the critical paradigm. Or, as I have suggested (Fish 1998), if interested in the artistry of practice, it can be conducted from within the artistic/holistic paradigm. This focuses on the appreciation of practice, rather as one knowledgeable in art might appreciate (recognise the characteristics of and the quality in) a particular painting. This involves critique, not negative criticism.

Equally important is the relationship of the researcher to that being researched. Educational evaluation is a form of, and is sometimes referred to as, practitioner research. Here, there is an acknowledgement that the researcher is "part of the world s/he is researching", and "has a history and a future in that culture" (Reed & Proctor 1995, p. 5). Such practitioners consider their practice critically within the history and traditions of the practical work of their profession. They will seek to utilise any evidence from a wide range of sources to help them understand their practice better. Since it is about understanding practice with a view to refining or developing it, this is also, demonstrably, a form of professional – or staff – development. It should be remembered that teachers seriously improve their practice in the light of enhanced educational understanding, not in response to mandates from outside.

EVALUATING CLINICAL EDUCATION, MENTORING AND PROFESSIONAL SUPERVISION

The above arguments place emphasis on facilitating the practitioner's exploration of (and thus ability to articulate, and defend or improve) intelligent conduct in clinical supervision, rather than on activities designed to measure and reshape behaviour. Depending on the overall interest, the interpretative, critical or artistic paradigms will provide the overall shape.

The educator (clinical supervisor) must be involved in the collection of evidence for evaluating the educational provision offered within the practice. Since good practice is context-specific; it cannot be well evaluated by "evaluation protocols" that seek to monitor the effectiveness of clinical supervision sessions and merely serve to impose uniformity of thinking about them. Indeed, a brief look at examples of such shows them to be at the level of generality, which fails to cast any light upon the quality of the educational interaction (Driscoll 2000, p. 187). The supervisor should therefore custom-design each evaluation, drawing on the principles of educational research, in which the evidence comes from a range of perspectives. The following headings offer prompts in this process.

The clinical supervisor should show evidence of having reconsidered:

- his/her own values, beliefs and intentions for the supervision
- the very aims of the programme/provision (and their appropriateness), and how they have shaped the educational provision offered
- the content of the programme/provision in the light of the supervisee's values, beliefs, intentions and comments on the process
- the context for learning (political, social, management, educational) and whether it is sympathetic to promoting learning
- the processes of teaching and learning and the quality of the learning opportunities provided
- whether there has been effective engagement with and participation by the supervisee
- how well the quality of learning has been facilitated in terms of workloads
- whether the expectations by the supervisor of the supervisee were appropriate and if they encouraged achievement
- the assessment processes (whether they enabled learners to demonstrate achievements; how formative assessment related to the final summative assessment)
- the evidence available for whether the supervisee's achievements met the required standards
- the quality and level of support provided for supervisee
- the arrangements for, and the quality of, admission and induction procedures of supervisee
- the arrangements for, and the quality of, educational supervision for the supervisee
- the appropriateness of the variety of technical, administrative, accommodation and resources support.

The perspectives consulted should include the following:

- the educator's own views/behaviours/research material
- the supervisee's views in oral and written feedback

- the administrative procedures
- the assessment results
- relevant evidence from any relevant audit procedures
- documents related to the curriculum and to inspection reports.

The investigative methods and means used to collect evidence should include:

- supervisees' narratives (reflections on practice – both oral and written)
- documentary analysis of curriculum documents and reports
- supervisees' assessment papers (where relevant)
- the health care educator's own reflective writing (enquiries into practice using critical incidents and reflective frameworks)
- comments from other colleagues
- interviews with supervisees conducted by supervisor and others
- formal (anonymous) supervisee evaluations.

ENDPIECE

Educational evaluation is an exploratory enterprise from which we cannot cease, and which, to summarise the spirit of T. S. Eliot's (1980) words in section V of *Little Gidding*, will enable us (endlessly) to return to the beginning of our clinical supervision and to come to know it for the first time. Perhaps the intrigue of that is what will motivate us to engage in all of it!

Acknowledgement

I am indebted to Carr & Hartnet 1996 for prompting my bulleted comments under "aims of education".

REFERENCES

Bishop V 1998 What is going on? Results of a questionnaire. In: Bishop V (ed) Clinical supervision in practice: some questions, answers and guidelines. Macmillan, London

Bowles N, Young C 1999 An evaluative study of clinical supervision based on Proctor's three function interactive model. Journal of Advanced Nursing 30(4):958–964

Butterworth T 1998 Evaluation research in clinical supervision: a case example. In: Butterworth T, Burnard P, Faugier J (eds) Clinical supervision and mentorship in nursing, 2nd edn. Stanley Thornes, Cheltenham

Carr W, Hartnett A 1996 Education and the struggle for democracy: the politics of educational ideas. Open University Press, London

Cotton A 2001 Clinical supervision UK style: good for nurses and nursing? Contemporary Nurse 11:60–70

Cutcliffe J, Butterworth T, Proctor B 2001 (eds) Fundamental themes in clinical supervision. Routledge, London

de Cossart L 2004 Patient assessment and surgical risk. In: Patterson-Brown S (ed) A companion to specialist surgical practice: core topics in general and emergency surgery, 3rd edn. Elsevier, Edinburgh

Driscoll J 2000 Practising clinical supervision: a reflective approach. Baillière Tindall, Edinburgh

Eliot T S 1980 Collected poems. Faber, London

Fish D 1995 Quality mentoring for student teachers: a principled approach to practice. David Fulton, London

Fish D 1998 Appreciating practice in the caring professions: refocusing professional development and practitioner research. Butterworth-Heinemann, Oxford

Fish D, Coles C 1998 Developing professional judgement in healthcare: learning through the critical appreciation of practice. Butterworth-Heinemann, Oxford

Fowler J (ed) 1998 The handbook of clinical supervision – your questions answered. Quay Books, Salisbury

Golby M 1993 Editorial comments. In: Golby M (ed) A reader provided for MEd students at Exeter University (limited publication). Fairway Press, Exeter

Harris P 1989 The nurse stress index. Work and Stress 3(4):335–336

Kemmis S 1995 Prologue: theorizing educational practice. In: Carr W (ed) For education: towards critical educational enquiry. Open University Press, London

Oakeshott M 1966 On human conduct. Routledge, London

O'Neill O 2002 A question of trust. Cambridge University Press, Cambridge

Power M 1997 The audit society: rituals of verification. Oxford University Press, Oxford

Proctor B 1986 Supervision: a co-operative exercise in accountability. In: Marken M, Payne M (eds) Enabling and ensuring supervision in practice. National Youth Bureau, Council for Education and Training in Youth and Community Work, Leicester

Reed J, Proctor S 1995 Practitioner research in healthcare: the inside story. Chapman and Hall, London

Schön D 1987 Changing patterns of enquiry in work and living (the Thomas Cubitt lecture). Journal of the Royal Society of Arts CXXXV(5367):226–233

Winstanley J 2001 Developing methods for evaluating clinical supervision. In: Cutcliffe J, Butterworth T, Proctor B (eds) Fundamental themes in clinical supervision. Routledge, London

Yegdich T 1999 Lost in the crucible of supportive clinical supervision: supervision is not therapy. Journal of Advanced Nursing 29(5):1265–1275

FURTHER READING

For those who wish to pursue the development of measures to evaluate supervision (like the Maslach burnout inventory; the Minnesota job satisfaction scale; the Cooper coping skills scale; the Swindon staff support service model), the following readings will be useful:

Bishop V 1998 What is going on? Results of a questionnaire. In: Bishop V (ed) Clinical supervision in practice: some questions, answers and guidelines. Macmillan, London, p 22–39

Carson J 1998 Instruments for evaluating clinical supervision. In: Bishop V (ed) Clinical supervision in practice: some questions, answers and guidelines. Macmillan, London, p 163–178

Carson J, Booth K, Butterworth T 1998 Clinical supervision, stress management and social support. In: Butterworth T, Burnard P, Faugier J (eds) Clinical supervision and mentorship in nursing, 2nd edn. Nelson Thornes, Cheltenham

McSherry R, Bassett C 2002 Developing and implementing a strategy to measure and evaluate the impact of practice development at a team or organizational level. In: Practice development in the clinical setting. Nelson Thornes, Cheltenham, p 26–54

Winstanley J 2001 Developing methods for evaluating clinical supervision. In: Cutcliffe J, Butterworth T, Proctor B (eds) Fundamental themes in clinical supervision. Routledge, London

Chapter 21

Transforming practice

CHAPTER CONTENTS

Transformation: "the act, process or instance of being changed, completely or extensively, in composition, structure, nature, character or condition"
(composite definition from the Macquarie and Oxford dictionaries)

PART 1 Transforming practice through teaching, learning and supporting relationships
Miranda Rose and Dawn Best

INTRODUCTION

In essence, this text is about the centrality of relationships in teaching and learning: the relationships between students and clinical educators; between mentors and mentees; between professionals and professional supervisors;

and between peers and colleagues. Many of the authors in this book have argued that getting the relationships *right* is the major *work* in the education/supervision domain. Some authors (McAllister (Chapter 17), Neville (Chapter 16) and Rose (Chapter 19)) have emphasised the importance of these relationships in sustaining us in our work and in challenging us to grow and find meaning in what we do. In this chapter, we further argue that getting the relationships *right* leads not just to better teaching and learning processes and outcomes, but to opportunities for powerful personal and system-level transformation. We do not use this word, *transformation*, lightly. We understand that it is a word that evokes powerful and potentially life-changing concepts. We argue that such opportunity exists in teaching, learning and supervisory practice. Further, we argue that today's economically driven health care systems need transformative processes more than they ever have before. We start with an account of an experience of educational transformation, as we hope this will help readers to understand our view of transformation.

A STORY OF TRANSFORMATION

Many experienced clinical educators and supervisors will have seen examples of transformation in their students. Some of the transformations we see are contained within the boundaries of clinical behaviour, and may on reflection appear *small*. Some, however, with seemingly minimal input from the clinical educator or supervisor, extend well beyond professional boundaries and are large-scale and life-changing. This story (a composite from our experience of several individuals) reflects the latter end of the continuum and may help to underscore the variability in terms of how we understand *success*.

Sophie came to me in my role as the clinical education coordinator for our university department at the time. She appeared at my door in tears and visibly distressed. Sophie had excelled in high school and easily sailed through the first three and a half years of her degree. She obtained high grades in all the academic and clinical placement subjects she had attempted and was on track for graduating successfully following a final 12-week clinical placement. In my office, Sophie, in tears, recounted how she had made her way to the first day of her final clinical placement and suddenly broke down crying in the car and had felt a great sense of panic and ill ease. She had driven home and called her clinical educator to say that she was too unwell to attend the clinic that day. The next day, she again went off to her clinic, this time managing to get to the clinic door before she began to feel unwell and faint. Again she went home and called in sick to the clinic. On the third day, she couldn't leave the house as she felt too panicked, too sickened. At the end of that first week, Sophie rang me and asked if she could see me about her clinical placement.

Clearly, Sophie was experiencing some kind of panic attacks, perhaps driven by performance anxiety. It was puzzling that she had performed so well in all of her previous clinics and that there were no obvious reasons (changes in home life, relationships, health) as to why she was experiencing the difficulty right now. Sophie expressed that she was devastated by her behaviour and feelings of being out of control. She was certainly catastrophising the situation, expressing that the situation was hopeless, that she was useless, and that she would just have to leave the course right now. This was the first time in her 22 years of life that she had not coped with/been *good* at something – and it scared her terribly. We agreed that the degree of distress she was experiencing required professional support and arranged for her to see the university student counsellor that afternoon. We also agreed that, until she felt well again, we would just take the clinical placement *off the agenda*. We made a time to catch up again the following week.

Over the following 8 months, Sophie experienced the highs and deep lows of personal counselling, while she examined what factors were contributing to her inability to *complete the degree*. It became apparent that she was in a very dependent relationship with her parents and that she was psychologically not ready to be an independent adult, which graduating from her degree represented. Sophie and I continued to meet every month during this period to check in with each other and to talk about her next placement. There were many times when Sophie expressed absolute desperation about her situation and a sense that she would never complete the degree and graduate to work in her chosen field. I kept expressing my view that the curly, windy roads to a place can be far more interesting and prepare us far better for the destination than the straight, direct and rapid routes.

She expressed such embarrassment at her public failure and felt there was so much loss of face and shame associated with her actions. I just kept challenging her view and asked who she would rather be treated by if she needed professional help – a clinician who had always experienced life in a positive and care-free way or a clinician who had personally experienced loss and stress, and gained wisdom through hardship and the resulting deep self-understanding. I offered her positive regard and a sense that her journey was just that, a difficult, scary, but extremely worthwhile journey. When we talked about her experiences we did not frame them in pathology, psychological disorder or aberrance. We framed them as an opportunity for growth and deepening. Of course, I am sure these frameworks were also present and probably of far more significance in what was occurring in her personal counselling, the content of which we never discussed.

It became very clear that we would need a gradual and gentle reintroduction to any clinical activity if she was to have a positive experience again. Sophie did eventually go back to clinic and, after a couple of false starts, completed and passed the final unit. Her clinical educators reinforced the view of opportunity for growth and offered positive regard and respect for her process. Her graduation was a major life event for her and her family. After graduation, she took a job quite some distance from the university and I lost contact with her. About 4 years later she wrote to me, a most beautiful and moving letter. She was happily employed in the profession and undertaking challenging and rewarding work. She expressed her gratitude to me for having faith in her process and for encouraging her to see the positive sides of adversity. She was transformed through this process.

Such opportunities may frequently be available to us as educators and supervisors. They may present to us simply, for example, as students requiring more time in a placement because they are not reaching competency in the prescribed number of days or a student developing an illness during the placement. Perhaps some of us are more comfortable with dealing with physical reasons for poor progress (such as common physical illnesses) as compared to psychological reasons (such as anxiety attacks). Conceivably, our high work loads and our perception of our role may act as barriers to seeing these possibilities for growth and transformation. However, it is important not to underestimate the significance of the relationship component in these teaching and learning opportunities.

HOW WE GOT HERE/OUR TRANSFORMATIONS

Our first book about clinical education, published in 1996, drew on the outcomes of a wonderful collaboration between a group of highly motivated and experienced individuals from the fields of occupational therapy, physiotherapy, speech pathology and education, working together in the Faculty of Health Sciences at La Trobe University in Australia. The members of the collaborative team developed a shared motivation to enhance the clinical education programmes of their respective disciplines. The team came together in 1989, because the members sensed that through cross-discipline activity something greater than the sum of their individual disciplines would emerge. The highly successful multi-discipline certificate course, Quality Supervision, resulted in 1990 (and is still running today) from their collaborative efforts. The text *Quality Supervision: Theory and practice for clinical supervisors* (Best & Rose 1996) built on the course structure and the teaching and learning experiences of the group and was used as the prime text for the course participants. We understand that the text has had wide appeal (particularly in Australia and the United Kingdom) and has been of great use to busy practising clinicians attempting to enhance their educational practice.

Many people over the past decade have asked why the Quality Supervision group/team has been so successful. On reflection, we believe that, right from the outset, the group recognised and celebrated differences (personal and professional) and provided a safe environment in which to build relationships. The group practised a great tolerance for others and for difference. One of the ground rules for the group was a shared emphasis on the importance of process as well as product. That is, time and space (sometimes team members' homes and outdoor hot tubs!) were valued as important variables in any project or plan that was under discussion. New members to the group were sometimes dismayed at the amount of time allocated for planning or reviewing course programmes and plans. The new members explained that they just wanted to get through things quickly and return to other pressing business (of which there has always been plenty). However, the group knew that developing anything of quality takes time. We also knew that quality relationships, in this mixed-discipline group, where we struggled to find a shared vocabulary, framework or set of principles for practice, were essential if the group was going to get beyond a superficial regurgitation of ideas already available in the literature.

We also believed that in any of our teaching activities it would be best to model whatever it was that we were asking of or suggesting to our course participants. Thus, reflective practice was always part of our group process, debriefing after course sessions, peer-critique about our own teaching sessions in the course, reflecting-in-action and out aloud for course participants to hear and see, modelling risk-taking behaviours and "not getting it right/perfect in public", and discussing our limitations and our own places of learning and learning journeys.

From 1994 the group expanded to include disciplines and staff from two other universities in Melbourne (Monash and Deakin) and five other disciplines (pharmacy; dietetics; radiography; podiatry; prosthetics and orthotics). Such multi-discipline and cross-university collaboration provided even greater challenges but ultimately provided a rich backdrop for the development of ideas and personal growth for all group members. Even though each current group member has enormous work load and time pressures, time for Quality Supervision activity is somehow always prioritised because we all know that it is essentially nourishing and sustaining.

During this same period, the Quality Supervision group took some risks and convened supervision conferences and seminars that invited local and international people working and researching in the areas of clinical education, mentoring and professional supervision to come together and learn from each other's disciplines and perspectives. We had a strong belief that our own knowledge and practice in clinical education could only be enhanced by understanding these broader related contexts and from learning from the experience of others. Thus, we set about bringing together the three related but apparently separate academic disciplines of clinical education, professional supervision and mentoring. There appeared to be minimal actual dialogue occurring amongst the three disciplines – given that their ideas and research were being published in disparate journals and texts and there was a lack of obvious reference to each discipline's body of work.

The results of the three disciplines coming together *in conference* were extremely positive, with the participant views being overwhelmingly encouraging and the team members' experiences affirmed. Again, the experience of risk (in inviting three somewhat unfamiliar disciplines together to a conference) and then the resulting nourishment, sustenance and growth have consolidated our view that reaching out and developing authentic relationships is the single most important issue in achieving growth and change. The enriching process of collaborative relationship is the lived, embodied experience of our group and what we bring to our educative and at times *transformative* activities.

THE CURRENT CONTEXT

There are many differences between the climate that prevailed when we wrote Best & Rose (1996) and when we wrote this current text in 2004. One significant difference in our local Australian context is the recognition that clinical education is a vital professional activity that maintains, protects and potentially develops the professions. Further, there is now a strong recognition that preparation for the role of clinical educator is both essential and a valued commodity worthy of time and financial expenditure. In 1990, when we first launched the Quality Supervision course, there was an expression of horror and outrage from some sectors of our disciplines, first that such a course was necessary and second that there would be a charge for undertaking such studies. We began slowly, with an initial intake of 25 participants. By 1995, this had risen to 60 participants, peaking in 2001 with 160 participants.

For the past three years we have capped the participant numbers at 120 (with a waiting list of 60 or more), in order to maintain a quality teaching and learning environment. We believe that the large rise in participant numbers reflects the growing awareness and value that professionals now place on clinical education as a discipline in its own right. We are not yet at the point where professionals are expected to be accredited clinical educators before they work with students but we can now see how this may come about in the near future.

A move to accrediting clinical facilities (hospitals, clinics, community health centres, etc.) and their staff offering clinical education is even more likely in an environment where university programmes are increasingly paying their external, non-university-employed clinical educators to educate the students on placements. Thus, the universities may begin to exert pressure in terms of the quality of the educational experiences the students receive. Further, the students themselves are paying more and more for their degrees and programmes in Australia as a user-pays system is implemented, and perhaps the students are now expecting more from their expenditure. In parallel, there is a movement occurring in Australian universities to replace the Bachelors degree programmes with graduate-entry Masters courses as the entry-level preparation for professional practice. Along with this move are the increasing demands that mature-age and full-fee-paying students enrolled in graduate-entry programmes tend to exert.

While the educational climate has changed over the past 15 years, it is apparent that individuals (both educators and students) are still seeking personal fulfillment in their work and studies (see Chapter 17). However, a tension exists between the current economic marketplace and institutional forces that create systems where employees are reduced to being merely instruments or mechanistic parts. In such mechanistic systems, the complexity and richness of the human experience are not really factored in. Such mismatch between the expectations of the employees of the system and the expectation of the humans working in the system may result in significant stress and burnout. A recent study of Canadian speech pathologists revealed an alarming burnout rate, with 76.1% of respondents experiencing some form of burnout (Potter & Lagacé 1995). Stress levels in speech pathologists working in acute health care centres have been found to be high, with 67% of respondents reporting moderate to severe levels of stress (Green & Brown 1984, as cited in Tatham et al 1989). Clinicians are being pushed to focus on throughput and measurable, reductionist outcomes, and we believe this is also a powerful motivational and shaping force in the educational actions of clinicians. Thus, clinicians require even greater preparation, tools and awareness in order to find ways to cope with the system forces and develop humanistic and transformative educational practices.

THE FUTURE

In looking toward the future, we anticipate changes that will have considerable influence on educational practice and experiences. An ageing population demands increased levels of service delivery and escalating health care costs (Duckett 2000), putting pressure on health workers to change their service delivery models. Further, the nature of the health professions themselves will need to respond as they struggle to provide adequate levels of care for the growing number of individuals seeking services. For example, in Australia there is a move toward educating less specialised, less educated, generic health care workers who would work under the specialist supervision of a qualified physiotherapist, occupational therapist or speech pathologist, thereby reducing the overall costs of providing the increased numbers of services. Such structural change to the workforce will have many ramifications for clinical education, professional supervision and mentoring practices.

There may be increasing pressures placed on health care workers as their roles become more complex and as the system expects greater outcomes from less and less resource. Thus, we anticipate that overall there will be a greater need for mentoring and professional supervision. We hope that service providers may move to a situation where the importance of professional supervision is recognised and formal structures are put in place to encourage clinicians to seek supervision and to subsidise or pay for it.

Shorter clinical placements may be a forced response to the increased demand for clinical placements from dwindling placement resources. Shorter placements will place considerable pressure on the educational experiences and outcomes for all parties. As has been discussed elsewhere in this text (see Chapters 5 and 6), if inadequate time is provided for students in placements, it will be extremely difficult for them to acquire the required knowledge, skills and attitudes. Perhaps there will also be a greater use of non-traditional placements (placements in areas of work not traditionally encompassed within the professional boundaries, placements without clinical educators or supervisors being present) and cross-discipline placements as a way of coping with limited resources. Certainly, as Roe-Shaw (see Chapter 13) discusses, we anticipate that there will be greater use of online and distance support for students on placements at considerable distance from their home university and local supports.

Finally, the professions will, we imagine, be forced to review the possibility of taking structural responsibility for the acquisition and evaluation of clinical competence in its membership by, for example, instituting a professional training or apprenticeship-type year after individuals have graduated from university preparatory programmes. While this model has existed in the United States of America for many years, it has not been favoured in Australia.

OUR HOPES

We believe that wisdom comes through knowing the system (context) and the self, and in talking to people who offer support. Some of us only truly know ourselves through saying what it is we think/believe/know to another, that is, *how we know* (a dialogical approach to knowing; see Wertsch 1991). The relationship between student and clinical educator, mentor and mentee, or supervisor and professional can bring mutual benefits for both and can sustain both. Ultimately, these relationships can be transformational and as such deserve our attention, conscious preparation and valuing.

It is our hope that this book provides a connection for the reader to others. We hope the words, concepts and frameworks in this text facilitate the reader to see the potential for connection to others, whether they be students or peers or supervisors. Most of all, we hope that people reading this text will gain a greater awareness, or a renewed awareness, of how these special relationships and connections help to re-energise and sustain us in our daily work and life.

Acknowledgements

Thank you to Joseph P Agan for introducing us to the language and concepts of dialogical approaches. Thank you to the inspirational students, teachers and mentors we have had along the way, who enabled transformative practice: Bernie Neville, Katie Kirby, Louise Brown, Janet Doyle, Jennifer Oates, Helen Edwards, Joy Higgs, Jacinta Douglas.

REFERENCES

Best D, Rose M 1996 Quality supervision. Theory and practice for clinical supervisors. W B Saunders, London

Duckett S 2000 The Australian health care system. Oxford University Press, South Melbourne

Potter R, Lagacé P 1995 The incidence of professional burnout among Canadian speech-language pathologists. Journal of Speech Language Pathology and Audiology 19:181–186

Tatham A, Clough B, Maxwell V 1989 Stress in speech therapy. Stress Medicine 5:259–264

Wertsch J 1991 Voices of the mind: a sociocultural approach to mediated action. Harvard University Press, Cambridge, MA

PART 2 Transforming practice through teaching, learning and supporting relationships: a perspective from the UK

Della Fish

As a teacher and teacher educator, I am very pleased to be associated with a publication that places education so firmly at the heart of clinical supervision and mentoring. I believe that for UK readers it should prove very timely, as they struggle to learn alongside colleagues from other professions in the brave new interprofessional world.

Education does have to be carefully nurtured in professions where it is *not* the primary expertise (as in all health care professions). In the UK, as elsewhere, the current climate is not sympathetic to, and current resources are not plentifully available for, what governments everywhere unwisely see as an inessential luxury. This book's publication is timely for UK readers. It stakes out the arguments for seeing investment in education as imperative. We must not lose sight of this in the lemming-like dash for the innovations and novelties that are dangled in front of us as special to, and vital for, the 21st century.

Education needs expert teachers. And teaching is a profession of itself. Indeed, in the UK many people have taken a four-year undergraduate course to prepare to enter it. This is because teachers themselves are part of the means to their educational ends, and thus have to be prepared as people, as well as experts in educational ideas and methods.

As the story at the beginning of this chapter shows, good teachers draw upon their own self-knowledge of personal values and beliefs and how these come together in an educational philosophy. They draw on their personality, their experience, their imagination (to see the world through the eyes of their learners), their compassion and patience, and their capacity for risk-taking (without which there is no creativity). And they also, importantly, draw on their educational understanding and an awareness of the moral dimensions of their practice.

Educational understanding involves the recognition of fundamental principles for fostering learning. These include the acknowledgement that, and commitment to ensure that, good learning should:

- be conducted in a sheltered and supportive context
- be transformative (in that it changes understanding and by this means changes conduct)
- be active and interactive
- be intrinsically motivating
- be life-long
- take place within the context of nurturing relationships
- be transacted through rich communications
- recognise that the role of the learner's talk is central.

This list has been adapted from Collins et al (2002), who provide reference to research in education that provides considerable evidence to support the importance of these educational tenets.

Some literature in the UK is beginning also to recognise the importance of what Aristotle taught us to call practical wisdom. He referred to this as the supreme intellectual virtue. It is about "knowing which general ethical principles to apply in a particular situation" (Carr 1995, p. 71). The teacher who possesses practical wisdom is the professional who "sees the particularities of the [learner's] practical situation in the light of their ethical significance and acts consistently on this basis", to achieve the greatest good for that particular learner. The exercise of practical wisdom is made manifest in a practitioner who has:

> a knowledge of what is required in a particular moral situation and a willingness to act so that this knowledge can take concrete form. It is a comprehensive moral capacity which combines practical knowledge of the good with sound judgement about what, in a particular situation, would constitute an appropriate expression of this "good".
>
> (Carr 1995, p. 71).

The combination of these factors (of personal attributes, together with educational understanding and practical wisdom) is what makes for a quality teacher. And quality health care teachers in the clinical setting are what make for quality health care. In these days of reduced resources and excessive accountability (see O'Neill 2002, and Chapter 20) the courage of such teachers to continue to be themselves in this way is our only real insurance against quick-fix "professional development", which seeks to change behaviour (the surface) but ignores the beliefs, values, theories and assumptions that drive practitioners' actions (see also Chapter 20).

There is encouragement for exploring such educational ideas and activities in the UK, through the practitioner research journals, and through movements like the Centre for Action Research and the British Educational Research Association. But these provide platforms for educator-researchers across all professions and sectors, and the opportunities they offer are not taken up very fully by those from health care. It remains to be seen whether the newly emerging National Health Service University will provide support for exploring and developing this kind of education specifically in health care.

Education is about growth (for teacher and learner), and about being and aspiring to become. The cultivation metaphor, so beloved of UK primary education in the mid 20th century, still has currency. Professionals must continue to have access to this kind of genuine education. Its significance needs recognition, its position needs to be privileged, and above all, its priority must be underscored in according quality time to it. In these respects, this book will (very properly) support the aspirations of some UK readers – and no doubt challenge the beliefs and actions of others.

REFERENCES

Carr W 1995 For education: towards critical educational inquiry. Open University Press, Maidenhead
Collins J, Harkin J, Nind M 2002 Manifesto for learning. Continuum Books, London
O'Neill O 2002 A question of trust. Cambridge University Press, Cambridge

PART 3 Transforming practice through teaching, learning and supporting relationships: a perspective from the USA
Marisue Pickering

Reading Rose & Best's introductory statements about the "centrality of relationships in teaching and learning" propelled me back to 1960 when I began work on a master's degree in speech-language pathology at Boston University. A major influence in the department at that time was Professor Albert T. Murphy who later was to write:

> *While knowledge of scientific fact and method are important, where clinical relationships are concerned, the personal relationship with the patient is more important than facts, even scientifically respectable ones. The speech-language pathologist has a relationship with each client, and improvement in the clinical condition is influenced by all the clinician's attitudes.*

(Murphy 1982, p. 454).

Murphy's view about clinical relationships was not solitary; see, for example, Emerick & Hood (1974). Additionally, as I have noted elsewhere (Pickering 1984a), the importance of the interpersonal relationship within the supervisory process was emphasised by numerous authors in the 1960s, 1970s and early 1980s. By the mid-1980s, many clinical educators would have agreed with Rose & Best about the importance of "getting the relationships *right*". Discussions by McCready et al (1984) and Pickering (1984b) are illustrative.

Similarly, clinical educators in the USA would be able to provide stories about transformation, as exemplified by a qualitative research study of the late 1980s (Pickering 1989–1990). This examination of the supervisory process as "an experience of interpersonal relationships and personal growth" (p. 16) quotes a master's-level student as stating, "I feel I have learned about myself and my abilities through her [the clinical educator's] guidance. She has allowed me to stand on my own and has offered me suggestions … generally she has let me grow" (p. 16). Clinical educators also found the process growth-producing. As one educator stated, "To me, growth is the ultimate goal as well as an on-going process in the supervisory interaction–growth of client, of clinician, and of supervisor" (Pickering 1989–1990, p. 23).

The fact that in the USA the current focus of clinical education discourse is on other topics (see my commentary for Chapter 1) does not diminish the significance of the supervisory relationship and the reality of growth and transformation within that relationship. This fact does suggest that, at this time, discussion of this basic element of clinical education is more likely to come from texts such as this present one, rather than from work produced in the USA.

CURRENT CONTEXT

Rose & Best posit a current Australian context where systemic forces, many of which are economic, create a mechanistic orientation where the "complexity and richness of the human experience is not really factored in". I think such factoring in is almost always a challenge for our field. Further, the idea that social institutions (including the workplace) place impositions on human growth is not new. Holifield (1983, p. 260), in reviewing post-World War II attitudes, places Erich Fromm, Karen Horney and Carl Rogers in a group of psychologists and social critics holding such views.

The issue for communication sciences and disorders (CSD) practitioners is that going beyond those speech behaviours with which we are so familiar always means taking time to develop our own practitioner-based values and skills relative to the human experience – not a small or insignificant task. Then, even after we develop our own humanistic values and skills, we need to be proactive in using them within our professional contexts. This probably means constant negotiation with a prevailing institutional work ethic and environment that may be antithetical to those values, as Rose & Best suggest.

Evidence-based practice (EBP) provides a mini case scenario for looking at both the current context in the USA and a possible tension between the needs of the marketplace and the values of humanistic practices. The context is this: one cannot be in CSD at this time without knowing about EBP. Discussions on the topic are regular features of our professional newspaper. The American Speech-Language-Hearing Association (ASHA) has in place a major committee whose task is to develop a plan to incorporate EBP into various association endeavours. Additionally, online resources are readily available (ASHA 2004). As one writer states, EBP "is increasingly being recognised as the preferred way to conduct practice in speech-language pathology" (Schlosser 2004, p. 6).

Is there a tension between the values of humanistic practice and the needs of a marketplace and a field that expect EBP? One recent writer has entered into this discussion by examining myths about EBP (Dollaghan 2004). A point is made that within EBP "the experiences, values, and preferences of ourselves and our patients can and should contribute to our clinical decisions" (Dollaghan 2004, p. 4). A subsequent author has taken the discussion a step further by arguing the primacy of relevant stakeholder perspectives when making a decision about the specifics of clinical practice (Schlosser 2004). As the field sorts out what it means by EBP and its place in clinical decision-making, clinical educators will be expected to provide leadership to students in their own EBP clinical decision-making.

EBP is an arena where clinical educators in the USA will need, as Rose & Best state about clinical educators in Australia, "preparation, tools and awareness" if they want to continue to develop practices that are both humanistic and transformative. Clinical educators will play a major role in incorporating into EBP a humanistic perspective, drawing on concepts such as those noted in this and other texts.

THE FUTURE

An initiative of potential future interest and significance for CSD concerns the exploration into healing approaches different from those usually employed by the medical establishment and allied health fields. The Boston Healing Landscape Project, located in the Department of Pediatrics at the Boston University School of Medicine, is working across disciplinary boundaries to understand and respond better to healing approaches in a variety of immigrant communities (Boston Healing Landscape Project 2004).

I find it exciting that physicians, religion scholars, anthropologists, sociologists, students and community intellectuals and practitioners are coming together to study the complexity of health and healing and the complexity of cultural understandings of illness. If CSD clinical educators believe in the richness of human experience and value humanistic and transformative interactions, then in-depth explorations – even when they originate outside our field – of how people view their health and their healing can only enhance our future understanding of teaching and learning.

REFERENCES

ASHA 2004 Resources on evidence-based practice. Online. Available: http://www.asha.org/about/publications/leader-online/archives/2003/q3/f030909b.htm 23 Aug 2004

Boston Healing Landscape Project 2004 Online. Available: http://www.bmc.org/pediatrics/special/bhlp/ 23 Aug 2004

Dollaghan C 2004 Evidence-based practice myths and realities. The ASHA Leader 9(7):4–5,12

Emerick L L, Hood S B 1974 The clinician–client relationship. Charles C Thomas, Springfield

Holifield E B 1983 A history of pastoral care in America. Abingdon Press, Nashville

McCready V, Shapiro D, Kennedy K 1984 Identifying hidden dynamics in supervision: four scenarios. In: Crago M, Pickering M (eds) Supervision in human communication disorders. Little, Brown, Boston, p 169–201

Murphy A T 1982 The clinical process and the speech-language pathologist. In: Shames G H, Wiig E H (eds) Human communication disorders. Charles E Merrill, Columbus, p 453–474

Pickering M 1984a Interpersonal communication in speech-language pathology supervisory conferences: a qualitative study. Journal of Speech and Hearing Disorders 49(2):189–195

Pickering M 1984b Interpersonal communication and the supervisory process: a search for Ariadne's thread. In: Crago M, Pickering M (eds) Supervision in human communication disorders. Little, Brown, Boston, p 203–225

Pickering M 1989–1990 The supervisory process: an experience of interpersonal relationships and personal growth. National Student Speech Language Hearing Association Journal 17:17–28

Schlosser R W 2004 Evidence-based practice in AAC: 10 points to consider. The ASHA Leader 9(12):6–7, 10–11

PART 4 Transforming practice through teaching, learning and supporting relationships: a perspective from Canada

Paul Hagler

THOUGHTS ON HOW WE GOT HERE AND WHERE WE ARE GOING

For the most part, we got here on the shoulders of dedicated people who saw a need to know more about the clinical education and supervision processes and did something about it. An outstanding example is Dr Jean Anderson, who wrote the first text in the area of speech-language pathology (1988) and was awarded a US Federal Office of Education training programme grant to educate speech-language pathologists at the doctoral level in the area of clinical supervision. At that time, we borrowed our theories from social work, education and clinical psychology, and we borrowed our investigative methods from cultural anthropology and experimental psychology. We were ill-equipped but diligent. We knew intuitively that the relationship was important, but occasionally we took a wrong turn along the path to understanding it.

For example, we tried to change participants' behaviours to align them with sound theory without first finding out if the theory worked. Inertia and logistics plagued us. The worst inertia was on the part of the ponderous old dinosaurs who, never having met Sophie, asked why we were trying to fix a process that wasn't broken. One logistical barrier that haunts us today is the heavy course load in most educational programmes. Even when administrators, professors, students and professional association liaisons all agree on the desirability of required coursework in clinical education/supervision, they don't know where to squeeze it in. Most educational programmes in Canada are no longer two academic years; they are two calendar years. No one wants entry-level educational programmes to be longer than they already are. Sometimes it seems we have not progressed much in 20 years. On the other hand, it is amazing to have accomplished as much as we have. We owe a great deal to the pioneers in clinical education who paved the way and pointed us in the right direction.

We are forever emphasising the importance of the relationship, and it is true that getting it *right* is the biggest challenge we face in the education/ supervision domain. When it *is* right, it sustains us in our work and helps us grow and find gratification in what we do. When it is wrong, it is a demoralising experience that leaves learner and teacher alike wanting to run away and never return. Even when the relationship is right, there is still something to nourish the cynic in some of us. Typically, if things are right, it is because the individuals are compatible people with a common goal, not because one or both of them is especially adept at working through problems in the relationship. The human animal, by nature, is almost as quarrelsome as sparrows at a crowded birdfeeder. To get everyone through the rough spots, it takes at least one participant in a relationship who possesses well-developed inter-personal and supervisory skills.

Unfortunately, we are still relying too much on our innate interpersonal skills to make the clinical education process successful. We do not require clinical education/supervision course work, at least not enough of it, in our professional education programmes. We do not screen for basic skills when recruiting new clinical educators, supervisors and mentors. We are unable to do so because we need everyone who steps forward, and we do not offer a professional credential in this important area. In short, we do not yet equip new graduates and professionals with the skills they need to get going when the going gets tough. However, I think that day will be here before we know it.

We are going to witness a heightened sense of need, perhaps even an urgent need, to educate current and future professionals about clinical edu-cation and supervision. My crystal ball tells me two factors will combine to cause this. One valid factor is the observation by Rose & Best that con-sumers, in a user-pay system, tend to expect more in exchange for their expenditure. That factor will combine with another phenomenon to ensure change. The second factor is that the workplace is showing an ever-decreasing tolerance of unacceptable conduct. Twenty years ago, we wrote rules of con-duct for employees to avert sexual harassment in the workplace. Failure to have such rules in place and failure to take appropriate action when prob-lems arose brought the legal system down on the heads of major employers in North America, including, in one case, Canada's national defence system. The fines were large, and the response was not only immediate, it was national in scope. Ten years ago, we rewrote those rules to include any type of harassment, and, at about the same time, we wrote rules for the ethical conduct of research with human subjects. As an aside, it is interesting that rules for the ethical conduct of research with animals predated similar rules for humans – but at least we got there.

With predictable fervour for implementing a right-minded plan, we have gone a little overboard with a few of the details here in Canada, but for the most part, researchers and ethics review boards want to do the right thing. People involved in teaching/learning relationships also want to do the right thing but, like researchers, not everyone always does. Things sometimes go off track, and when they do, we have a prescribed, multi-level, administra-tive hierarchy through which the aggrieved party can appeal. For example, if the complainant is a student and the accusation relates to course work, most universities have about five internal administrative levels to which the student can grieve. If all those steps fail to produce the desired result, the student can still go to the courts. Of course, everyone along the way under-stands where the problem could end up and naturally wants to avoid that.

In the end, responsibility for doing the right thing is passed along to the per-son on the front lines. The point is this: when it comes to conduct in the work-place, we have lofty expectations of one another, and on some matters, those expectations have become formal policies. These policies tend to have teeth, too. Failure to abide by them can result in serious reprimand or even dismissal. It is reasonable to believe that some day in the near future a clinical educator or professional supervisor will be taken to task (perhaps even to court) for "conduct unbecoming" and if the individual's conduct is embarrassing or costly enough for the employer, a new policy will be written in an effort to avert all future problems of that type. The upshot will be a substantially heightened effort on the part of clinical educators and supervisors in professional settings to prepare themselves for their jobs and to nurture their relationships with their learners. Likewise, as with sexual harassment and research ethics, it will be incumbent upon employers to do everything within their powers to ensure that consumers of the future have no legitimate complaints.

Australia's Quality Supervision group views its expansion to include five other disciplines – pharmacy, dietetics, radiography, podiatry, prosthetics and orthotics – as instrumental in the group's overall success. Even in the absence of a parallel, national special-interest group, a similar interdisciplinary scenario has evolved in some educational environments in Canada, where the typical alliances are among audiology, occupational therapy, physical therapy and speech-language pathology – with some recent movement to include pharmacy, dental hygiene and nursing. There are regional differences in the combination of disciplines, but which ones is less important than the fact that multiple disciplines are working together to understand better and implement sound practices and to support one another. We, too, organise conferences and seminars to enable people working and researching in the areas of clinical education, mentoring and professional supervision to learn from one another. This will continue to be essential if we are to grow our knowledge base and present a united front on critical issues. A united front can be immensely helpful if policy changes are required, because it is extremely difficult for upper-level administrators to ignore a chorus of insistent voices from multiple disciplines advocating change.

Like Australia, Canada faces a move by service providers to keep costs down by employing assistants to help clinical professionals. The implications for clinical education, professional supervision and mentoring practices are immense. For example, university-based clinical practicum coordinators worry about who will oversee the clinical education of these new assistants. If clinical professionals have to oversee the assistants' clinical education, perhaps the professionals will accept fewer professional students. If working assistants supervise student assistants, perhaps the student assistants will not receive as good an education. How much monitoring of assistants' activities is adequate? Where do the assistants' scopes of practice start and stop? Is patient/client safety an issue? Will assistants take professionals' jobs? I didn't say these made sense.

These questions and others continue to arise, even though many of them have been answered. Rose & Best are correct that pressure on health care workers to take on more complex responsibilities with fewer resources will heighten the need for good mentoring and professional supervision. However, these same phenomena may also deter health care workers from accepting students for clinical placements and new co-workers for professional supervision or mentoring. Professionals are becoming weary of increasing responsibilities, long hours, pay cuts and generally feeling unappreciated, so requests for extra commitments are sometimes met with growls of protest.

How to address dwindling clinical placement options seems to be a chronic universal problem. Let us hope we do not have to go to shorter placements as a solution. Reduced time in practicum placements will almost certainly compromise our ability to prepare graduates to hit the ground running in their post-graduation jobs. If that happens, I foresee a groundswell of complaints from employers. One potentially viable partial response is greater use of non-traditional and cross-discipline placements. In Canada, occupational therapy has implemented this practice quite effectively, but for some reason the rest of us fail to understand, the other rehabilitation professions have not followed suit. Online and distance continuing education opportunities for working professionals abound in Canada, but comparable support for students during their clinical placements is not being used much at all.

CONCLUSION

Again, the parallels are many, and the differences are relatively few. This book will definitely connect the reader to others who share in the joys and challenges of clinical education, professional supervision and mentoring. It most assuredly will provide a heightened awareness of how these relationships not only sustain us at work but also enable us to grow. Ideally, it will be a required text for countless health sciences students enrolled in credit courses on clinical education. The international and interdisciplinary perspectives provide reassurance to many of us that we are not alone. This includes researchers, educators, administrators, service providers, officers of professional associations and students. All of us who read this text will gain from the information between its covers.

REFERENCE

Anderson J 1988 The supervisory process in speech-language pathology. Little, Brown, Boston

Index

Note: Page numbers in bold refer to figures, tables or illustrations.